Northern Plant Lore

A Field Guide to The Ancestral Use of Plants in Northern Europe

Eoghan Odinsson

Ancient Herblore, Modern Science, Healthy Families

Visit my website at www.eoghanodinsson.com

Printed in the United States of America

First Printing: May 2012

ISBN-13: 978-0-9878394-5-9
ISBN-10: 0987839454

Library and Archives Canada Cataloguing in Publication

Odinsson, Eoghan, 1969-
      Northern plant lore : a field guide to the ancestral use of plants in Northern Europe / Eoghan Odinsson.

"Ancient herblore, modern science, healthy families".
Includes bibliographical references and index.
ISBN 978-0-9878394-5-9

1. Medicinal plants--Europe, Northern--History.
2. Materia medica, Vegetable--Europe, Northern--History.
3. Traditional medicine--Europe, Northern--History.
4. Ethnopharmacology--Europe, Northern--History. I. Title.

RS176.O35 2012   615.3'210948   C2012-903302-2

By The Same Author

Dedication

In memory of my grandfather, Albert Bernard Lecky (Grampy).

"I had rather be on my farm than be emperor of the world"

- George Washington

Foreword

The practise of herbal medicine has a long history and is common to every human culture. Each society learns to make best use of the resources available to it, and to develop combinations of treatment in order to deal with complex medical problems.

This splendid new book by a respected author in the world of Germanic lore offers a unique amalgam of traditional and modern knowledge presented in a handy and easily referenced format. Not only does Odinsson provide details of the plants' preferred habitat and notes in their cultivation, he also draws on some encyclopaedic references to flesh out the botanical aspects with culinary uses and historical notes.

The book also includes a number of recipes which make recreating the cultural world of societies long gone a more immediate experience for those who would like to try these materials at first hand. Even the use of vegetable dyestuffs is included.

It is easy for us to overlook the importance which cultivated plants had in the life of agricultural communities, whose existence depended on a careful management of resources which had to be replenished with a great deal of labour. Wheat and other types of grain had to be winnowed and threshed, then ground to make flour for bread - or else it was allowed to ferment and turned into that liquid food we call 'beer' or 'ale'. These drinks could be flavoured with hops to make them bitter, or with gale.

The wealth of information presented with concision and clarity makes this book indispensible for the medical herbalist with a general or specific interest in the medicinal or therapeutic action of traditional ingredients.

Stephen Pollington
Essex, 2012

Preface

I wrote this book out of a love of all things that grow, for the musty smell of the forest after a rain, for the mighty trees that grace the land, and with the hope that we can re-acquaint ourselves with these profound treasures.

I'm the first generation on my mother's side of the family that didn't grow up on the farm. I spent summers on the farm, played with the calves and new kittens each year, but I was not a farmer, nor did I have any connection to the earth, at least not in the sense that my grandfather and his forefathers did.

Many of us are long removed from the farm, but I still remember warming my feet in front of the wood stove with my grandmother in the chilly spring mornings – the wood stove was used for cooking as well as heating the house. It's these little vignettes that I hang on to when I visit the cities, and it's those sentiments that were the motivation behind writing this book.

Maybe it's not practical for us all go back to the farm, but I would at least like to reconnect with the skills our forefathers had. One such opportunity is to reclaim our knowledge of plants and herbs for medicinal purposes. This is knowledge accumulated over thousands of years – we have documents[1] with Anglo Saxon herb lore dating back around 1100 years. Despite the antiquity of this knowledge, or perhaps because of it, many of us dismiss herbal remedies as folksy nonsense. Perhaps we shouldn't be so hasty.

The active ingredient in willow bark, once prescribed by Hippocrates[2], is salicin, which is converted in the body into salicylic acid. The discovery of salicylic acid would eventually lead to the development of the acetylated form, acetylsalicylic

---

[1] The Lacnunga ('Remedies') is a collection of miscellaneous Anglo-Saxon medical texts and prayers, written mainly in Old English and Latin. It is found, following other medical texts, in London, British Library Manuscript Harley 585, a codex probably compiled in England in the late tenth or early eleventh century. Many of its herbal remedies are also found, in variant form, in Bald's Leechbook, another Anglo-Saxon medical compendium.

[2] Hippocrates of Cos (ca. 460 BC – ca. 370 BC) was an ancient Greek physician of the Age of Pericles (Classical Athens), and is considered one of the most outstanding figures in the history of medicine. He is referred to as the father of Western medicine

acid, also known as "aspirin", when it was isolated from a plant known as meadowsweet.

In my first book, *Northern Lore*, I started the process of studying the old herbal practices and compared them to modern medical research. In that book I presented a sampling of ten remedies that were used by our ancestors and had proven medical efficacy (i.e. they worked). In this book, as promised, I'll continue to present the findings of that research in an easily accessible format.

As is the case when you undertake any large project, you must set boundaries, and so I did when writing this book. My goal was to review the herb and plant lore used by our ancestors in England, as documented in the *The Lacnunga Manuscript*, *The Old English Herbarium Manuscript V, and Bald's Leechbook,* then determine which of those cures worked. I relied upon Stephen Pollington's excellent translation and analysis of these works in his book *"Leechcraft: Early English Charms, Plant Lore and Healing".* This served as a master list of all documented herbal and plant based medicinal ingredients known to our ancestors.

The second step was to examine which of those ingredients had proven medical efficacy. I decided to use the *"The Complete German Commission E Monographs: Therapeutic Guide to Herbal Medicines"* as my guide, as this was a comprehensive study, with the results published in one convenient volume.

The German Commission E Monographs are a guide to therapeutic herbal medicine with 380 monographs evaluating the safety and efficacy of herbs for licensed medical prescribing in Germany. The commission itself was formed in 1978, and no longer exists.

The monographs were published between 1984 and 1994 in the *Bundesanzeiger. The Commission E Monographs* were imported into the United States with considerable fanfare in 1998 by The American Botanical Council. They were unequivocally endorsed in a foreword by the late Varro Tyler, a well-known professor of pharmacognosy at Purdue University. Tyler states in his foreword that:

"...safety data were reviewed by the Commissioners according to a "doctrine of absolute proof" and efficacy according to a "doctrine of reasonable certainty."

The third and last component of *Northern Plant Lore*, was to add the rich folklore available to us in Maud Grieve's *A Modern Herbal.*

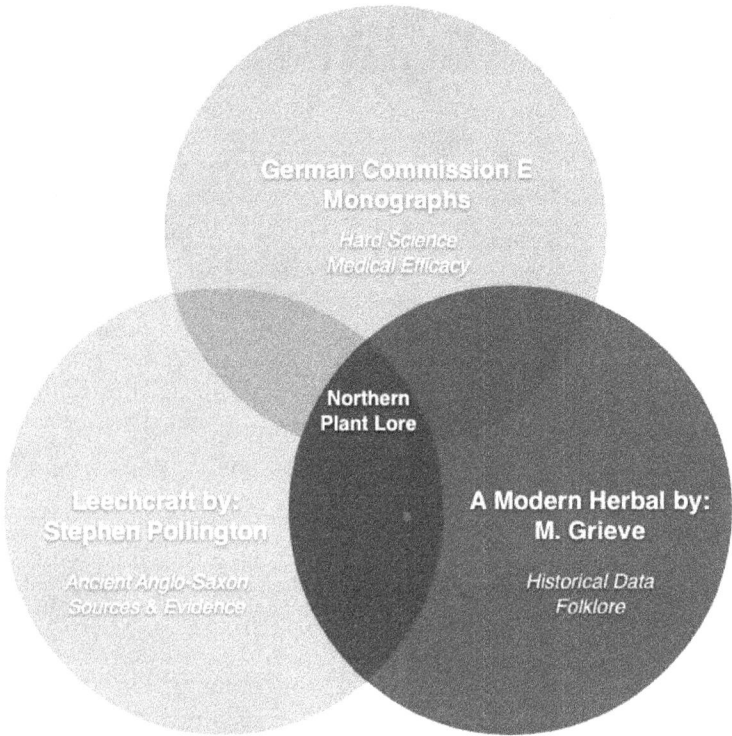

German Commission E
Monographs

Hard Science
Medical Efficacy

Northern
Plant Lore

Leechcraft by:
Stephen Pollington

Ancient Anglo-Saxon
Sources & Evidence

A Modern Herbal by:
M. Grieve

Historical Data
Folklore

Figure 1 - The main references for "Northern Plant Lore"

Disclaimer

I wrote and published this book for entertainment purposes. I'm a researcher and writer, NOT a professional Herbalist or Physician; please see your doctor if you have any health concerns.

Acknowledgement

I first want to thank my son Shea who worked very hard over his summer break as my intern and helped immensely with research and editing. This was a wonderful adventure for both of us, and this is his book as much as mine.

Thanks to my lovely wife Melinda for her editing precision, without which polishing, my books would be rough and ragged indeed.

As busy as he is, Researcher and Author of Anglo-Saxon History and Culture, Stephen Pollington was very kind in agreeing to write the Foreword of this book, and frankly without his extensive work on "Leechcraft: Early English Charms, Plant-Lore and Healing", this book would not have been possible. Cheers Stephen!

Thanks to Ed Greenwood of www.botanical.com for allowing me to use his electronic version of M. Grieve's "A Modern Herbal". Ed spent countless hours inputting the text of this old and excellent book into electronic form, and as a result, I was able to include a lot of that great historical material in Northern Plant Lore.

I would like to give recognition to Project Gutenberg's founder, Michael S. Hart, who passed away September 6, 2011. Project Gutenberg has digitized over 36,000 books that have become public domain, and offer them free of charge.

About the Author

Canadian born Eoghan Odinsson is an award winning journalist and author with a lifelong passion for the knowledge of our Northern forefathers – or "folk lore" - literally, the knowledge of our people.

Graduating from the University of Aberdeen in Scotland with his Masters of Science degree, he subsequently taught for the University, and was a dissertation advisor for graduate students.

In addition to his academic background, Eoghan also holds a Black Belt in Chito-Ryu Karate, and has taught Martial Arts in Canada and the USA.

Eoghan has just returned from a ten-year stretch working in the Washington D.C. area, and is now back in his native Ottawa Valley where he lives with his wife, son and three dogs.

Table of Contents

Introduction

In a raging predawn Canadian blizzard, a policeman struggled to drag my pregnant mother through six foot snow drifts to get her into the hospital. By this time she was well into labor. It was a Thursday – Thor's day. That's how I came into the world.

I suppose it's no surprise then that I've been fascinated by our Northern Culture for my entire life. I'm proud of the tenacity and resourcefulness my ancestors embodied which brought me into this world. For thousands of years our Northern forefathers endured biting cold, limited resources and invading empires. Despite this, their culture flourished and their legacy endured; my passion is this legacy and its echoes into our modern world.

Modern man and woman are quick to embrace new technologies which make their lives more convenient, and safer; rightly so. I want the best for my family. Modern medicine is one such convenience for which I am quite thankful. We have accomplished much in the way of curing diseases and caring for the sick and infirm, but too often it seems we believe in this modern application of medicine at the exclusion of our old ways.

The Ancient Romans favored old and established practices over new and innovative. *"Mos maiorum,"* or *"custom of our ancestors,"* was a phrase often used to refer to the older ways being better, or for maintaining the status quo. Although I don't believe we should exclude the new and innovative, I feel there should be harmony between the continuum of old and new.

In industrialized Northern nations we increasingly rely on corporate pharmaceutical giants whose only mandate is profit, to provide us what we need to keep our families healthy. Given that by some estimates it costs companies $500 million dollars, and can take 15 years to prove a new compound safe for American markets via FDA approval, many cures go unexplored as to their full potential and are labeled "supplements".

Why is this such a costly process? One glaring reason, felt most acutely in the United States, is that fear of potential lawsuits and the ensuing cost, is factored into every business decision - this makes most research a non-starter. Why haven't we demanded such legislation be addressed? Surely it's possible to change the laws so that our people can take better advantage of cures and remedies? In North America the conflict of interest, and risk to our well being, is so basic and obvious, yet seemingly ignored. Our own laws, which are supposed to protect us from harm, may in fact be denying our families the best care available.

Maybe researching historical cures that have been proven by modern science is one way for us to take control of our own health - one small step, so to speak.

I look forward to taking this journey with you.

How to Use This Book

This book's goal is to reconnect you with the knowledge of the Anglo-Saxons, and to highlight some modern scientific findings connected with the plants and herbs they used.

Please keep in mind that the HISTORICAL NOTES are almost entirely from M. Grieves famous book, *A Modern Herbal*, and was written nearly a hundred years ago. Where it talks about modern medicine or science, remember that this was modern in the context of someone living a hundred years ago; I includeed it for the rich descriptions and lore.

Quick Reference

The charts on the following pages are intended to help you quickly find a plant or herb related to either a specific ailment, or referenced by specific physiological categories.

Treatments by Categories

Physiological Category	Physiological Condition	Indicated Herb(s)
Cardiovascular	Atherosclerosis	Onion
	Cardiac Insufficiency	Hawthorn, Lily of the Valley
	Cardiac Symptoms	Motherwort
	Circulatory Disorders	Butcher's Broom, Rosemary
	Cor Pulmonade	Lily of the Valley
	Geriatric Vascular Changes	Garlic, Hawthorn, Onion
	Hypercholesteremia	Garlic
	Tachycardia	Motherwort
Dermatological	Ano-genital Irritation	Oak Bark
	Burns	St. John's Wort
	Irrigation, Mouth	Mallow
	Itching	Butcher's Broom
	Seborrhea	Heartsease
	Skin, Injury or Irritation	Agrimony, Oak Bark, plantain
Endocrinology, Reproductive System, Obstetrics / Gynecology, Prostate	Pelvic Cramps	Yarrow
	Premenstrual Syndrome (PMS)	Yarrow
Gastrointestinal	Appetite, Loss of	Centaury, Chicory, Dandelion, Fenugreek, Horehound, Onion, Wormwood, Yarrow
	Bloating, Feeling of Abdominal Fullness	Caraway, Dandelion, Fennel
	Colon, Irritable (Irritable Bowel Syndrome)	Flax
	Constipation	Buckthorn, Flax
	Diarrhea	Agrimony, Lady's Mantle, Oak Bark, Tormentil
	Diverticulitis	Flax
Gastrointestinal	Dyspepsia	Artichoke, Caraway, Centaury, Chicory, Coriander, Dandelion, Dill, Fennel, Horehound, Mistletoe, Radish, Rosemary, Sage, Wormwood, Yarrow, St. John's Wort
	Flatulence	Caraway, Dandelion, Fennel, Horehound

	Gastric Mucosa, Inflammation of	Marsh Mallow
	Hemorrhoids	Butcher's Broom
	Inflammation, Gastrointestinal Tract	Marsh Mallow
Hematology, lymphatic, Cancer	Malignant Tumors	Mistletoe
Liver and Gallbladder	Biliary Dyskinesia	Dandelion, Radish, Wormwood
	Biliary Spasm	Celandine
	Cholelithiasis	Radish
Neurology, Psychiatry	Anxiety	Hop, Valerian
	Depression	St. John's Wort
	Mood Disturbance	Hop
	Perspiration, Excessive	Sage
	Restlessness	Hop, Valerian
	Sleep Disturbances, Insomnia	Hop, Valerian
Respiratory (Lower and Upper Respiratory Tract Including Ears, Nose, Throat, Sinuses)	Catarrh, Upper Respiratory Tract	Coltsfoot, Fennel, Ivy, Primrose, Radish, Soapwort, Thyme, Watercress
	Colds and Flu	Elder
	Cough	Coltsfoot, Mallow, Marsh Mallow
	Inflammation, Oral or Pharyngeal	Blackthorn, Coltsfoot, Mallow, Marsh Mallow, Myrrh, Oak Bark, plantain, Rose, Sage
	Mucous Membrane, Irritation	Mallow, Marsh Mallow
Rheumatological, Orthopedic, Muscles, Contusions	Arthritis	Mistletoe
	Bruises, Contusions	Comfrey, St. John's Wort
	Edema, Post-traumatic	Horsetail
	Leg Cramps	Butcher's Broom
	Ligaments, Pulled	Comfrey
	Muscle Pain	St. John's Wort
	Rheumatism	Birch Leaf, Rosemary
Urinary Tract System (Kidney, Ureter, Bladder)	Diuretic	Dandelion
	Kidney Stones and Gravel	Asparagus, Birch Leaf, Horsetail, Lovage, Parsley

Treatments by Conditions:

Physiological Condition	Indicated Herb(s)
Ano-genital Irritation	Oak Bark
Anxiety	Hop, Valerian
Appetite, Loss of	Centaury, Chicory, Dandelion, Fenugreek, Horehound, Onion, Wormwood, Yarrow
Artherosclerosis	Onion
Arthritis	Mistletoe
Biliary Dyskinesia	Dandelion, Radish, Wormwood
Biliary Spasm	Celandine
Bloating, Feeling of Abdominal Fullness	Caraway, Dandelion, Fennel
Bruises, Contusions	Comfrey, St. John's Wort
Burns	St. John's Wort
Cardiac Insufficiency	Hawthorn, Lily of the Valley
Cardiac Symptoms	Motherwort
Catarrh, Upper Respiratory Tract	Coltsfoot, Fennel, Ivy, Primrose, Radish, Soapwort, Thyme, Watercress
Cholelithiasis	Radish
Circulatory Disorders	Butcher's Broom, Rosemary
Colds and Flu	Elder
Colon, Irritable (Irritable Bowel Syndrome)	Flax
Constipation	Buckthorn, Flax
Cor Pulmonade	Lily of the Valley
Cough	Coltsfoot, Mallow, Marsh Mallow
Depression	St. John's Wort
Diarrhea	Agrimony, Lady's Mantle, Oak Bark, Tormentil
Diuretic	Dandelion
Diverticulitis	Flax
Dyspepsia	Artichoke, Caraway, Centaury, Chicory, Coriander, Dandelion, Dill, Fennel, Horehound, Mistletoe, Radish, Rosemary, Sage, Wormwood, Yarrow, St. John's Wort
Edema, Post-traumatic	Horsetail
Flatulence	Caraway, Dandelion, Fennel, Horehound
Gastric Mucosa, Inflammation of	Marsh Mallow
Geriatric Vascular Changes	Garlic, Hawthorn, Onion
Hemorrhoids	Butcher's Broom
Hypercholesteremia	Garlic
Inflammation, Gastrointestinal Tract	Marsh Mallow
Inflammation, Oral or Pharyngeal	Blackthorn, Coltsfoot, Mallow, Marsh Mallow, Myrrh, Oak Bark, plantain, Rose, Sage
Irrigation, Mouth	Mallow
Itching	Butcher's Broom
Kidney Stones and Gravel	Asparagus, Birch Leaf, Horsetail, Lovage, Parsley

Leg Cramps	Butcher's Broom
Ligaments, Pulled	Comfrey
Malignant Tumors	Mistletoe
Mood Disturbance	Hop
Mucous Membrane, Irritation	Mallow, Marsh Mallow
Muscle Pain	St. John's Wort
Pelvic Cramps	Yarrow
Perspiration, Excessive	Sage
Premenstrual Syndrome (PMS)	Yarrow
Restlessness	Hop, Valerian
Rheumatism	Birch Leaf, Rosemary
Seborrhea	Heartsease
Skin, Injury or Irritation	Agrimony, Oak Bark, plantain
Sleep Disturbances, Insomnia	Hop, Valerian
Tachycardia	Motherwort

Plant Monographs

The monographs on the following pages provide details on each plant and herb. You'll find pictures, quick facts, cultivation information, and detailed historical profile for most plants.

Agrimony

Rosaceae Potereae

239. Agrimonia Eupatoria

Quick Facts

Latin/Linnaen:	*Agrimonia Eupatoria L.*
Family:	*Rosaceaee*
Old English :	Garclife, Garcliue, Garclive
Synonyms:	Burr Marigold, Church Steeples, Cocklebur, Common Agrimony, Harvest Lice, Liverwort, Philanthropos, Rat's Tail, Stickwort, White Tansy
Action:	Astringent
Parts Used:	Dried above ground parts.
Indicated For:	**Internal**: Mild, non-specific, acute diarrhea; inflammation of oral and pharyngeal mucosa. **External:** Mild, superficial inflammation of the skin.
Dosage:	**For Internal application**: Average daily dosage of 3g. of herb, or equivalent preparations.
Preparation:	Crushed Herb or Herb Powder for tisanes, or other natural preparations for internal or external use. infusions, decoctions or tinctures.
Cautions:	
Other Ues:	**Tissane**: make a sweetly scented and honey-flavored tea. Use 250ml or a cup of boiling water to steep 5 to 10 ml-about 1 to 2 teaspoons of powdered agrimony, if this is unavailable, use 15 ml-or three teaspoons of lightly crushed fresh agrimony leaves in 250 ml. Let the herb diffuse slowly into the water. **Brewing**: Add the fresh flowers of the agrimony to home brewed beer as an herbal taste enhancer. **Dye:** A deep yellow dye can be made from the leaves and stems harvested in the fall. Harvesting earlier in the year will yield a buff yellow. **Crafts**: Any sweet-smelling plant sachets and potpourris can be improved by including fragrant agrimony flowers in the mix. **Tanning**: Owing to its presence of tannin, its use has been recommended in dressing leather.

Description

The whole of Agrimonia Eupatoria is dark green with numerous soft hairs. The soft hairs aid in the plant's seed pods sticking to any animal or person coming in contact with the plant. The flower spikes have a spicy odor like apricots.

Agrimonia Eupatoria is a food plant for the caterpillars of the snout moth Endotricha flammealis.

The common agrimony grows as a deciduous, perennial herbaceous plant and reached heights of up to 100 centimeters. Its roots are deep rhizomes, from which spring the stems. It is characterized by its typical serrated edged pinnate leaves.

The short-stemmed yellow flowers appear from June to September in long, spike-like, racemose inflorescences. The single flower has an urn-shaped curved flower cup; the upper edge has several rows of soft, curved hook-shaped bristles, 1 to 4 millimeters long. The hermaphrodite flower has fivefold radial symmetry. There are five sepals present. There are five yellow, rounded petals. The petals and the five to 20 stamens rise above the tip of the flower cup. The two medium-sized carpels in the flower cups are sunk into, but not fused with it.

Cultivating & Harvesting

Hardiness Zone:	**6-10**
Soil pH:	Neutral
Soil type:	Average, well-drained soil
Cultivation:	Grow in containers where minimum temperatures go below 41 degrees F. Separate suckers when 2 to 6 inches high.
Sunlight:	Full sun to light shade
Habitat:	Europe / Asia / Africa: This is a common wayside plant which you would expect to find on roadside verges and grassy cliffs. It is very common throughout England, Wales and Ireland but not so often seen in the highlands and far North of Scotland.

The flowers with their abundant pollen supply attract hoverflies, flies and honey bees. The pollinated flowers develop fruits with burs. These attach to passing grazing animals such as cattle, sheep and deer and are spread over a large area.

Historical Notes

Agrimony has been stated to have medical and magical properties since the time of Pliny the elder. It is ruled astrologically by Cancer, according to Nicholas Culpeper. Common folklore held that it could cure musket wounds, and ward off witchcraft.

The name Agrimony is from Argemone, a word given by the Greeks to plants which were healing to the eyes, the name Eupatoria refers to Mithridates Eupator, a king who was a renowned concoctor of herbal remedies. The magic power of Agrimony is mentioned in an old English medical manuscript:

'If it be leyd under mann's heed,

He shal sleepyn as he were deed;

He shal never drede ne wakyn

Till fro under his heed it be takyn.'

Agrimony was one of the most famous vulnerary herbs. The Anglo-Saxons, who called it Garclive, taught that it would heal wounds, snake bites, warts, etc.

Bald's Leechbook advised the use of Agrimony as a cure for male impotence - saying it should be boiled in milk, and that it could excite a man who was "insufficiently virile;" it also states that when boiled in Welsh beer it would have the opposite effect.

Historical Medicinal Uses - For Entertainment ONLY

In traditional herbal medicine it was recommended as a cure for insomnia, often being incorporated in herbal pillows. It was also believed to be able to draw out splinters.

Modern herbalists (circa 1900) prescribe it for disorders of the kidneys, liver and bladder, and for irritable bowel syndrome. It is a mild astringent.

A. gryposepala, the plant's North American relative, also has traditional medical uses.

In the time of Chaucer, when we find its name appearing in the form of Egrimoyne, it was used with Mugwort and vinegar for 'a bad back' and 'alle woundes': and one of these old writers recommends it to be taken with a mixture of pounded frogs and human blood, as a remedy for all internal haemorrhages. It formed an ingredient of the famous arquebusade water as prepared against wounds inflicted by an arquebus, or hand-gun, and was mentioned by Philip de Comines, in his account of the battle of Morat in 1476. In France, the eau de arquebusade is still applied for sprains and bruises, being carefully made from many aromatic herbs. It was at one time included in the London Materia Medica as a vulnerary herb, but modern official medicine does not recognize its virtues, though it is still fully appreciated in herbal practice as a mild astringent and tonic, useful in coughs, diarrhoea and relaxed bowels. By pouring a pint of boiling water on a handful of the dried herb - stem, leaves and flowers - an excellent gargle may be made for a relaxed throat, and a teacupful of the same infusion is recommended, taken cold three or four times in the day for looseness in the bowels, also for passive losses of blood. It may be given either in infusion or decoction.

There are several other plants, not actually related botanically to the Common Agrimony, that were given the same name by the older herbalists because of their similar properties. These are the Common Hemp Agrimony, *Eupatorium Cannabinum* (Linn.) called by Gerard the Common Dutch Agrimony, and by Salmon, in his English Herbal (1710), *Eupatorium Aquaticum mas*, the Water Agrimony- also the plant now called the Trifid Bur-Marigold, *Bidens tripartita* (Linn.), but by older herbalists named the Water Hemp, Bastard Hemp and Bastard Agrimony. The name Bastard Agrimony has also been given to a species of true Agrimony, *Agrimonium Agrimonoides*, a native of Italy, growing in moist woods and among bushes.

Artichoke (Cardoon)

Quick Facts

Latin/Linnaen:	*Scolymus Cardunculus*
Family:	*Compositae*
Old English :	None
Synonyms:	None
Action:	Choleretic
Parts Used:	Leaf
Indicated For:	Dyspeptic problems
Dosage:	Unless othewise prescribed: Average daily dosage: Drug, 6g; Equivalent preparations.
Mode of Administration:	Dried, cut leaves, pressed juice of fresh plant, and other galenical preparations for internal use.
Cautions:	Known allergies to artichokes and other composites. Obstruction of bile ducts. In case of gallstones, use only after consultations with a physician.
Other Uses:	**Tea** - Artichokes can also be made into an herbal tea. It affords some of the qualities of the whole vegetable, acting as a diuretic and improving liver function. Artichoke tea is produced as a commercial product in the Da Lat region of Vietnam.
	Liqueur - Artichoke is the primary flavor of the 33-proof (16.5%-alcohol) Italian liqueur Cynar produced exclusively by the Campari Group. It can be served over ice as an aperitif or as a cocktail mixed with orange juice, especially popular in Switzerland.

Description

The Artichoke, or Cardoon, *Cynara Scolymus* & *Cynara Cardunculus,* is a perennial thistle-like plant which is member of the aster family, *Asteraceae,* (or archaic: daisy family, *Compositae*). It is a naturally occurring variant of the same species as the globe artichoke, and has many cultivated varieties. It is native to Southern Europe around the Mediterranean, where it was domesticated in ancient times.

It grows to 1.4–2 metres (4.6–6.6 ft) tall, with arching, deeply lobed, silvery, glaucous-green leaves 50–82 centimetres (20–32 in) long. The flowers develop in a large head from an edible bud about 8–15 centimetres (3.1–5.9 in) diameter with numerous triangular scales; the individual florets are purple. The edible portion of the buds consists primarily of the fleshy lower portions of the involucral bracts and the base, known as the "heart"; the mass of immature florets in the center of the bud is called the "choke" or beard. These are inedible in older larger flowers.

Cultivation

Hardiness Zone:	6-10
Soil pH:	6.0-7.0
Soil type:	Light, well drained soil
Cultivation:	Can be seed propagated; start indoors 8-12 weeks before last frost. Divisions can be planted after last frost. Tender perennial.
Sunlight:	Full sun-partial shade
Habitat:	Native to the Mediterranean, now grows as a weed in grassland areas.

Cardoon stalks can be covered with small, nearly invisible spines that can cause substantial pain if they become lodged in the skin. Several spineless cultivars have been developed to overcome this, but care in handling is recommended for all types.

Cardoon requires a long, cool growing season (about five months), but it is frost-sensitive. It also typically requires substantial growing space per plant, so is not much grown save where it is a regional favorite.

The cardoon is highly invasive and is able to adapt to dry climates. It has become a major weed in the pampas of Argentina and California; it is also considered a weed in Australia.

Historical Notes

The earliest description of the cardoon comes from the fourth century BC Greek writer Theophrastus. The cardoon was popular in Greek, Roman, and Persian cuisine. Cardoons remained popular in medieval and early modern Europe, and were common in the vegetable gardens of colonial America. They fell from fashion only in the late 19th century. In Europe, cardoon is still cultivated in France (Provence, Savoie, Lyonnais), Spain and Italy. In the Geneva region, where Huguenot refugees introduced it about 1685, the local variety cardy is considered a culinary specialty. "Before Cardoons are sent to table, the stalks or ribs are blanched by tying them together and wrapping them round with straw, which is also tied up with cord, and left so for about three weeks".

Gastronomy

Cardoons also are common vegetables in Northern Africa, often used in Algerian or Tunisian couscous.

While the flower buds can be eaten much as the artichoke, more often the stems are eaten after being braised in cooking liquid. Battered and fried, the stems are also traditionally served at St. Joseph's altars in New Orleans.

The stalks, which look like large celery stalks, can be served steamed or braised. They have an artichoke-like flavor. Cardoons are available in the market only in the winter months. In the U.S.A., it is rarely found in stores, but available in farmers' markets, where it is available through May, June, and July. The main root can also be boiled and served cold. Acclaimed chef Mario Batali calls the cardoon one of his favorite vegetables and says they have a "very sexy flavor."

Cardoons are also an ingredient in one of the national dishes of Spain, the cocido madrileño, a slow-cooking, one-pot, meat and vegetable dinner simmered in broth.

In the Abruzzi region of Italy, Christmas lunch is traditionally started with a soup of cardoons cooked in chicken broth with little meatballs (lamb or more rarely, beef), sometimes with the further addition of egg (which scrambles in the hot soup - called stracciatella) or fried chopped liver and heart.

It requires so much room that it is little grown in small gardens, and as a crop can hardly pay for the enormous extent of ground that it claims.

Artichoke Bottoms

If dried, they must be soaked, then stewed in weak gravy, and served with or without forcemeat in each. Or they may be boiled in milk, and served with cream sauce; or added to ragouts, French pies, etc.

To Dress Artichokes

Trim a few of the outside leaves off, and cut the stalk even. If young, half an hour will boil them. They are better for being gathered two or three days, first. Serve them with melted butter, in as many small cups as there are Artichokes, to help with each.

To keep Artichokes for the Winter

Artichoke bottoms, slowly dried, should be kept in paper bags.

RECIPES

Artichokes à la Barigoule

Trim some small Artichokes, and with the handle of an iron tablespoon scoop out all the fibrous part inside, Put about a pound of clean hog's-lard into a frying-pan on the fire, and when quite hot, fry the bottom of the Artichokes in it for about 3 minutes; then turn them upside down, and fry the tips of the leaves also, drain them upon a cloth to absorb all the grease, and fill them with a similar preparation to that directed for tomatoes a la Provencale; tie them up with a string, and place them in a large stewpan or <u>fricaudeaupan</u>; moisten with a little good stock; put the lid on; place them in the oven to simmer for about an hour; remove the strings, fill the centre of each Artichoke with some Italian sauce; dish them up with some of the sauce, and serve.

Artichokes à la Lyonnaise

Pull off the lower leaves without damaging the bottoms of the Artichokes, which must be turned smooth with a sharp knife; cut the Artichokes into quarters, remove the fibrous parts, trim them neatly, and parboil them in water with a little salt. Then put them in a saucepan on a slow fire to simmer very gently for about three-quarters of an hour, taking care that they do not burn; when done they should be of a deep yellow colour and nicely glazed. Dish them up in the form of a dome, showing the bottom of the Artichokes only; remove any leaves that may have broken off in the sautapan; add a spoonful of brown gravy or sauce, 2 pats of butter and some lemon-juice, simmer this over the fire, stirring it meanwhile with a spoon; and when the butter has been mixed in with the sauce, pour it over the Artichokes, and serve.

Asparagus

Asparagus officinalis L. Gemeiner Spargel.

Quick Facts

Latin/Linnaen:	*Asparagus officinalis*
Family:	*Asparagaceae*
Old English :	None
Synonyms:	None
Action:	Diuretic effect
Parts Used:	Root
Indicated For:	Irrigation therapy for inflammatory disease of the urinary tract and for prevention of kidney stones.
Dosage:	Unless otherwise prescribed: Daily dosage: 45-60g of rhizome; equivalent preparations.
Preparation:	Cut rhizomes for teas, as well as other galenical preparations for internal use. Note: Irrigation therapy: Be sure to provide adequate fluids.
Cautions:	Inflammatory kidney diseases. Note: No irrigation therapy if edema exists because of functional heart or kidney disorders. In rare cases, allergic skin reactions.
Other Uses:	

Description

Asparagus officinalis is a spring vegetable, a flowering perennial plant species in the genus *Asparagus*. It was once classified in the lily family, like its Allium cousins, onions and garlic, but the *Liliaceae* have been split and the onion-like plants are now in the family *Amaryllidaceae* and asparagus in the *Asparagaceae*. *Asparagus officinalis* is native to most of Europe, northern Africa and western Asia, and is widely cultivated as a vegetable crop.

Asparagus is an herbaceous, perennial plant growing to 100–150 centimetres (39–59 in) tall, with stout stems with much-branched feathery foliage. The "leaves" are in fact needle-like cladodes (modified stems) in the axils of scale leaves; they are 6–32 millimetres (0.24–1.3 in) long and 1 millimetre (0.039 in) broad, and clustered 4–15 together. The root system is adventitious and the root type is fasciculated. The flowers are bell-shaped, greenish-white to yellowish, 4.5–6.5 millimetres (0.18–0.26 in) long, with six tepals partially fused together at the base; they are produced singly or in clusters of 2–3 in the junctions of the branchlets.

Plants native to the western coasts of Europe (from northern Spain north to Ireland, Great Britain, and northwest Germany) are treated as Asparagus officinalis subsp. prostratus (Dumort.) Corb., distinguished by its low-growing, often prostrate stems growing to only 30–70 centimetres (12–28 in) high, and shorter cladodes 2–18 millimetres (0.079–0.71 in) long. It is treated as a distinct species, Asparagus prostratus Dumort, by some authors. A remarkable adaptation is the edible asparagus, while in the Macaronesian Islands several species, (Asparagus umbellatus, Asparagus scoparius, etc.), are preserved the original form, a leafy vine; in the Mediterranean, the asparagus genus has evolved into thorny species.

Cultivation

Hardiness Zone:	4-10
Soil pH:	4.3-8.2 saline soil
Soil type:	Light/Medium/Heavy well drained soil
Cultivation:	Easy to grow, can start the asparagus bed from seed, but plants reach the cutting stage quicker if 1 year old roots are used. Perennial.
Sunlight:	Sun-semi shade
Habitat:	Native to most of Europe, northern Africa and western Asia. Thrives in soils which are too saline for normal plants.

Asparagus is usually dioecious, meaning male and female flowers on separate plants, but occasionally hermaphrodite flowers are found. The fruit of the asparagus plant is a small red berry which is poisonous to humans.

Tomatoes are a useful companion plant for asparagus. Tomato plants repel the asparagus beetle and the asparagus repels root nematodes which are harmful to tomatoes.

An asparagus plant can be productive for up to 20 years.

Historical Notes

This well-known table delicacy may be found wild on the sea-coast in the South-west of England, especially near the Lizard, in the Isle of Anglesea, otherwise it is a rare native. In the southern parts of Russia and Poland the waste steppes are covered with this plant, which is there eaten by horses and cattle as grass. It is also common in Greece, and was formerly much esteemed as a vegetable by the Greeks and Romans. It appears to have been cultivated in the time of Cato the Elder, 200 years B.C., and Pliny mentions a species that grew near Ravenna, of which three heads would weigh a pound.

About 20,000 years ago, asparagus was eaten near Aswan in Egypt. It has been used as a vegetable and medicine, owing to its delicate flavour, diuretic properties, and more. It is pictured as an offering on an Egyptian frieze dating to 3000 BC. In ancient times, it was known in Syria and in Spain. Greeks and Romans ate it fresh when in season and dried the vegetable for use in winter; Romans would even freeze it high in the Alps, for the Feast of Epicurius. Emperor Augustus reserved the Asparagus Fleet for hauling the vegetable, and coined the expression "faster than cooking asparagus" for quick action.

There is a recipe for cooking asparagus in the oldest surviving book of recipes, Apicius's third century AD De re coquinaria, Book III.

Asparagus drew little medieval attention until al-Nafzawi's The Perfumed Garden celebrates its aphrodisiacal power, which the Indian Ananga Ranga attributes to special phosporus elements that also counteract fatigue, and by 1469 it was cultivated in French monasteries. Asparagus appears to have been hardly noticed in England until 1538, and in Germany until 1542.

France's Louis XIV had special greenhouses built for growing it. The finest texture and the strongest and yet delicate taste is in the tips. The points d'amour ("love tips") were served as a delicacy to Madame de Pompadour. Asparagus became available to the New World around 1850, in the United States

The virtues of Asparagus are well known as a diuretic and laxative; and for those of sedentary habits who suffer from symptoms of gravel, it has been found very beneficial, as well as in cases of dropsy. The fresh expressed juice is taken medicinally in tablespoonful doses.

Prussian Asparagus, which is brought to some English markets, is not a species of Asparagus at all, but consists of the spikes of Ornithogalum pyrenaicum, which grows abundantly in hedges and pastures (especially in the locality of Bath).

Culpepper tells us 'The decoction of the roots (Asparagus) boiled in wine, and taken is good to clear the sight, and being held in the mouth easeth the toothache.' He also tells us it helps those sinews that 'are shrunk by cramps and convulsions, and helpeth the sciatica.'

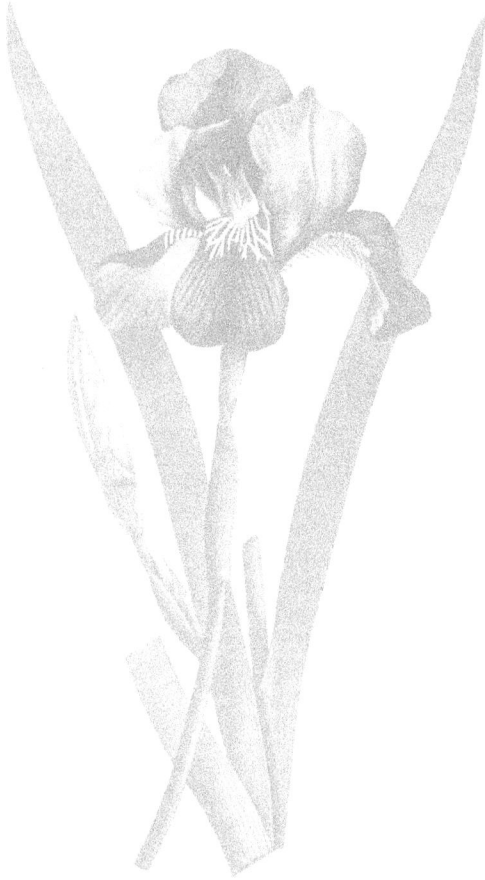

Birch Leaf

XVI. 5.   76. Betulaceae.

104. Betula verrucosa Ehrhart. Weiße Birke.

Quick Facts

Latin/Linnaen:	*Betula Pendula*
Family:	*Betulaceae*
Old English :	None
Synonyms:	White Birch, Bouleau (Fr.)
Action:	Diuretic
Parts Used:	Leaves
Indicated For:	Irrigation therapy for bacterial and inflammatory diseases of the urinary tract and for kidney gravel; supportive therapy for rheumatic ailments.
Dosage:	Unless otherwise prescribed: Average daily dosage: 2-3g of herb several times a daily; equivalent preparations.
Preparation:	Comminuted herb or dry extracts for teas, as well as other galenical preparations and freshly pressed plant juices or oral use. Note: For irrigation therapy, observe copious fluid intake.
Cautions:	Note: No irrigation therapy if edema exists due to impaired heart and kidney function.
Other Uses:	Extensive – See Historical Notes

Description

Betula pendula (Silver Birch) is a widespread European birch, though in southern Europe it is only found at higher altitudes. Its range extends into southwest Asia in the mountains of northern Turkey and the Caucasus. The closely related Betula platyphylla in northern Asia and Betula szechuanica of central Asia are also treated as varieties of Silver Birch by some botanists, as B. pendula var. platyphylla and B. pendula var. szechuanica respectively

It is a medium-sized deciduous tree, typically reaching 15–25 m tall (exceptionally up to 39 m), with a slender trunk usually under 40 cm diameter (exceptionally to 1 m diameter), and a crown of arched branches with drooping branchlets. The bark is white, often with black diamond-shaped marks or larger patches, particularly at the base. The shoots are rough with small warts, and hairless, and the leaves 3–7 cm long, triangular with a broad base and pointed tip, and coarsely double-toothed serrated margins. The flowers are wind-pollinated catkins, produced before the leaves in early spring, the small (1–2 mm) winged seeds ripening in late summer on pendulous, cylindrical catkins 2–4 cm long and 7 mm broad.

It is distinguished from the related Downy Birch (B. pubescens, the other common European birch) in having hairless, warty shoots (hairy and without warts in Downy Birch), more triangular leaves with double serration on the margins (more ovoid and with single serrations in Downy Birch), and whiter bark often with scattered black fissures (greyer, less fissured, in Downy Birch). It is also distinguished cytologically, Silver Birch being diploid (with two sets of chromosomes), whereas Downy Birch is tetraploid (four sets of chromosomes). Hybrids between the two are known, but are very rare, and being triploid, are sterile. The two have differences in habitat requirements, with Silver Birch found mainly on dry, sandy soils, and Downy Birch more common on wet, poorly drained sites such as clay soils and peat bogs. Silver birch also demands slightly more summer warmth than does Downy birch, which is significant in the cooler parts of Europe. Many North American texts treat the two species as conspecific (and cause confusion by combining the Downy Birch's alternative vernacular name 'White Birch', with the scientific name B. pendula of the other species), but they are regarded as distinct species throughout Europe.

It commonly grows with the mycorrhizal fungus Amanita muscaria in a mutualistic relationship. This applies particularly to acidic or nutrient poor soils. Other mycorrhizal associates include Leccinum scabrum and Cantharellus cibarius. Old trees are often killed by the decay fungus Piptoporus betulinus, and the branches often have witch's brooms caused by the fungus Taphrina betulina.

Cultivation

Hardiness Zone:	2-7
Soil pH:	Below 6.5
Soil type:	Can tolerate poor soil.
Cultivation:	Can be cultivated by seed or transplant.
Sunlight:	Sun
Habitat:	Northern Europe, southern Europe only at high altitudes. Naturalized in Canada. Requires a cool climate.

The Silver Birch is a fast growing, but short lived deciduous tree. It is a good tree to grow near a compost pile because it aids in the fermentation process. It is a shallow rooted tree that may need water during dry periods.

Historical Notes

The name is a very ancient one, probably derived from the Sanscrit bhurga, 'a tree whose bark is used for writing upon.' From its uses in boat-building and roofing it is also connected with the A.S. beorgan, 'to protect or shelter.' The Birch was also known as Beth or Beith to our Gaelic ancestors, and as Bedwen by the Welsh.

Coleridge speaks of it as the 'Lady of the Woods.' It is remarkable for its lightness, grace, and elegance, and after rain it has a fragrant odour.
The young branches are of a rich red brown or orange brown, and the trunks usually white, especially in the second species of B. alba, B. verrucosa. B. pubescens is darker, and has downy instead of warted twigs.

The wood is soft and not very durable, but being cheap, and the tree being able to thrive in any situation and soil, growing all over Europe, is used for many humble purposes, such as bobbins for thread mills, herring-barrel staves, broom handles, and various fancy articles. In country districts the Birch has very many uses, the lighter twigs being employed for thatching and wattles. The twigs are also used in broom making and in the manufacture of cloth. The tree has also been one of the sources from which asphyxiating gases have been manufactured, and its charcoal is much used for gunpowder.

Other Uses

Oiled Paper - The white epidermis of the bark is separable into thin layers, which may be employed as a substitute for oiled paper in a variety of uses.

Oiling Leather - It yields oil of Birch Tar, and the peculiar, well-known odour of Russia leather is due to the use of this oil in the process of dressing. It likewise imparts durability to leather, and it is owing to its presence that books bound in Russia leather are not liable to become mouldy. The production of Birch Tar oil is a Russian industry of considerable importance.

Insect Repellant - It is also distilled in Holland and Germany, but these oils are appreciably different from the Russian oil. It has the property of keeping away insects and preventing gnatbites when smeared on the hands.

Tanning - Birch bark only contains about 3 per cent tannic acid, but is extensively used for tanning, wherever there are large birch forests, throughout Northern Europe. As it gives a pale colour to the skin, it is used for the preliminary and the final stages of tanning. It contains betulin and betuls camphor. The leaves contain betulorentic acid.

Solvent - Birch Tar oil is almost identical with Wintergreen oil. It is not completely soluble in 95 per cent acetic acid, nor in aniline, but Turpentine oil dissolves it completely.

Birch Wine -When the stem of the tree is wounded, a saccharine juice flows out which is susceptible, with yeast, of vinous fermentation. A beer, wine, spirit and vinegar are prepared from it in some parts of Europe. Birch Wine, concocted from this thin, sugary sap of the tree, collected from incisions made in the trees in March, honey, cloves and lemon peel being added and then the whole fermented with yeast, makes a very pleasant cordial, formerly much appreciated. From 16 to 18 gallons of sap may be drawn from one large tree, and a moderate tapping does no harm.

Birch Wine Recipe

- 🌿 1 gallon birch sap
- 🌿 1 3/4 lbs granulated sugar
- 🌿 1/2 oz. citric acid
- 🌿 1/8 tsp tannin
- 🌿 1 tsp yeast nutrient
- 🌿 1 pkt Reisling or Graves wine yeast

First measure the specific gravity of the sap with a hydrometer to determine exactly how much sugar to add to achieve a starting specific gravity of 1.085-1.090. In an enamel- or teflon-coated pot, stir the required amount of sugar into the birch sap and bring to a boil. Immediately remove from the heat and stir until all sugar, citric acid and yeast nutrient is dissolved. When cool, stir in the tannin and pitch the activated yeast. Cover the primary and stir daily for 8-10 days. Transfer to a secondary and fit airlock. Ferment to dryness (6-8 weeks), rack into a sanitized secondary, refit the airlock and bulk age 6 months, checking airlock from time to time to make sure it doesn't dry out. Rack, sweeten if desired and bottle.

Historical Medicinal Uses - For Entertainment ONLY

Various parts of the tree have been applied to medicinal uses. The young shoots and leaves secrete a resinous substance having acid properties, which, combined with alkalies, is said to be a tonic laxative. The leaves have a peculiar, aromatic, agreeable odour and a bitter taste, and have been employed in the form of infusion (Birch Tea) in gout, rheumatism and dropsy, and recommended as a reliable solvent of stone in the kidneys. With the bark they resolve and resist putrefaction. A decoction of them is good for bathing skin eruptions, and is serviceable in dropsy. The oil is astringent, and is mainly employed for its curative effects in skin affections, especially eczema, but is also used for some internal maladies. The inner bark is bitter and astringent, and has been used in intermittent fevers. The vernal sap is diuretic.

Moxa is made from the yellow, fungous excrescences of the wood, which sometimes swell out from the fissures.

Other Species

B. benta (Cherry Birch, Black Birch, Sweet Birch, Mahogany Birch, or Mountain Mahogany) is an American variety, with richlymarked wood suitable for the use of cabinet and pianoforte makers. The liquor is used in Kamschatka without previous fermentation. The cambium, or the layer between the wood and the bast, is eaten in the spring, cut into strips like vermicelli, and the bark is stimulant, diaphoretic, and astringent, in a warm infusion. In decoction or syrup it forms an excellent tonic for dysentery, and is said to be useful in gravel and female obstructions.

B. trophylla is a syn. of Rhus Aromatica, or Fragrant Sumach.

B. papyracea, or Paper Birch, is largely used for canoe-making in America.

B. nana, or Smooth Dwarf Birch, rarely grows above 3 feet in height. The leaves are said to dye a better yellow than the Common Birch; the seeds are a principal food of ptarmigan in Lapland; Moxa is prepared from it and regarded as an effective remedy in all painful diseases.

Blackthorn

394. *Prunus spinosa* L.   Schlehdorn.

Quick Facts

Latin/Linnaen:	*Prunus Spinosa*
Family:	*Rosaceae*
Old English :	Slahþorn
Synonyms:	Sloe-thorn
Action:	Astringent
Parts Used:	Berry
Indicated For:	Mild inflammations of the oral and pharyngeal mucosa.
Dosage:	Unless otherwise prescribed: Daily dosage: 2-4g drug; equivalent preparation.
Preparation:	Comminuted herb for teas and other galenical preparations for mouth rinses.
Cautions:	None
Other Uses:	**Dye**: If gathered before ripe, the berries furnish a yellow dye, used formerly for staining maps or paper. The bark also affords a yellow dye.
	Pigment: When ripe, if mixed with gum-arabic and limewater, they form the pigment 'Sap or bladder green,' so well known to water-colour painters.

Description

Prunus spinosa (blackthorn or sloe) is a species of Prunus native to Europe, western Asia, and locally in northwest Africa. It is also locally naturalised in New Zealand and eastern North America.

Prunus spinosa is a deciduous large shrub or small tree growing to 5 m tall, with blackish bark and dense, stiff, spiny branches. The leaves are oval, 2–4.5 cm long and 1.2–2 cm broad, with a serrated margin. The flowers are 1.5 cm diameter, with five creamy-white petals; they are produced shortly before the leaves in early spring, and are hermaphroditic and insect-pollinated. The fruit, called a "sloe", is a drupe 10–12 millimetres (0.39–0.47 in) in diameter, black with a purple-blue waxy bloom, ripening in autumn, and harvested -- traditionally, at least in the UK, in October or November after the first frosts. Sloes are thin-fleshed, with a very strongly astringent flavour when fresh.

Prunus spinosa is frequently confused with the related P. cerasifera (cherry plum), particularly in early spring when the latter starts flowering somewhat earlier than P. spinosa. They can be distinguished by flower colour, creamy white in P. spinosa, pure white in P. cerasifera. They can also be distinguished in winter by the more shrubby habit with stiffer, wider-angled branches of P. spinosa; in summer by the relatively narrower leaves of P. spinosa, more than twice as long as broad;[1][4] and in autumn by the colour of the fruit skin -- purplish-black in P. spinosa and yellow or red in P. cerasifera.

The foliage is sometimes eaten by the larvae of Lepidoptera, including emperor moth, willow beauty, white-pinion spotted, common emerald, November moth, pale November moth, mottled pug, green pug, brimstone moth, feathered thorn, brown-tail, yellow-tail, short-cloaked moth, lesser yellow underwing, lesser broad-bordered yellow underwing, double square-spot, black and brown hairstreaks, hawthorn moth (Scythropia crataegella) and the case-bearer moth Coleophora anatipennella. Dead blackthorn wood provides food for the caterpillars of the concealer moth Esperia oliviella.

Cultivation

Hardiness Zone:	4
Soil pH	Prefers alkaline soil
Soil type	All well drained soils except acidic. Tolerant of maritime exposure.
Cultivation:	Division of suckers during dormant season. Seed reproduction is slow, can take 18 months. Softwood cuttings.
Sunlight:	Sunny to part sun.

Habitat:	Sunny edge of woodland, hedge. Britain and Europe

Historical Notes

The expression "sloe-eyed" for a person with dark eyes comes from the fruit, and is first attested in A. J. Wilson's 1867 novel Vashti. The word "sloe" comes from Old English slāh.

Buckthorn (Alder)

Quick Facts

Latin/Linnaen:	*Rhamnus cathartica*
Family:	*Rhamnaceae*
Old English :	ðefeðorn, þefan, þorn
Synonyms:	Common Buckthorn, Purging Buckthorn, Highwaythorn, Waythorn, Hartsthorn, Ramsthorn, Black Dogwood. Frangula Bark
Action:	Laxative
Parts Used:	Berries, Bark
Indicated For:	Constipation
Dosage:	Unless otherwise prescribed: 20-30 mg hydroxyanthracene derivatives daily, calculated as glycofrangulin A. The individually correct dosage is the smallest dosage necessary to maintain a soft stool.
Preparation:	**Bark:** Tea, decoction, cold maceration or elixir.
	Berry: Crushed drug for infusions, boiling, cold macerations or elixirs.
Cautions:	Some patients may suffer from gastrointentinal cramps. If this occurs, the dose should be reduced. In the case of chronic use/overuse: loss of electrolytes, especially loss of potassium.
	Contraindications: Obstruction of the bowel or intestines, acute inflammatory conditions of the bowels such as Crohn's disease, colitis, apendicitis; abdominal pain of unknown origin; children under 12 years; pregnancy.
Other Uses:	None known

Description

Rhamnus cathartica is a deciduous shrub or small tree growing up to 10 m tall, with grey-brown bark and spiny branches. The leaves are elliptic to oval, 2.5–9 cm long and 1.2–3.5 cm broad; they are green, turning yellow in autumn, and are arranged somewhat variably in opposite to subopposite pairs or alternately. The flowers are yellowish-green, with four petals; they are dioecious and insect pollinated. The fruit is a globose black drupe 6–10 mm diameter containing two to four seeds; it is mildly poisonous for people, but readily eaten by birds, which disperse the seeds in their droppings.

It is generally about the same size as the Common Buckthorn, but is distinguished from it by its less bushy and more tree-like habit, by the absence of thorns on its branches and by its larger and entire, not toothed, feather-veined leaves, which are all arranged alternately on the stem, none opposite to one another. The flowers are produced not only from the wood of the preceding year, but also on the shoots of the current year, and have a five-parted calyx, while that of the Common Buckthorn is four-cleft. They bloom in May and are of an inconspicuous green. Their fruit, which is ripe in September, is not unlike that of the Common Buckthorn, but the berry has only two, or at most three, roundish, angular seeds, instead of four. Bees are likewise constant visitors of the flowers of this species, and goats eat the leaves voraciously.

Cultivation

Hardiness Zone:	3-8
Soil pH:	Neutral-Alkaline
Soil type:	High calcium content
Cultivation:	Easily grown by seed.
Sunlight:	Sun-part sun
Habitat:	Native to Europe, northwest Africa, western Asia. It is adaptable to many environments; woodlands, wood edges, prairies and open fields.

The Common Buckthorn, *Rhamnus cathartica*, is shade-tolerant, moderately fast-growing and short-lived. This species is a tough, durable tree which adapts to urban or suburban environments, and virtually any area it is dispersed in. It is widely regarded as a major invasive species whose shade prevents the establishment of native trees or shrubs. It has become the target of efforts to eradicate it from home sites, parks and woodland areas. It is difficult to control because it sprouts vigorously and repeatedly from the root collar following cutting, girdling, or burning, though it can be controlled by applying concentrated herbicide to the cut stem. (Check your local laws to be sure that cultivation is permitted.)

Historical Notes

Buckthorn was well known to the AngloSaxons and is mentioned as Hartsthorn or Waythorn in their medical writings and glossaries dating before the Norman Conquest. The Welsh physicians of the thirteenth century prescribed the juice of the fruit of Buckthorn boiled with honey as an aperient drink.

In place of the violently-acting juice of the berries of the Common Buckthorn, a fluid extract prepared from the bark of the closely allied and milder Alder Buckthorn or Black Alder (Rhamnus Frangula, Linn.) has been proved a very satisfactory substitute. Frangula bark is official both in the United States and the British Pharmacopoeia. Its use has been, however, somewhat neglected and the much advertized Cascara Sagrada (R. purshianus) has greatly taken its place, though it is a less agreeable aperient.

Historical Medicinal Uses - For Entertainment ONLY

The dried bark collected from the young trunk and moderately-sized branches in early summer and kept at least one year before being used. It is stripped from the branches and dried either on sunny days, out of doors, in halfshade, or by artificial heat, on shelves or trays, in a warm, well-ventilated room.

The dried bark varies considerably in appearance, according to the age of the branch or stem from which it has been taken. Young bark, which is to be preferred, occurs in narrow, single or double quills and is of papery texture, about 1/25 inch thick. It is of a greyish or blackish-brown colour outside, with numerous small, whitish corky warts. When gently scraped, the inner layers are seen to be crimson in colour. The inner surface of the bark is smooth, of a pale, yellowish brown and very finely striated. The fracture is short. Older bark is rougher externally, thicker and usually in single quills or channelled pieces.

The bark is nearly inodorous; its taste is pleasant, sweetish and slightly bitter. When masticated, it colours the saliva yellow. This milder English Buckthorn acts likewise as a tonic to the intestine and is especially useful for relieving piles. Lozenges of the Alder Buckthorn are dispensed under the name of 'Aperient Fruit Lozenges.' The juice of the berries, though little used, is aperient without being irritating.

Country people used to take the bark boiled in ale for jaundice.

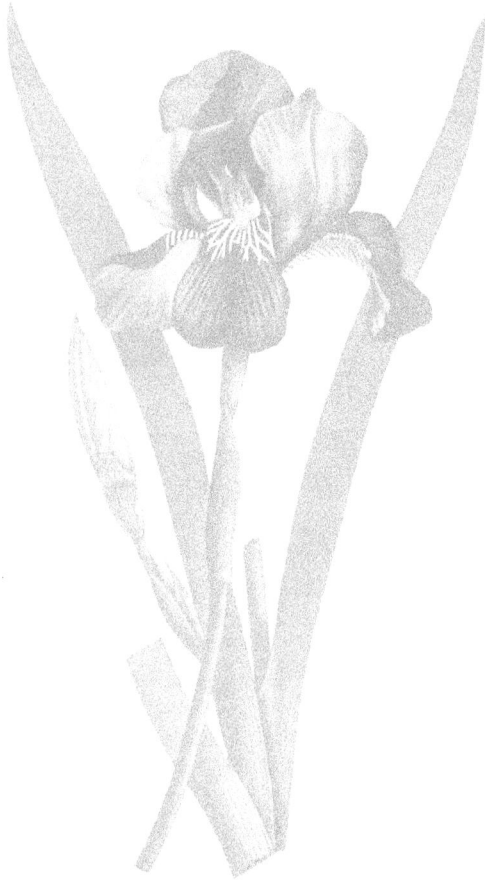

Butcher's Broom

114. *Ruscus aculeatus L.* Stechender Mäusedorn.

Quick Facts

Latin/Linnaen:	*Ruscus aculeatus*
Family:	*Asparagaceae*
Old English :	Cneowolen
Synonyms:	Knee Holly, kneeholm, knee hull, pettigree, and sweet broom Kneeholy. Jew's Myrtle.
Action:	Increase in venous tone, Electrolyte-like reaction on the cell wall of capillaries, Antiphlogistic, Diuretic.
Parts Used:	Roots
Indicated For:	Supportive therapy for discomforts of chronic venous insufficiency, such as pain and heaviness, as well as cramps in the legs, itching, and swelling. Supprotive therapy for complaints of hemorrhoids, such as itching and burning.
Dosage:	Unless otherwise prescribed: Daily dosage: Raw extract, equivalent to 7-11 mg total ruscogenin (determined as the sum of neoruscogenin and ruscogenin obtained after fermentation or acid hydrolysis).
Preparation:	Extracts and their preparations for internal use.
Cautions:	In rare cases, gastric disorders or nausea may occur.
Other Uses:	None known

Description

Ruscus aculeatus is a low evergreen Eurasian shrub, with flat shoots known as cladodes that give the appearance of stiff, spine-tipped leaves. Small greenish flowers appear in spring, and are borne singly in the centre of the cladodes. The female flowers are followed by a red berry, and the seeds are bird-distributed, but the plant also spreads vegetatively by means of rhizomes. *Ruscus aculeatus* occurs in woodlands and hedgerows, where it is tolerant of deep shade, and also on coastal cliffs. It is also widely planted in gardens, and has spread as a garden escape in many areas outside its native range.

Butcher's broom has been known to enhance blood flow to the brain, legs, and hands. It has been used to relieve constipation and water retention and improve circulation. Since Butcher's broom tightens blood vessels and capillaries, it is used to treat a common condition known as varicose veins (Bouskela, Cyrino, and Marcelon).

It is also used for hemorrhoids. In a 1999 open-label (not blinded) clinical trial, the herb was tested as a hemorrhoid treatment and showed statistically significant positive results. It also showed reduction in venous insufficiency in two other studies. It was approved by the German Commission E guidelines for hemorrhoids treatment. It is occasionally prescribed for varicose veins which can be a complication of pregnancy. However, since it is classified as a natural product, there is no evidence or trials to suggest complete safety for the fetus. A qualified healthcare practitioner should be consulted prior to using this compound during pregnancy.

A study published in 1999 suggested that Butcher's Broom may also improve symptoms of postural hypotension without increasing supine blood pressure. Suggested mechanisms to explain this include stimulation of venous alpha 1 and 2 adrenoreceptors and decreased capillary permiability.

Cultivation

Hardiness Zone:	7-9
Soil pH:	6-8
Soil type:	Is tolerant of poor soil, prefers dry soil.
Cultivation:	By seed, root division or cuttings.
Sunlight:	Prefers shade.
Habitat:	Hedgerows and woodlands

Butcher's Broom is very hardy, thriving in almost any soil or situation, and is often planted in shrubberies or edges of woods, on account of its remaining green after the deciduous trees have shed their leaves.

Propagation is generally effected by division of the roots in autumn. The shrub may also be propagated by seed, but quicker results are obtained by the other method. When planted under trees it soon spreads into large clumps.

Historical Notes

Butcher's Broom, a low, shrubby, evergreen plant, which occurs not infrequently in woods and waste and bushy places, especially in the south of England, is sometimes called Knee Holly, though it is in no way allied to the true Holly, being a member of the Lily tribe. It is, however, entirely different in appearance to the bulbous plants we regard as the characteristic representatives of this group, it being, in fact, the only Liliaceous shrub known in England, and the only representative of its genus among our flora, the other species of the genus, Ruscus, being mostly native to northern Africa.

The name Knee Holly appears to have been given it from its rising to about the height of a man's knee (though occasionally specimens are found growing about 3 feet high), and from its having, like the true Holly, prickly leaves, which are also evergreen.

There is no other British plant exhibiting any similarity to the Butcher's Broom. Its tough, green, erect, striated stems, which are destitute of bark, send out from the upper part many short branches, plentifully furnished with very rigid leaves, which are really a mere expansion of the stem, and terminate each in a single sharp spine. The small greenish-white flowers are solitary growing from the centre of the leaves and blossom in the early spring. They are dioecious, i.e. stamens and pistils are on different plants, as is also mostly the case with the Holly and Mistletoe. The corolla is deeply six-cleft, the stamens, in the one kind of flower, connected at the base, the style, in the fertile flowers, surrounded by a nectary. The fertile flowers are succeeded by scarlet berries as large as cherries, which are ripe in September, and remain attached to the plant all the winter and cause it often to be picked for room decoration.

Another member of the same family is Ruscus racemosus or Alexandrinus, a favourite evergreen shrub with the leaf-like branches unarmed, and the racemes of small flowers terminal. It is the original of the 'poets' laurel' so often seen in classic prints. It too has red berries - smaller than those of the Butcher's Broom.

Other species are R. androgynous, a native of the Canaries, which bears its flowers along the edges of the so-called leaves; R. Hypophyllum, in which the flowers are borne on the underside of the flattened branches; and R. Hypoglossum, also from southern Europe, in which the flowers are on the upper side under a bract-like branchlet.

The young shoots of Butcher's Broom have often been eaten like those of the Asparagus, a plant to which it is closely allied. The matured branches used to be bound into bundles and sold to butchers for sweeping their blocks, hence the name: Butcher's Broom. It is frequently made into besoms in Italy. One of the names given the plant, 'Jew's Myrtle,' points to its use for service during the Feast of Tabernacles. 'Pettigree' is another old popular name, the meaning of which is not clear.

Parkinson tells us that Butcher's Broom was used to preserve 'hanged meate' from being eaten by mice, and also for the making of brooms, 'but the King's Chamber is by revolution of time turned to the Butcher's stall, for that a bundle of the stalkes tied together serveth them to cleanse their stalls and from thence have we our English name of Butcher's broom.'

Historical Medicinal Uses - For Entertainment ONLY

Culpepper says it is 'a plant of Mars, being of a gallant cleansing and opening quality. The decoction of the root drank, and a poultice made of the berries and leaves applied, are effectual-in knitting and consolidating broken bones or parts out of joint. The common way of using it is to boil the root of it, and Parsley and Fennel and Smallage in white wine, and drink the decoction, adding the like quantity of Grassroot to them: The more of the root you boil the stronger will the decoction be; it works no ill effects, yet I hope you have wit enough to give the strongest decoction to the strongest bodies.'

The root or rhizome is used and is collected in autumn. The root is thick, striking deep into the ground. When dry, it is brownish grey, 2 to 4 inches long and

1/3 inch in diameter, having somewhat crowded rings and rounded stem scars on the upper surface and many woody rootlets below. If a transverse section be made, a number of vascular bundles in the central portion are to be seen. The root has no odour, but its taste is sweetish at first and then slightly acrid.

The whole herb is also collected, being dried in the same manner as Holly leaves.

Butcher's Broom was said to be a diaphoretic, diuretic, deobstruent and aperient, and was much recommended by Dioscorides and other ancient physicians as an aperient and diuretic in dropsy, urinary obstructions and nephritic cases.

A decoction of the root is the usual form of administration, and it is still considered of use in jaundice and gravel. One pint of boiling water to 1 OZ. of the twigs, or 1/2 oz. of the bruised fresh root has also been recommended as an infusion, which may be taken as tea.

In scrofulous tumours, advantage has been realized by administering the root in doses of a drachm every morning.

The decoction, sweetened with honey, is said to clear the chest of phlegm and relieve difficult breathing.

The boughs have been employed for flogging chilblains.

Caraway

Quick Facts

Latin/Linnaen:	*Carum carvi*
Family:	*Apiaceae*
Old English :	Cymen
Synonyms:	Cumin, Meridian Fennel, Persian Cumin
Action:	Antispasmodic, Antimicrobial
Parts Used:	Oil and Seed
Indicated For:	Dyspeptic problems, such as mild, spastic condition of the gastrointestinal tract, (**seed**: bloating and fullness)(**oil**: flatulence and fullness)
Dosage:	Unless otherwise prescribed: Daily dosage: 1.5-6g of seeds; equivalent preparations. Oil, unless otherwise prescribed: Daily dosage: 3-6 drops.
Preparation:	Essential oil and its galenical preparations for internal use. Freshly crushed seeds for infusions as well as for other galenical preparations for internal use.
Cautions:	
Other Uses:	Caraway is another member of the group of aromatic, umbelliferous plants characterized by carminative properties, like Anise, Cumin, Dill and Fennel. It is grown, however, less for the medicinal properties of the fruits, or so-called 'seeds,' than for their use as a flavouring in cookery, confectionery and liqueurs .

Description

Caraway (Carum carvi) also known as meridian fennel, or Persian cumin is a biennial plant with smooth, furrowed stems growing 1 1/2 to 2 feet high, hearing finely cut leaves, and umbels of white flowers which blossom in June. The fruits which are popularly and incorrectly called seeds - and which correspond in general character to those of the other plants of this large family, are laterally compressed, somewhat horny and translucent, slightly curved, and marked with five distinct, pale ridges. They evolve a pleasant, aromatic odour when bruised, and have an agreeable taste.

The plant is similar in appearance to a carrot plant, with finely divided, feathery leaves with thread-like divisions, growing on 20–30 cm stems. The main flower stem is 40–60 cm tall, with small white or pink flowers in umbels. Caraway fruits are crescent-shaped achenes, around 2 mm long, with five pale ridges.

The leaves possess similar properties and afford an oil identical with that of the fruit. The tender leaves in spring have been boiled in soup, to give it an aromatic flavour.

The plant is distributed throughout the northern and central parts of Europe and Asia, though where it occurs in this country it is only considered a naturalized species, having apparently escaped from cultivation.

Cultivation

Hardiness Zone:	3-10
Soil pH:	5.8-7.5
Soil type:	Well drained soil rich in organic matter.
Cultivation:	Sow seeds directly, as the caraway has a long tap root which is difficult to transplant. To have ongoing seeds, sow 2 years in a row. It will likely self seed after that.
Sunlight:	Full sun
Habitat:	The plant is distributed throughout the northern and central parts of Europe and Asia.

Caraway can be either a biennial or annual plant. Annual caraway requires an extended growing season. Caraway does best in clean, weed free conditions. It resembles Queen Anne's Lace, so be sure not to mistake it for a weed. Peas and strawberries are good companion plants. The long taproot of the Caraway breaks up and conditions the soil for shallow rooted plants.

The plant prefers warm, sunny locations and well-drained soil rich in organic matter. In warmer regions it is planted in the winter months as an annual. In temperate climates it is planted as a summer annual or biennial. There is however a polyploid variant (with four haploid sets=4n) of this plant that was found to be perennial.

Historical Notes

The roots are thick and tapering, like a parsnip, though much smaller and are edible. Parkinson declared them, when young, to be superior in flavour to Parsnips. Mixed with milk and made into bread, they are said to have formed the 'Chara' of Julius Ceasar, eaten by the soldiers of Valerius.

Caraway was well known in classic days, and it is believed that its use originated with the ancient Arabs, who called the 'seeds' Karawya, a name they still bear in the East, and clearly the origin of our word Caraway and the Latin name Carvi, although Pliny would have us believe that the name Carvi was derived from Caria, in Asia Minor, where according to him the plant was originally found. In old Spanish the name occurs as Alcaravea.

Caraway is frequently mentioned by the old writers. Dioscorides advised the oil to be taken by pale-faced girls. In the Middle Ages and in Shakespeare's times it was very popular.

'The seed,' says Parkinson, 'is much used to be put among baked fruit, or into bread, cakes, etc., to give them a rellish. It is also made into comfites and taken for cold or wind in the body, which also are served to the table with fruit.'

In Henry IV, Squire Shallow invites Falstaff to 'a pippin and a dish of caraways.' The custom of serving roast apples with a little saucerful of Caraway is still kept up at Trinity College, Cambridge, and at some of the old-fashioned London Livery Dinners, just as in Shakespeare's days - and in Scotland to this day a saucerful is put down at tea to dip the buttered side of bread into and called 'salt water jelly.'

The scattering of the seed over cakes has long been practised, and Caraway-seed cake was formerly a standing institution at the feasts given by farmers to their labourers at the end of the wheat-sowing. The little Caraway comfits consist of the seeds encrusted with white sugar. In Germany, the peasants flavour their cheese, cabbage, soups, and household bread with Caraway, and in Norway and Sweden, polenta-like, black, Caraway bread is largely eaten in country districts.

The oil extracted from the fruits is used as an ingredient of alcoholic liquors: both the Russians and the Germans make from Caraway a liqueur, 'Kummel,' and Caraway enters into the composition of l'huile de Venus and other cordials.

A curious superstition was held in olden times about the Caraway. It was deemed to confer the gift of retention, preventing the theft of any object which contained it, and holding the thief in custody within the invaded house. In like manner it was thought to keep lovers from proving fickle (forming an ingredient of love potions), and also to prevent fowls and pigeons from straying. It is an undoubted fact that tame pigeons, who are particularly fond of the seeds, will never stray if they are given a piece of baked Caraway dough in their cote.

Habitat

One marked peculiarity about Caraway is that it is indigenous to all parts of Europe, Siberia, Turkey in Asia, Persia, India and North Africa, and yet it is cultivated only in a few comparatively restricted areas. It grows wild in many parts of Canada and the United States, but is nowhere grown there as a field or garden crop. Its cultivation is restricted to relatively small areas in England, Holland, Germany, Finland, Russia, Norway and Morocco, where it constitutes one of the chief agricultural industries within its narrow confines. It has so far received comparatively little attention in England, where it is grown only in Essex, Kent and Suffolk, upon old grassland broken up for the purpose. Holland cultivates the main crop, producing and exporting far larger quantities than any other country. It is cultivated most extensively there in the provinces of Groningen and North Holland, in which more than half the acreage is found. In the whole country about 20,000 acres are devoted to this crop, each acre yielding about 1,000 lb., whereas while Caraway is grown commercially throughout Germany, Austria, France and parts of Spain, the character and amounts produced are very variable, and the yield per acre varies only from 400 to 700 lb., and these countries do not produce much more than they require for home consumption. Morocco produces a grade of Caraway that comes regularly into the English and American markets, but is somewhat inferior in quality. Dutch Caraway is preferred among consumers in the United States, and the bulk used there comes from Holland.

During the last year or two (circa 1913) there has been a scarcity of Caraway, owing partly to the fact that the extensive area of land in Holland usually employed for the cultivation of the plant was devastated by floods towards the close of 1915. Much dill seed is now being sold in its place. Quite lately, a small grower reported that she had netted L. 5 (pounds sterling) from growing Caraway on a corner of what otherwise would have been waste ground.

Etymology

The etymology of caraway is complex and poorly understood. Caraway has been called by many names in different regions, with names deriving from the Latin cuminum (cumin), the Greek karon (again, cumin), which was adapted into Latin as carum (now meaning caraway), and the Sanskrit karavi, sometimes translated as "caraway" but other times understood to mean "fennel." The Italian finocchio meridionale (meridian fennel) suggests these shared roots, while cumino tedesco (German cumin) again points towards cumin--though caraway also has its own name in Italian, caro. Other languages share similar peculiarities, with the Norwegian name "karve", Yiddish borrowing the German Kümmel (caraway) as kimmel to mean caraway, yet using the semitic term kamoon for cumin, which is Kreuzkümmel in German.

English usage of the term caraway dates back to at least 1440, and is considered by Skeat to be of Arabic origin, though Katzer believes the Arabic al-karawya (cf. Spanish alcaravea) to be derived from the Latin carum.

Celandine

Chelidonium majus L.

Quick Facts

Latin/Linnaen:	*Chelidonium Majus*
Family:	*Papaveraceae*
Old English :	Cilðenige, Celðenie, Celeðonie
Synonyms:	Greater celandine, wartwort
Action:	There is evidence of a mildly antispasmodic, papaverine-like action on the upper digestive tract. Cytostatic, nonspecific immune stimulation.
Parts Used:	Herb
Indicated For:	Spastic discomfort of bile ducts and gastrointestinal tract.
Dosage:	Unless otherwise prescribed: average daily dosage 2-5g of herb, equivalent to 12-30mg total alkaloids calculated as chelidonine.
Preparation:	Cut herb, herb powder or dried extracts for liquid and solid medicinal forms for internal use.
Cautions:	
Other Uses:	None known

Description

Chelidonium majus (greater celandine; in Europe tetterwort, although in America the same name refers to bloodroot) is an herbaceous perennial plant, the only species in the genus Chelidonium. It is native to Europe and western Asia and introduced widely in North America.

While the greater celandine belongs to the poppy family, the lesser celandine belongs to the buttercup family.

Greater celandine has an erect habit, and reaches 30 to 120 cm high. The leaves are lobed and wavy-edged (crenate), 30 cm long. The sap is a yellow to orange latex, which can be hard to remove from hands and clothing. The plant is highly irritating and allergenic.

The flowers consist of four yellow petals, each about 1 cm long, with two sepals. A double-flowered variety occurs naturally. The flowers appear from late spring to summer in umbelliform cymes of about 4 flowers.

The seeds are small and black, borne in a long capsule. Each has an elaiosome, which attracts ants to disperse the seeds (myrmecochory).

It is considered an aggressive invasive plant in natural areas (both woods and fields). Control is mainly via pulling or spraying the plant before seed dispersal.

Cultivation

Hardiness Zone:	5-8
Soil pH:	4-8, but prefers 6.5
Soil type:	Prefers moist soil
Cultivation:	Easily propagated by seed, can become invasive.
Sunlight:	Shade to full sun
Habitat:	Native to Europe

Historical Notes

This plant is undoubtedly the true Celandine, having nothing in common with the Lesser Celandine except the colour of its flowers. It was a drug plant in the Middle Ages and is mentioned by Pliny, to whom we owe the tradition that it is called Chelidonium from the Greek chelidon (a swallow), because it comes into flower when the swallows arrive and fades at their departure. (The English name Celandine is merely a corruption of the Greek word.) Its acrid juice has been employed successfully in removing films from the cornea of the eye, a property which Pliny tells us was discovered by swallows, this being a double reason why the plant should be named after these birds.

Gerard says:

'the juice of the herbe is good to sharpen the sight, for it cleanseth and consumeth away slimie things that cleave about the ball of the eye and hinder the sight and especially being boiled with honey in a brasen vessell, as Dioscorides teacheth.'

It is one of the twenty-four herbs mentioned in Mercer's Herbal. In the fourteenth century, a drink made with Celandine was supposed to be good for the blood. Clusius, the celebrated Dutch botanist, considered that the juice, dropped into small green wounds, effected rapid cure, and when dropped into the eye would take away specks and stop incipient suffusions. The old alchemists held that it was good to 'superstifle the jaundice,' because of its intense yellow colour.

Centaury

Centaurium minus. 1. Blüthe 2. Frucht 3. Saame. Tausendgulden Kraut.

Quick Facts

Latin/Linnaen:	*Centaurium erythraea*
Family:	*Gentianaceae*
Old English :	Curmealle, Curmelle
Synonyms:	Bloodwort, gentian, fillwort, feverwort
Action:	Increase in gastric juice secretion.
Parts Used:	Herb
Indicated For:	Loss of appetite, peptic discomfort.
Dosage:	Unless otherwise prescribed: Average daily dosage: 6g of drug; equivelant preparations. Extract: Daily dosage: 1-2g
Preparation:	Ground herb for teas and other bitter tasting preparations for internal use.
Cautions:	
Other Uses:	None known.

Description

Centaurium erythraea is a species of flowering plant in the gentian family known by the common names common centaury and European centaury. This centaury is a widespread plant of Europe and parts of western Asia and northern Africa. It has also naturalised in parts of North America and throughout eastern Australia, where it is an introduced species. This is an erect biennial herb which reaches half a meter in height. It grows from a small basal rosette and bolts a leafy, erect stem which may branch. The triangular leaves are arranged oppositely on the stem and the erect inflorescences emerge from the stem and grow parallel to it, sometimes tangling with the foliage. Each inflorescence may contain many flowers.

The petite flower is pinkish-lavender and about a centimeter across, flat-faced with yellow anthers. The fruit is a cylindrical capsule.

It flowers from June until September.

The European centaury is used as a medical herb in many parts of Europe. The herb, mainly prepared as tea, is thought to possess medical properties beneficial for patients with gastric and liver diseases. It is also a powerful antioxidant. The active ingredients of the centaury are mainly phenolic acids as ferulic and sinapic acids. The plant also contains amounts of sterols as brassicasterol and stigmasterol.

Centaury varies a great deal according to) its situation, and some botanists enumerate several distinct species, namely: E. pulchella (Dwarf Centaury), a minute plant, 2 to 8 inches high, with an exceedingly slender stem and a few stalked flowers (often only one); this is found on the sandy seashore, especially in the West of England, and has been picked at Newquay, Cornwall; E. littoralis (Dwarf Tufted Centaury), a stunted plant, with broad leaves, and flowers crowded into a kind of head; this occurs on turfy sea-cliffs, and E. latifolia (Broadleaved Centaury), which has even broader leaves than the last, and bears its flowers in forked tufts, the main stem being divided into three branches. There are other minute differences, for which the student may consult more scientific works.

Besides the English species, others from the south of Europe, the Azores, etc., with yellow or pink flowers, are occasionally grown in gardens.

Cultivation

Hardiness Zone:	4-9
Soil pH	6.1-7.8
Soil type	Light sandy soil
Cultivation:	Sow from seed directly outdoors in fall.
Sunlight:	Sun to partial shade
Habitat:	Native of north Africa, western Asia and Europe. Grows in dry pastures and chalky cliffs. Naturalized in North America.

Historical Notes

The name of the genus to which it is at present assigned, Erythraea, is derived from the Greek erythros (red), from the colour of the flowers. The genus was formerly called Chironia, from the Centaur Chiron, who was famous in Greek mythology for his skill in medicinal herbs, and is supposed to have cured himself with it from a wound he had accidentally received from an arrow poisoned with the blood of the hydra. The English name Centaury has the same origin. The ancients named the plant Fel Terrae, or Gall of the Earth from its extreme bitterness. The old English name of Felwort is equivalent in meaning to this, and is applied to all the plants of the Gentian family. It is also thought to be the 'Graveolentia Centaurea' of Virgil, to which Lucretius gives the more significant epithet of tristia, in reference to this same intense bitterness. As this bitterness had a healing and tonic effect attributed to it, we sometimes find the Centaury called Febrifuga and Feverwort. It is known popularly also as Christ's Ladder, and the name Centaury has become corrupted in Worcestershire to 'Centre of the Sun.'

We find a reference to it in Le Petit Albert. Fifteen magical herbs of the Ancients are given:

'The eleventh hearbe is named of the Chaldees, Isiphon . . . of Englishmen, Centory . . . this herbe hath a marvellous virtue, for if it be joined with the blood of a female lapwing, or black plover, and put with oile in a lamp, all that compass it about shall believe themselves to be witches, so that one shall believe of another that his head is in heaven and his feete on earth; and if the aforesaid thynge be put in the fire when the starres shine it shall appeare yt the sterres runne one agaynste another and fyghte.' (English translation, 1619.)

Also in a translation of an old mediaeval Latin poem of the tenth century, by Macer, there is mention of Centaury (with other herbs) as being powerful against 'wykked sperytis.'

Of all the bitter appetizing wild herbs which serve as excellent simple tonics, the Centaury is the most efficacious, sharing the antiseptic virtues of the Field Gentian and the Buckbean.

The whole herb is used, and usually collected in July, when just breaking into flower and dried. The plant has a slight odour, which disappears when dried.

The Field Gentian is dried in the same manner.

Centaury contains a bitter principle, Erythro-centaurin, which is colourless, crystalline, non-nitrogenous, reddened by sunlight; a bitter glucoside, Erytaurin; Valeric acid, wax, etc.

The dried herb is given in infusion or powder, or made into an extract. It is used extensively in dyspepsia, for languid digestion with heartburn after food, in an infusion of 1 OZ. of the dried herb to 1 pint of water. When run down and suffering from want of appetite, a wineglassful of this infusion Centaury Tea - taken three or four times daily, half an hour before meals, is found of great benefit. The same infusion may also be taken for muscular rheumatism.

Culpepper tells us that:

'the herbe is so safe that you cannot fail in the using of it, only give it inwardly for inward diseases, use it outwardly for outward diseases. 'Tis very wholesome, but not very toothsome. It helps those that have the dropsy, or the green-sickness, being much used by the Italians in powder for that purpose. It kills worms ... as is found by experience.... A dram of the powder taken in wine, is a wonderful good help against the biting and poison of an adder. The juice of the herb with a little honey put to it, is good to clear the eyes from dimness, mists and clouds that offend or hinder sight. It is singularly good both for green and fresh wounds, as also for old ulcers and sores, to close up the one and cleanse the other, and perfectly to cure them both, although they are hollow or fistulous; the green herb, especially, being bruised and laid thereto. The decoction thereof dropped into the ears, cleanses them from worms . . . and takes away all freckles, spots, and marks in the skin, being washed with it.'

The Saxon herbalists prescribed it largely for snake-bites and other poisons, and it was long celebrated for the cure of intermittent fevers, hence its name of Feverwort.

The herb formed the basis of the once famous Portland Powder, which was said to be a specific for gout.

Centaury is given with Barberry Bark for jaundice. It has also been much employed as a vermifuge, and a decoction of the plant is said to destroy body vermin.

The green herb, bruised, is reputed to be good as an application to wounds and sores.

Chicory

Cichorium Intybus L. Gemeine Wegewarte.

Quick Facts

Latin/Linnaen:	*Cichorium intybus*
Family:	*Asteraceae*
Old English :	Eofola
Synonyms:	Endive, Blue Sailors, Succory, Coffeeweed, Wild Succory. Hendibeh, Barbe de Capucin
Action:	Mildly choleretic
Parts Used:	Flowering herbs, leaves and roots.
Indicated For:	Loss of appetite, dyspepsia
Dosage:	Unless otherwise prescribed: Average daily dosage: 3g of herb; equivelant preparations.
Preparation:	2 teaspoons of root or herb to one cup of cold water. Boil and strain.
Cautions:	Allergies to chicory and other composites. In case of gallstones, use only after consultation with a physician. In rare cases, allergic skin reactions.
Other Uses:	**Food:** Fresh greens can be used in a salad, They may be cut and used from young plants, but are generally blanched, as the unblanched leaves are bitter. This forced foliage is termed by the French Barbe de Capucin and forms a favourite winter salad, much eaten in France and Belgium. A particularly fine strain is known as Witloof, in Belgium, where smallholders make a great feature of this crop and excel in its cultivation. The young blanched heads also form a good vegetable for cooking, similar to Sea Kale. A common meal in Rome, 'puntarelle', is made with chicory sprouts.
	Beverages: Enormous quantities of the plant are cultivated on the Continent, to supply the grocer with the ground Chicory which forms an ingredient or adulteration to coffee. In Belgium, Chicory is sometimes even used as a drink without admixture of coffee. For this purpose, the thick cultivated root is sliced kiln-dried, roasted and then ground. It differs from coffee in the absence of volatile oil, rich aromatic flavour, caffeine and caffeotannic acid, and in the presence of a large amount of ash, including silica. When roasted, it yields 45 to 65 per cent of soluble extractive matter. Roasted Coffee yields only 21 to 25 per cent of soluble extract, this

difference affording a means of approximately determining the amount of Chicory in a mixture.

When infused, Chicory gives to coffee a bitterish taste and a dark colour. French writers say it is contra-stimulante, and serves to correct the excitation caused by the principles of coffee, and that it suits bilious subjects who suffer from habitual constipation, but is ill-adapted for persons whose vital energy soon flags, and that for lymphatic or bloodless persons its use should be avoided.

Description

Chicory is a perennial, with a tap root like the Dandelion. The stems are 2 to 3 feet high, the lateral branches numerous and spreading, given off at a very considerable angle from the central stem, so that the general effect of the plant, though spreading, is not rich and full, as the branches stretch out some distance in each direction and are but sparsely clothed with leaves of any considerable size. The general aspect of the plant is somewhat stiff and angular.

The lower leaves of the plant are large and spreading - thickly covered with hairs, something like the form of the Dandelion leaf, except that the numerous lateral segments or lobes are in general direction about at a right angle with the central stem, instead of pointing downwards, as in similar portions of the leaf of the Dandelion. The terminal lobe is larger and all the segments are coarsely toothed. The upper leaves are very much smaller and less divided, their bases clasping the stems.

The flowerheads are numerous, placed in the axils of the stem-leaves, generally in clusters of two or three. When fully expanded, the blooms are rather large and of a delicate tint of blue: the colour is said to specially appeal to the humble bee. They are in blossom from July to September. However sunny the day, by the early afternoon every bloom is closed, its petal-rays drawing together. Linnaeus used the Chicory as one of the flowers in his floral Clock at Upsala, because of its regularity in opening at 5 a.m. and closing at 10 a.m. in that latitude.

Cultivation

Hardiness Zone:	3-9
Soil pH:	5.5-6.8
Soil type:	Tolerant of poor well drained soil.
Cultivation:	Easily started from seed.
Sunlight:	Full sun
Habitat:	Grows freely along roadsides, Native to Europe.

Chicory is a hardy biennial plant with a tap root. It has been used as a forage plant in Europe and New Zealand for hundreds of years. The tap root makes it drought tolerant. Chicory can be cultivated for its leaves or root.

Chicory is a hardy perennial and will grow in almost any soil. For use as a salad, the plant may be easily cultivated in the kitchen garden. Sow the seed in May or June, in drills about 1 inch deep, about 12 inches apart, and thin out the young plants to 6 or 8 inches apart in the rows; when well up, water in very dry weather.

For blanching, dig up in October as many as may be needed, and after cutting off the leaves, it is well to let the roots be exposed to the air for a fortnight or three weeks; they should then be planted in deep boxes or pots of sand or light soil, leaving 8 inches between the soil and the top of the box. A cover of some sort is put on the box to exclude the light and the box put into a warm place, either in a warm green-house, under the stage, or, being so hardy, they may be successful in a moderately warm cellar and shed from which frost is excluded. Deprived of light, the young oncoming leaves become blanched and greatly elongated, and in this state are cut and sent to the market. If light is totally debarred, as it should be, the produce will be of a beautiful creamy white colour, soft and nearly destitute of the bitter flavour present when the plants are grown in the open air.

Historical Notes

Wild Chicory or Succory is not uncommon in many parts of England and Ireland, though by no means a common plant in Scotland. It is more common on gravel or chalk, especially on the downs of the south-east coast, and in places where the soil is of a light and sandy nature, when it is freely to be found on waste land, open borders of fields and by the roadside, and is easily recognized by its tough, twig-like stems, along which are ranged large, bright blue flowers about the size and shape of the Dandelion. Sir Jas. E. Smith, founder of the Linnean Society, says of the tough stems: 'From the earliest period of my recollection, when I can just remember tugging ineffectually with all my infant strength at the tough stalks of the wild Succory, on the chalky hills about Norwich....'

It has been suggested that the name Succory came from the Latin succurrere (to run under), because of the depth to which the root penetrates. It may, however be a corruption of Chicory, or Ctchorium, a word of Egyptian origin, which in various forms is the name of the plant in practically every European language. The Arabian physicians called it 'Chicourey.' Intybus, the specific name of the Chicory, is a modification of another Eastern name for the plant - Hendibeh. The Endive, an allied but foreign species (a native of southern Asia and northern provinces of China) derives both its common and specific names from the same word. The Endive and the Succory are the only two species in the genus Cichorium. There is little doubt that the Cichorium mentioned by Theophrastus as in use amongst the ancients was the wild Chicory, since the names by which the wild plant is known in all the languages of modern Europe are merely corruptions of the original Greek word, while there are different names in the different countries for the Garden Endive.

Succory was known to the Romans and eaten by them as a vegetable or in salads, its use in this way being mentioned by Horace, Virgil, Ovid, and Pliny.

On the Continent, Chicory is much cultivated, not only as a salad and vegetable, but also for fodder and more especially for the sake of its root, which though woody in the wild state, under cultivation becomes large and fleshy, with a thick rind, and is employed extensively when roasted and ground, for blending with coffee.

In (England), Chicory has been little grown. There was an attempt in 1788 to introduce its cultivation here as fodder, it being grown largely for that purpose in France, especially for sheep, but it would seem not to have met with success and has not been grown as a farm crop, though it furnishes abundance of good fodder at a time when green food is scarce, growing very quickly, two cuttings being possible in the first year and three in subsequent years, the produce being said to be superior on the whole to Lucerne. Although this plant, being succulent, seldom dries well for hay in this country, it seems valuable as fresh food for horses, cows and sheep: rabbits are fond of it. There has been an attempt since the war (WWI) to re-introduce the cultivation of Chicory, and it has been successfully grown at the experimental farm of the University College of North Wales at Bangor, and at Kirton, Lincolnshire, for the first time for forty years, was reported in March, 1917, to be yielding 20 tons per acre.

When grown for a forage crop, it should be sown during the last week in May, or first week in June, in drills about 15 inches apart, the plants being afterwards singled to from 6 inches to 8 inches in the row. About 5 lb. of seed will be needed for the acre. If sown too early the plant is likely to bolt. So grown, the crop of leaves can be cut in autumn to be fed to stock of all kinds, such as poultry, rabbits, cows, etc., and in following years, if the crop is kept clean, the foliage may be mown off three or four times. So grown it should of course never be allowed to seed.

On the Continent, especially in Belgium, the young and tender roots are boiled and eaten with butter like parsnips, and form a very palatable vegetable.

The fresh root is bitter, with a milky juice, which is somewhat aperient and slightly sedative, suiting subjects troubled with bilious torpor, whilst, on good authority, the plant has been pronounced useful against pulmonary consumption.

Historical Medicinal Uses - For Entertainment ONLY

A decoction of 1 OZ. of the root to a pint of boiling water, taken freely, has been found effective in jaundice, liver enlargements, gout and rheumatic complaints, and a decoction of the plant, fresh gathered, has been recommended for gravel.

Syrup of Succory is an excellent laxative for children, as it acts without irritation.

An infusion of the herb is useful for skin eruptions connected with gout.

The old herbalists considered that the leaves when bruised made a good poultice for swellings, inflammations and inflamed eyes, and that 'when boiled in broth for those that have hot, weak and feeble stomachs doe strengthen the same.' Tusser (1573) considered it - together with Endive - a useful remedy for ague, and Parkinson pronounced Succory to be a 'fine, cleansing, jovial plant.'

Chicory when taken too habitually, or freely, causes venous passive congestion in the digestive organs within the abdomen and a fullness of blood in the head. If used in excess as a medicine it is said to bring about loss of visual power in the retina.

From the flowers water was distilled to allay inflammation of the eyes. With violets, they were used to make the confection, 'Violet plates,' in the days of Charles II.

The seeds contain abundantly demulcent oil, whilst the petals furnish a glucoside, which is colourless unless treated with alkalies, when it becomes of a golden yellow. The leaves have been used to dye blue.

SWINE'S CHICORY (Arnoseris pusilla, Gaertn.), also known as Lamb's Succory, is a cornfield weed belonging to a closely related genus. All its leaves are radical, and it has small heads of yellow flowers on leafless, branched flower-stalks. It has no therapeutic uses.

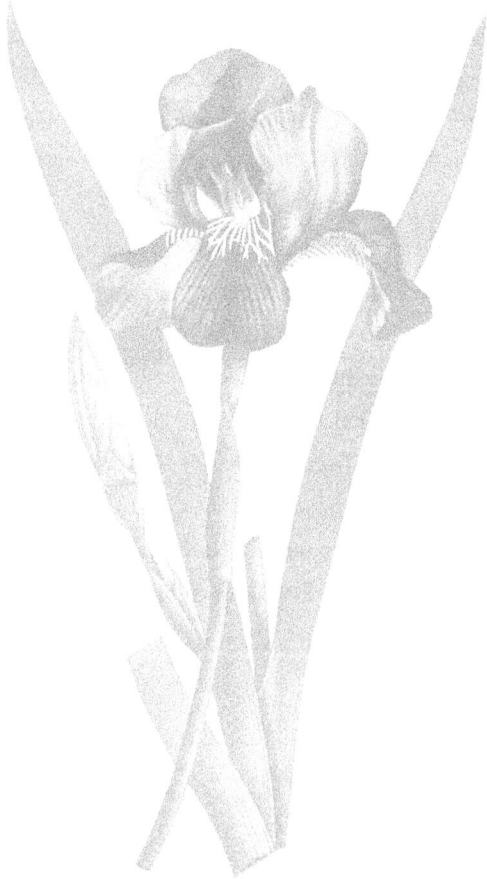

Coltsfoot

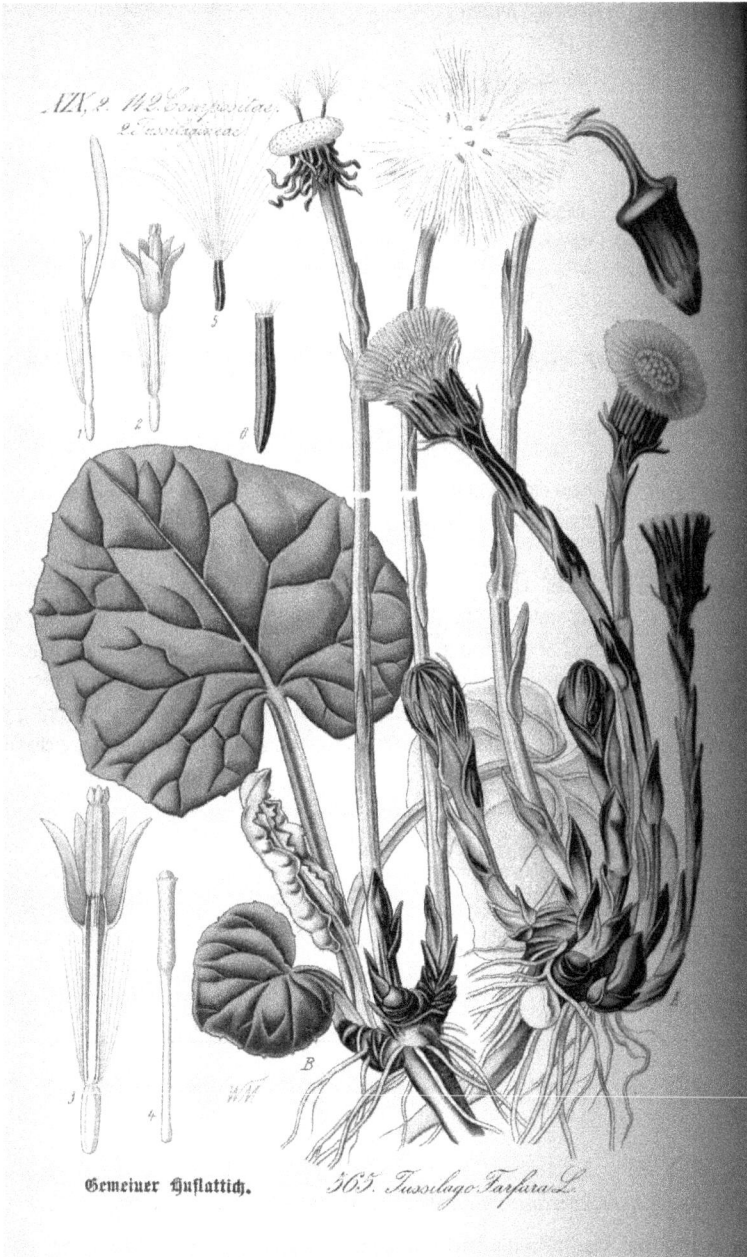

Gemeiner Huflattich.   365. Tussilago Farfara L.

Quick Facts

Latin/Linnaen:	*Tussilago farfara*
Family:	*Asteraceae*
Old English :	Clite
Synonyms:	Hallfoot, Foalswort, Coughwort, Horsehoof, Ass's Foot, Foalswort, Fieldhove, Bullsfoot, Donnhove, (French) Pas d'âne.
Action:	Inhibits inflammation, Furthers the formation of callus, Antimitotic
Parts Used:	Leaf
Indicated For:	Acute catarrh of the respiratory tract with cough and hoarseness, acute, mild inflammation of the oral and pharyngeal mucosa.
Dosage:	Unless otherwise prescribed: Daily dosage: 4.5 - 6 g of drug; equivalent preparations. The daily dosage of coltsfoot tea (drug) and of tea mixtures must not exceed micro g pyrrolizidine alkaloids with 1,2 unsaturated necine structure, including their N-oxides. The daily dosage for extracts and pressed juice from fresh plants must not be more than 1 micro g of total pyrrolizidine alkaloids with 1,2 unsaturated necine structure, including their N-oxides.
Preparation:	Comminuted drug for infusions, pressed plant juice or other galenical preparations for internal use.
Cautions:	Contraindications: Pregnancy, nursing.
Other Uses:	

Description

Tussilago farfara, commonly known as Coltsfoot, is a plant in the family *Asteraceae* that has traditionally had medicinal uses. However, the discovery of toxic pyrrolizidine alkaloids in the plant has resulted in liver health concerns. The name "tussilago" itself means "cough suppressant"

Coltsfoot is a perennial herbaceous plant that spreads by seeds and rhizomes. *Tussilago* is often found in colonies of dozens of plants. The flowers, which superficially resemble dandelions, appear in early spring before dandelions appear. The leaves, which resemble a colt's foot in cross section, do not appear usually until after the seeds are set. Thus, the flowers appear on stems with no apparent leaves, and the later appearing leaves then wither and die during the season without seeming to set flowers. The plant is typically between 10 - 30 cm in height.

Coltsfoot is native to several locations in Europe and Asia. It is also a common plant in North America and South America where it has been introduced, most likely by settlers as a medicinal item. The plant is often found in waste and disturbed places and along roadsides and paths. In some areas it is considered an invasive species.

Cultivation

Hardiness Zone:	4-9
Soil pH:	Neutral to alkaline
Soil type:	It grows on roadsides and can tolerate gravelly soils.
Cultivation:	It is able to be started by seed. It spreads in the wild by seed and rhizome growth.
Sunlight:	Sun to part sun
Habitat:	Native to Europe, north Africa and Asia. Naturalized to North America.

Coltsfoot is a low growing perennial plant. It is an invasive plant that is hard to control. It is recommended to plant in a pot which is buried in the ground to prevent the rhizomes from spreading.

Historical Notes

Coltsfoot grows abundantly throughout England, especially along the sides of railway banks and in waste places, on poor stiff soils, growing as well in wet ground as in dry situations. It has long-stalked, hoof-shaped leaves, about 4 inches across, with angular teeth on the margins. Both surfaces are covered, when young, with loose, white, felted woolly hairs, but those on the upper surface fall off as the leaf expands. This felty covering easily rubs off and before the introduction of matches, wrapped in a rag dipped in a solution of saltpetre and dried in the sun, used to be considered an excellent tinder.

The specific name of the plant is derived from Farfarus, an ancient name of the White Poplar, the leaves of which present some resemblance in form and colour to those of this plant. There is a closer resemblance, however, to the leaves of the Butterbur, which must not be collected in error; they may be distinguished by their more rounded outline, larger size and less sinuate margin.

After the leaves have died down, the shoot rests and produces in the following February a flowering stem, consisting of a single peduncle with numerous reddish bracts and whitish hairs and a terminal, composite yellow flower, whilst other shoots develop leaves, which appear only much later, after the flower stems in their turn have died down. These two parts of the plant, both of which are used medicinally, are, therefore, collected separately and usually sold separately.

The root is spreading, small and white, and has also been used medicinally.

An old name for Coltsfoot was Filius ante patrem (the son before the father), because the star-like, golden flowers appear and wither before the broad, sea-green leaves are produced.

The seeds are crowned with a tuft of silky hairs, the pappus, which are often used by goldfinches to line their nests, and it has been stated were in former days frequently employed by the Highlanders for stuffing mattresses and pillows.

The underground stems preserve their vitality for a long period when buried deeply, so that in places where the plant has not been observed before, it will often spring up in profusion after the ground has been disturbed. In gardens and pastures it is a troublesome weed, very difficult to extirpate.

The leaves, collected in June and early part of July, and, to a slighter extent, the flower-stalks collected in February.

Historical Medicinal Uses - For Entertainment ONLY

Medicinal Action and Uses: Demulcent, expectorant and tonic. One of the most popular of cough remedies. It is generally given together with other herbs possessing pectoral qualities, such as Horehound, Marshmallow, Ground Ivy, etc.

The botanical name, Tussilago, signifies 'cough dispeller,' and Coltsfoot has justly been termed 'nature's best herb for the lungs and her most eminent thoracic.' The smoking of the leaves for a cough has the recommendation of Dioscorides, Galen, Pliny, Boyle, and other great authorities, both ancient and modern, Linnaeus stating that the Swedes of his time smoked it for that purpose. Pliny recommended the use of both roots and leaves. The leaves are the basis of the British Herb Tobacco, in which Coltsfoot predominates, the other ingredients being Buckbean, Eyebright, Betony, Rosemary, Thyme, Lavender, and Chamomile flowers. This relieves asthma and also the difficult breathing of old bronchitis. Those suffering from asthma, catarrh and other lung troubles derive much benefit from smoking this Herbal Tobacco, the use of which does not entail any of the injurious effects of ordinary tobacco.

A decoction is made of 1 OZ. of leaves, in 1 quart of water boiled down to a pint, sweetened with honey or liquorice, and taken in teacupful doses frequently. This is good for both colds and asthma.

Coltsfoot tea is also made for the same purpose, and Coltsfoot Rock has long been a domestic remedy for coughs.

A decoction made so strong as to be sweet and glutinous has proved of great service in scrofulous cases, and, with Wormwood, has been found efficacious in calculus complaints.

The flower-stalks contain constituents similar to those of the leaves, and are directed by the British Pharmacopceia to be employed in the preparation of Syrup of Coltsfoot, which is much recommended for use in chronic bronchitis.

In Paris, the Coltsfoot flowers used to be painted as a sign on the doorpost of an apothecarie's shop.

Culpepper says:

'The fresh leaves, or juice, or syrup thereof, is good for a bad dry cough, or wheezing and shortness of breath. The dry leaves are best for those who have their rheums and distillations upon their lungs causing a cough: for which also the dried leaves taken as tobacco, or the root is very good. The distilled water hereof simply or with elder-flowers or nightshade is a singularly good remedy against all agues, to drink 2 OZ. at a time and apply cloths wet therein to the head and stomach, which also does much good being applied to any hot swellings or inflammations. It helpeth St. Anthony's fire (erysypelas) and burnings, and is singular good to take away wheals.'

One of the local names for Coltsfoot, viz. Donnhove, seems to have been derived from Donn, an old word for horse, hence Donkey (a little horse). Donnhove became corrupted to Tun-hoof as did Hay-hove (a name for Ground Ivy) to ale-hoof.

The plant is so dissimilar in appearance at different periods that both Gerard and Parkinson give two illustrations: one entitled 'Tussilago florens, Coltsfoot in floure,' and the other, 'Tussilaginous folia, the leaves of Coltsfoot,' or 'Tussilago herba sine flore.'

'Coltsfoot hath many white and long creeping roots, from which rise up naked stalkes about a spanne long, bearing at the top yellow floures; when the stalke and seede is perished there appear springing out of the earth many broad leaves, green above, and next the ground of a white, hoarie, or grayish colour. Seldom, or never, shall you find leaves and floures at once, but the floures are past before the leaves come out of the ground, as may appear by the first picture, which setteth forth the naked stalkes and floures, and by the second, which porttraiteth the leaves only.'

Pliny and many of the older botanists thought that the Coltsfoot was without leaves, an error that is scarcely excusable, for, notwithstanding the fact that the flowers appear in a general way before the leaves, small leaves often begin to make their appearance before the flowering season is over.

Pliny recommends the dried leaves and roots of Coltsfoot to be burnt, and the smoke drawn into the mouth through a reed and swallowed, as a remedy for an obstinate cough, the patient sipping a little wine between each inhalation. To derive the full benefit from it, it had to be burnt on cypress charcoal.

Comfrey

Tafel 9.

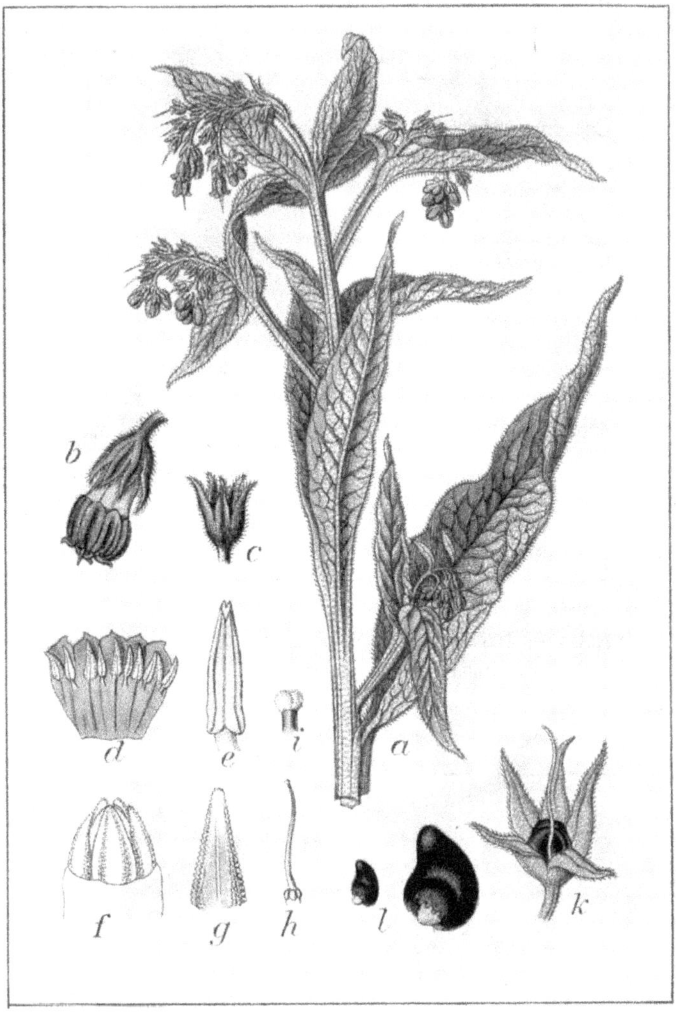

Echter Beinwell, Symphytum officinale.

Quick Facts - Herb and Leaf

Latin/Linnaen:	*Symphytum officinale or Symphyti herba / - follium*
Family:	*Boraginaceae*
Old English :	Galluc, Galloc
Synonyms:	Gallapple, All-heal, Knitback, Bruisewort, Comphrey
Action:	Antiinflammatory
Parts Used:	herb and leaf
Indicated For:	External: Bruises, sprains
Dosage:	Unless otherwise prescribed: Ointments and other preparations for external application with 5-20 percent dried drug; equivalent preparations.
	The daily applied dosage should not exceed 100 micro g of pyrrolizidine alkaloids with 1,2 - unsaturated necine structure, including their N - oxides
Preparation:	Comminuted herb and other galenical preparations for external use.
Cautions:	Note : Application should only occur on intact skin. During pregnancy use only after consultation with a physician
Other Uses:	

Quick Facts - Root

Latin/Linnaen:	*Symphyti radix*
Family:	*Boraginaceae*
Old English :	Galluc, Galloc
Synonyms:	Gallapple, All-heal, Knitback, Bruisewort, Comphrey
Action:	Antiinflammatory, Furthers the formation of callus, Antimitotic
Parts Used:	Root
Indicated For:	External: Bruises, pulled muscles and ligaments, sprains
Dosage:	Unless otherwise prescribed: Ointments or other preparations for external use are made up with 5-20 percent of the drug and prepared accordingly. The daily dose should not exceed more than 100 micro g pyrrolizidine alkaloids with 1,2 unsaturated necine structure, including its N-oxides
Preparation:	Crushed root, extracts, the pressed juice of the fresh plant for semi-solid preparations and poultices for external use.
Cautions:	Note: Application should only occur on intact skin; during pregnancy use only after consulting a phyiscian
Other Uses:	

Description

Comfrey (*Symphytum officinale L.*) is a perennial herb of the family *Boraginaceae* with a black, turnip-like root and large, hairy broad leaves that bears small bell-shaped flowers of various colours, typically cream or purplish, which may be striped. The leaves are oblong, and often differ in appearance depending upon their position on the stem: Lower leaves are broad at the base and tapered at the ends while upper leaves are broad throughout and narrow only at the ends. The root has a black exterior and fleshy whitish interior filled with juice.

It is native to Europe, growing in damp, grassy places, and is locally frequent throughout Ireland and Britain on river banks and ditches. Comfrey has a thick, hairy stem, and grows 2 - 5 feet tall.

More common is the hybrid between *S. officinale* and *S. asperum*, *Symphytum × uplandicum*, known as Russian Comfrey, which is widespread in the British Isles, and which interbreeds with *S. officinale*. Compared to *S. officinale*, *S. × uplandicum* is generally more bristly and has flowers which tend to be more blue or violet.

Comfrey has long been recognised by both organic gardeners and herbalists for its great usefulness and versatility; of particular interest is the 'Bocking 14' cultivar of Russian Comfrey. Bocking 14 is a sterile variety which can be propogated by root cuttings. This strain was developed during the 1950s by Lawrence D Hills, the founder of the Henry Doubleday Research Association (the organic gardening organisation itself named after the Quaker pioneer who first introduced Russian Comfrey into Britain in the 1910s) following trials at Bocking, near Braintree, the original home of the organization.

It is used as a fertilizer and also has many purported medicinal uses. The main species used now is *Symphytum × uplandicum* or Russian comfrey, a hybrid between *Symphytum officinale* (common comfrey) and *Symphytum asperum* (rough comfrey).

Cultivation

Hardiness Zone:	4-8
Soil pH:	All except strongly acidic.
Soil type:	Wet soil, but tolerant of dry.
Cultivation:	Root divisions and seed.
Sunlight:	Full sun to partial shade
Habitat:	Native to Europe, and now naturalized to all temperate regions around the globe.

Adding comfrey to your compost helps to heat it and adds nutrients. Use comfrey tea to water plants. The long tap root helps to break up soil and draw nutrients up from deep below the surface. Bocking 14 is a sterile variety, which can be divided, but will not spread by seed. Care should be used in selecting a site for comfrey, as it is very difficult to remove once planted. Comfrey leaves can be added to the soil before planting and will not draw the nitrogen out of the soil as will most other uncomposted plants.

Historical Notes

This well-known showy plant is a member of the Borage and Forget-me-not tribe, *Boraginaceae*.

The plant is erect in habit and rough and hairy all over. There is a branched rootstock, the roots are fibrous and fleshy spindle-shaped, an inch or less in diameter and up to a foot long, smooth, blackish externally, and internally white, fleshy and juicy.

The creamy yellow-flowered form is stated by Hooker to be *Symphytum officinale* proper, and the purple flowered he considered a variety and named it S. officinale, var patens. The botanist Sibthorpe makes a definite species of it under the name patens.

There is another species, *S. tuberosum*, found in wet places from North Wales, Stafford and Lincoln northwards into Scotland, and most common in the south of Scotland, though absent from Ireland.

In this form, the stem is scarcely branched and but slightly winged, the bases of the leaves being hardly at all continued down the stem. Though also covered with hairs, the latter are not so bristly. The root-stock is short and horizontal with slender root fibres. This is a much smaller plant, the stem rarely more than a foot high, rather slender and leafy. The lower radical leaves are much as in *S. officinale* in form, but with longer footstalks. The flowers, creamy-yellow in colour though about the same size as those of *S. officinale*, are in much smaller masses.

The Common Comfrey is abundantly met with in England, but is rare in Scotland; the tuberous Comfrey is commonly found in Scotland, but is seldom met with in England, the northern counties of England and North Wales being its extreme southern limit, so that except in the narrow zone of country common to both, there will be no possibility of mistaking the one species for the other.

The variety of *S. officinale*, with a purplish flower, is more common in many parts of the Continent than in England. The purple and yellowish flowers are not found mixed where the plants grow wild: the difference in colour is permanent in plants raised from seed.

[In the water-meadows which form such a well-known feature in South Wilts, especially in the valleys round about Salisbury, Common Comfrey is abundant, and the flowers vary in colour from creamy-white to a pretty rose-pink; while the purple sort is the commonest. - Note by a Wiltshire writer.]

A variety with flowers of a rich blue colour S. Asperimum, Prickly Comfrey, was introduced into this country from the Caucasus in 1811 as a fodder plant. This species is the largest of the genus, rising to 5 feet and more, with prickly stems and bold foliage, the leaves very large and oval, the hairs on them having bulbous bases. It was extensively recommended as a green food for most animals, it being claimed for it that it contained a considerable amount of flesh-forming substances, and was, moreover, both preventative and curative of foot and mouth disease in cattle. It has the advantage of producing large crops, two at least in a season, if cut before the flowers quite expand, and in favourable circumstances even more, so that 40 to 50 tons of green food per acre might be reckoned on. At the time of its introduction, a number of farmers and smallholders planted it. It was found, however that though horses, cattle and pigs would eat it, they never took kindly to it as forage. Horses in time of scarcity will eat it in small quantities in the green state, though do not care for it dried. It is a useful food in the green state for pigs of all ages, but it takes a little time for them to get used to it. Its feeding value, however, has been proved to be not so very much more than that of grass and though it grows luxuriantly in all moist situations, where the soil is pretty good, it is not adapted for either dry or poor land.

Formerly country people cultivated Comfrey in their gardens for its virtue in wound healing, and the many local names of the plant testify to its long reputation as a vulnerary herb - in the Middle Ages it was a famous remedy for broken bones. The very name, Comfrey, is a corruption of con firma, in allusion to the uniting of bones it was thought to effect, and the botanical name, Symphytum, is derived from the Greek symphyo (to unite).

As an ornamental plant, Comfrey is often introduced into gardens, from which it is very difficult to eradicate it when it has once established itself, a new plant arising from any severed portion of the root.

Historical Medicinal Uses - For Entertainment ONLY
Parts Used Medicinally

The root and leaves, generally collected from wild plants.

Comfrey leaves are sometimes found as an adulteration to Foxglove leaves, which they somewhat resemble, but may be distinguished by the smaller veins not extending into the wings of the leaf-stalk, and by having on their surface isolated stiff hairs. They are also more lanceolate than Foxglove leaves.

The chief and most important constituent of Comfrey root is mucilage, which it contains in great abundance, more even than Marshmallow. It also contains from 0.6 to 0.8 per cent of Allantoin and a little tannin. Starch is present in a very small amount.

Medicinal Action and Uses

Comfrey is demulcent, mildly astringent and expectorant. As the plant abounds in mucilage, it is frequently given whenever a mucilaginous medicine is required and has been used like Marshmallow for intestinal troubles. It is very similar in its emollient action to Marshmallow, but in many cases is even preferred to it and is an ingredient in a large number of herbal preparations. It forms a gentle remedy in cases of diarrhoea and dysentery. A decoction is made by boiling 1/2 to 1 OZ. of crushed root in 1 quart of water or milk, which is taken in wineglassful doses, frequently.

For its demulcent action it has long been employed domestically in lung troubles and also for quinsy and whooping-cough. The root is more effectual than the leaves and is the part usually used in cases of coughs. It is highly esteemed for all pulmonary complaints, consumption and bleeding of the lungs. A strong decoction, or tea, is recommended in cases of internal haemorrhage, whether from the lungs, stomach, bowels or from bleeding piles -to be taken every two hours till the haemorrhage ceases, in severe cases, a teaspoonful of Witch Hazel extract being added to the Comfrey root tea.

A modern medicinal tincture, employed by homoeopaths, is made from the root with spirits of wine, 10 drops in a tablespoonful of water being administered several times a day.

Comfrey leaves are of much value as an external remedy, both in the form of fomentations, for sprains, swellings and bruises, and as a poultice, to severe cuts, to promote suppuration of boils and abscesses, and gangrenous and ill-conditioned ulcers . The whole plant, beaten to a cataplasm and applied hot as a poultice, has always been deemed excellent for soothing pain in any tender, inflamed or suppurating part. It was formerly applied to raw, indolent ulcers as a glutinous astringent. It is useful in any kind of inflammatory swelling.

Internally, the leaves are taken in the form of an infusion, 1 OZ. of the leaves to 1 pint of boiling water.

Fluid extract: dose, 1/2 to 2 drachms.

The reputation of Comfrey as a vulnerary has been considered due partly to the fact of its reducing the swollen parts in the immediate neighbourhood of fractures, causing union to take place with greater facility. Gerard affirmed: 'A salve concocted from the fresh herb will certainly tend to promote the healing of bruised and broken parts.' Surgeons have declared that the powdered root, if dissolved in water to a mucilage, is far from contemptible for bleedings and fractures, whilst it hastens the callus of bones under repair. Its virtues as a vulnerary are now attributed to the Allantoin it contains. According to Macalister (British Medical

Journal, Jan. 6, 1912), Allantoin in aqueous solution in strengths of 0.3 per cent has a powerful action in strengthening epithelial formations, and is a valuable remedy not only in external ulceration, but also in ulcers of the stomach and duodenum. Comfrey Root is used as a source of this cell proliferant Allantoin, employed in the dealing of chronic wounds, burns, ulcers, etc., though Allantoin is also made artificially.

The following is from the Chemist and Druggist of August 13, 1921:

'Allantoin is a fresh instance of the good judgment of our rustics, especially of old times, with regard to the virtues of plants. The great Comfrey or consound, though it was official with us down to the middle of the eighteenth century, never had a very prominent place in professional practice; but our herbalists were loud in its praise and the country culler of simples held it almost infallible as a remedy for both external and internal wounds bruises, and ulcers, for phlegm, for spitting of blood, ruptures, haemorrhoids, etc. For ulcers of the stomach and liver especially, the root (the part used) was regarded as of sovereign virtue. It is precisely for such complaints as these that Allantoin, obtained from the rhizome of the plant, is now prescribed. One old Syrupus de Symphyto was a rather complicated preparation. Gerard has a better formula, also a compound, which he highly recommends for ulcers of the lungs. The old Edinburgh formula is the simplest and probably the best: Fresh Comfrey leaves and fresh plantain leaves, of each lb.ss.; bruise them and well squeeze out the juice, add to the dregs spring water lb.ij.; boil to half, and mix the strained liquor with the expressed juice; add an equal quantity of white sugar and boil to a syrup.'

Culpepper says:

'The great Comfrey ("great" to distinguish it from the "Middle Comfrey" - another name for the Bugle) restrains spitting of blood. The root boiled in water or wine and the decoction drank, heals inward hurts, bruises, wounds and ulcers of the lungs, and causes the phlegm that oppresses him to be casily spit forth.... A syrup made there of is very effectual in inward hurts, and the distilled water for the same purpose also, and for outward wounds or sores in the fleshy or sinewy parts of the body, and to abate the fits of agues and to allay the sharpness of humours. A decoction of the leaves is good for those purposes, but not so effectual as the roots. The roots being outwardly applied cure fresh wounds or cuts immediately, being bruised and laid thereto; and is specially good for ruptures and broken bones, so powerful to consolidate and knit together that if they be boiled with dissevered pieces of flesh in a pot, it will join them together again.'

He goes on to describe its curative effect on haemorrhoids and continues:

'The roots of Comfrey taken fresh, beaten small and spread upon leather and laid upon any place troubled with the gout presently gives ease: and applied in the same manner it eases pained joints and tends to heal running ulcers, gangrenes, mortifications, for which it hath by often experience been found helpful.'

The young leaves form a good green vegetable, and are not infrequently eaten by country people. When fully grown they become, however, coarse and unpleasant in taste. They have been used to flavour cakes and other food.

In some parts of Ireland Comfrey is eaten as a cure for defective circulation and poverty of blood, being regarded as a perfectly safe and harmless remedy.

Comfrey roots, together with Chichory and Dandelion roots, are used to make a well-known vegetation 'Coffee,' that tastes practically the same as ordinary coffee, with none of its injurious effects.

A strong decoction has been used on the Continent for tanning leather, and in Angora a sort of glue is got from the common Comfrey, which is used for spinning the famous fleeces of that country.

In that inimitable little book by Russell George Alexander, called A Plain Plantain, in which he quotes from an old MS. inscribed 'Madam Susanna Avery, Her Book, May ye 12th Anno Domini 1688,' we find the following reference to Comfrey: 'From the French conserve, Latin conserva - healing: conserves - to boil together; to heal. A Wound Herb.' 'The roots,' says a sixteenthcentury writer, 'heal all inwarde woundes and burstings,' and Baker (Jewell of Health, 1567) says: 'The water of the Greater Comferie druncke helpeth such as are bursten, and that have broken the bone of the legge.' In cookery, the leaves gathered young may be used as a substitute for Spinach; the young shoots have been eaten after blanching by forcing them to grow through heaps of earth.

Coriander

Coriandrum sativum L.

Quick Facts

Latin/Linnaen:	*Coriandrum Sativum*
Family:	*Apiaceae*
Old English :	Celendre
Synonyms:	None
Action:	Unkown
Parts Used:	Seed
Indicated For:	Dyspeptic complaints, loss of appetite.
Dosage:	Unless otherwise Prescribed: Average daily dosage: 3 g of drug; equivalent preparations.
Preparation:	Crushed and powdered drug, as well as other galenical preparations for internal use. Powder, dry extracts and other galenical preparations for internal use and external use.
Cautions:	
Other Uses:	**Culinary**: It is still much used in the East as a condiment, and forms an ingredient in curry powder. The fresh leaves are also used in soups and salads.

Description

Coriander (*Coriandrum sativum*), also called cilantro or dhania, is an annual herb in the family *Apiaceae*. Coriander is native to southern Europe and North Africa to southwestern Asia and is found occasionally in Britain in fields and waste places, and by the sides of rivers. It is frequently found in a semi-wild state in the east of England, having escaped from cultivation. It is a soft, hairless plant growing to 50 centimetres (20 in) tall. The leaves are variable in shape, broadly lobed at the base of the plant, and slender and feathery higher on the flowering stems. The flowers are borne in small umbels, white or very pale pink, asymmetrical, with the petals pointing away from the center of the umbel longer (5–6 mm) than those pointing towards it (only 1–3 mm long). The fruit is a globular, dry schizocarp 3–5 mm diameter. While in the English-speaking world (except for the U.S.) the leaves and seeds are known as coriander, in American culinary usage the leaves are generally referred to by the Spanish word cilantro.

Cultivation

Hardiness Zone:	Planted annually anywhere
Soil pH:	6.1-7.8
Soil type:	Well drained soil, potting mix if growing in pots.
Cultivation:	Plant seed directly as the root disturbance from transplanting causes bolting.
Sunlight:	Full sun if growing for seed
Habitat:	It is grown to a small extent in the Eastern counties of England, but more especially in Essex. It is also cultivated in various parts of Continental Europe, and in northern Africa, Malta and India.

Per M. Grieve's A Modern Herbal:

"Coriander likes a warm, dry, light soil, though it also does well in the somewhat heavy soil of Essex.

Sow in mild, dry weather in April, in shallow drills, about 1/2 inch deep and 8 or 9 inches apart, and cover it evenly with the soil. The seeds are slow in germinating. The seeds may also be sown in March, in heat, for planting out in May.

As the seeds ripen, about August, the disagreeable odour gives place to a pleasant aroma, and the plant is then cut down with sickles and when dry the fruit is threshed out.

The best land yields on an average 15 cwt. per acre. It is grown to a small extent in the Eastern counties, but more especially in Essex. It is also cultivated in various parts of Continental Europe, and in northern Africa, Malta and India."

Historical Notes

It is an annual, with erect stems, 1 to 3 feet high, slender and branched. The lowest leaves are stalked and pinnate, the leaflets roundish or oval, slightly lobed. The segments of the uppermost leaves are linear and more divided. The flowers are in shortly-stalked umbels, five to ten rays, pale mauve, almost white, delicately pretty. The seed clusters are very symmetrical and the seeds fall as soon as ripe. The plant is bright green, shining, glabrous and intensely foetid.

Gerard described it as follows:

'The common kind of Coriander is a very striking herb, it has a round stalk full of branches, two feet long. The leaves are almost like the leaves of the parsley, but later on become more jagged, almost like the leaves of Fumitorie, but a great deal smaller and tenderer. The flowers are white and grow in round tassels like Dill.'

The inhabitants of Peru are so fond of the taste and smell of this herb that it enters into almost all their dishes, and the taste is often objectionable to any but a native. Both in Peru and in Egypt, the leaves are put into soup.

The seeds are quite round like tiny balls. They lose their disagreeable scent on drying and become fragrant- the longer they are kept, the more fragrant they become.

Coriander was originally introduced from the East, being one of the herbs brought to Britain by the Romans. As an aromatic stimulant and spice, it has been cultivated and used from very ancient times. It was employed by Hippocrates and other Greek physicians.

The name Coriandrum, used by Pliny, is derived from koros, (a bug), in reference to the foetid smell of the leaves.

Pliny tells us that 'the best (Coriander) came from Egypt,' and from thence no doubt the Israelites gained their knowledge of its properties.

The Africans are said to have called this herb by a similar name (goid), which Gesenius derives from a verb (gadad), signifying 'to cut,' in allusion to the furrowed appearance of the fruit.

It is still much used in the East as a condiment, and forms an ingredient in curry powder.

In the northern countries of Europe, the seeds are sometimes mixed with bread, but the chief consumption of Coriander seed in this country is in flavouring certain alcoholic liquors, for which purpose it is largely grown in Essex. Distillers of gin make use of it, and veterinary surgeons employ it as a drug for cattle and horses. The fruit is the only part of the plant that seems to have any medical or dietetical reputation.

Confectioners form from the seeds little, round pink and white comfits for children.

It is included in the British Pharmacopceia, but it is chiefly used to disguise unpleasant medicine.

A power of conferring immortality is thought by the Chinese to be a property of the seeds.

Turner says (1551):

"Coriandre layd to wyth breade or barly mele is good for Saynt Antonyes fyre" (the *erysipelas: so called because it was supposed to have been cured by the intercession of St. Anthony). Coriander cakes are seldom made now.'*

Parts Used

The fruit (so-called seeds) are of globular form, beaked, finely ribbed, yellowish-brown 1/5 inch in diameter, with five longitudinal ridges, separable into two halves (the mericarps), each of which is concave internally and shows two broad, longitudinal oil cells (vittae). The seeds have an aromatic taste and, when crushed, a characteristic odour.

Constituents

Coriander fruit contains about 1 per cent of volatile oil, which is the active ingredient. It is pale yellow or colourless, and has the odour of Coriander and a mild aromatic taste. The fruit yields about 5 per cent of ash and contains also malic acid, tannin and some fatty matter.

Coriander fruit of the British Pharmacopoeia is directed to be obtained from plants cultivated in Britain, the fruit before being submitted to distillation being brushed or bruised.

The English-grown are said to have the finest flavour, though the Russian and German are the richest in oil. The Mogadore are the largest and brightest, but contain less oil, and the Bombay fruit, which are also large, are distinguished by their oval shape and yield the least oil of any.

Historical Medicinal Uses - For Entertainment ONLY

Medicinal Action and Uses: Stimulant, aromatic and carminative. The powdered fruit, fluid extract and oil are chiefly used medicinally as flavouring to disguise the taste of active purgatives and correct their griping tendencies. It is an ingredient of the following compound preparations of the Pharmacopceia: confection, syrup and tincture of senna, and tincture and syrup of Rhubarb, and enters also into compounds with angelica gentian, jalap, quassia and lavender. As a corrigent to senna, it is considered superior to other aromatics.

If used too freely the seeds become narcotic.

Coriander water was formerly much esteemed as a carminative for windy colic.

Preparations

Powdered fruit: dose, 10 to 60 grains. Fluid extract, 5 to 30 drops. B.P.: dose, 1/2 to 3 drops.

Cowslip / Primrose

472 Primula officinalis Jacquin.   Gebräuchlicher Himmelsschlüssel.

Quick Facts

Latin/Linnaen:	*Primula veris*
Family:	*Primulaceae*
Old English :	Cusloppe, Cūslyppe
Synonyms:	Primula officinalis L., Paigle, Cuy lippe, Herb Peter, Paigle, Peggle, Key Flower, Key of Heaven, Fairy Cups, Petty Mulleins, Crewel, Buckles, Palsywort, Plumrocks.
Action:	Secretolytic, Expectorant
Parts Used:	Flower/Root
Indicated For:	Flower: Catarrhs of the respiratory tract / Root : same
Dosage:	Flower: Daily dosage: 2-4g of drug; 2.5-7.5g of tincture equivalent preparation. Root: Daily dosage: 0.5-1.5 g of drug; 1.5-3g of tincture equivalent preparations
Preparation:	Flower: Comminuted herb for teas and other galenical preparations for internal use. Root: Comminuted drug for teas and cold macerations, as well as other galenical preparations for internal use.
Cautions:	Flower: Known allergies to primrose
	Stomach upsets and nausea can occur.
Other Uses:	**Culinary:** Cowslip leaves have been traditionally used in Spanish cooking as a salad green. Uses in English cookery includes using the flowers to flavour country wine and vinegars; sugared to be a sweet or eaten as part of a composed salad while the juice of the cowslip is used to prepare tansy for frying. The close cousin of the cowslip, the primrose (P. vulgaris), has often been confused with the cowslip and its uses in cuisine are similar with the addition of its flowers being used as a colouring agent in desserts.

Description

Primula veris (Cowslip; syn. *Primula officinalis* Hill) is a flowering plant in the genus *Primula*. The species is native throughout most of temperate Europe and Asia, and although absent from more northerly areas including much of northwest Scotland, it reappears in northernmost Sutherland and Orkney.

The common name cowslip derives from the Old English cūslyppe meaning "cow dung", probably because the plant was often found growing amongst the manure in cow pastures.

The species name veris means "of spring".

Folk names include Cowslip, Cuy lippe, Herb Peter, Paigle, Peggle, Key Flower, Key of Heaven, Fairy Cups, Petty Mulleins, Crewel, Buckles, Palsywort, Plumrocks.

Primula veris is a low growing herbaceous perennial plant with a rosette of leaves 5–15 cm long and 2–6 cm broad. The deep yellow flowers are produced in the spring between April and May; they are in clusters of 10-30 together on a single stem 5–20 cm tall, each flower 9–15 mm broad. Red-flowered plants occur rarely.

Cowslip is frequently found on more open ground than *Primula vulgaris* (primrose) including open fields, meadows, and coastal dunes and clifftops. The seeds are often included in wild-flower seed mixes used to landscape motorway banks and similar civil engineering earth-works where the plants may be seen in dense stands.

Similar species: It may be confused with the closely related *Primula elatior* (oxlip), which has a similar general appearance although the oxlip has larger, pale yellow flowers more like a primrose, and a corolla tube without folds.

Cultivation

Hardiness Zone:	4-9
Soil pH:	6.1-7.8
Soil type:	Well drained moist light soil

Cultivation:	Division or by seed
Sunlight:	Full sun-partial shade
Habitat:	Native to temperate Europe and Asia, often found in open fields.

Cowslip is a perennial that thrives in moist soil. Their flowers appear in late winter/early spring and make an attractive show if naturalized in lawns. Let them self-seed to encourage spreading before mowing.

Historical Notes

Many of the Primrose tribe possess active medicinal properties. Besides the Cowslip and the Primrose, this family includes the little Scarlet Pimpernel (*Anagallis*), as truly a herald of warm summer weather as the Primrose is of spring, the Yellow Loosestrife and the Moneywort (*Lysimachia vulgaris* and *Nummularia*), the handsome Water Violet (*Hottonia*) and the nodding Cyclamen or Sowbread, all of which have medicinal value to a greater or lesser degree. Less important British members of the group are the Chaffweed (*Centunculus minimus*), one of the smallest among British plants, the Chickweed Wintergreen (*Trientalis*), the Sea Milk-wort (*Glaux maritima*), which has succulent salty leaves and has been used as a pickle, and the Common Brookweed or Water Pimpernel (*Samolus*).

The botanical name of the order, *Primulaceae*, is based on that of the genus Primula, to which belong not only those favourite spring flowers of the country-side, the Primrose, Cowslip, and their less common relative the Oxlip, but also the delicately-tinted greenhouse species that are such welcome pot plants for our rooms in mid-winter.

Linnaeus considered the Primrose, Cowslip and Oxlip to be but varieties of one species, but in this opinion later botanists have not followed him, though in all essential points they are identical.

Quite early in the spring, the Cowslip begins to produce its leaves. At first, each is just two tight coils, rolled backwards and lying side by side; these slowly unroll and a leaf similar to that of a Primrose, but shorter and rounder, appears. All the leaves lie nearly flat on the ground in a rosette, from the centre of which rises a long stalk, crowned by the flowers, which spring all from one point, in separate little stalks, and thus form an 'umbel.' The number of the flowers in an umbel varies very much in different specimens.

We quote the following from Familiar Wild Flowers:

'It is a curious fact that the inflorescence of the Primrose is as truly umbellate as that of the Cowslip, though in the former case it can only be detected by carefully tracing the flower stems to their base, when all will be found to spring from one common point. In some varieties of the Primrose the umbel is raised on a stalk, as in the Cowslip. This form is sometimes called Oxlip; it is by some writers raised to the dignity of an independent position as a true and distinct species. . . . Primrose roots may at times be met with bearing both forms, one or more stalked umbels together with a number of the ordinary type of flower.'

The sepals of the flowers are united to form pale green crinkled bags, from which the corolla projects, showing a golden disk about inch across with scalloped edges, the petals being united into a narrow tube within the calyx. On the yellow disk are five red spots, one on each petal.

'In their gold coats spots you see,

These be rubies fairy favours

In those freckles lie their savours.'

The Midsummer Night's Dream refers to the old belief that the flower held a magic value for the complexion.

The origin of Cowslip is obscure: it has been suggested that it is a corruption of 'Cow's Leek,' leek being derived from the Anglo-Saxon word leac, meaning a plant (comp. Houseleek).

In old Herbals we find the plant called Herb Peter and Key Flower, the pendent flowers suggesting a bunch of keys, the emblem of St. Peter, the idea having descended from old pagan times, for in Norse mythology the flower was dedicated to Frcya, the Key Virgin, and was thought to admit to her treasure palace. In northern Europe the idea of dedication to the goddess was transferred with the change of religion, and it became dedicated to the Virgin Mary, so we find it called 'Our Lady's Keys' and 'Key of Heaven,' and 'Keyflower' remains still the most usual name.

The flowers have a very distinctive and fresh fragrance and somewhat narcotic juices, which have given rise to their use in making the fermented liquor called Cowslip Wine, which had formerly a great and deserved reputation and is still largely drunk in country parts, being much produced in the Midlands. It is made from the 'peeps,' i.e. the yellow petal rings, in the following way: A gallon of 'peeps' with 4 lb. of lump sugar and the rind of 3 lemons is added to a gallon of cold spring water. A cup of fresh yeast is then included and the liquor stirred every day for a week. It is then put into a barrel with the juice of the lemons and left to 'work.' When 'quiet,' it is corked down for eight or nine months and finally bottled. The wine should be perfectly clear and of a pale yellow colour and has almost the value of a liqueur. In certain children's ailments, Cowslip Wine, given in small doses as a medicine, is particularly beneficial.

Young Cowslip leaves were at one time eaten in country salads and mixed with other herbs to stuff meat, whilst the flowers were made into a delicate conserve. Cowslip salad from the petals, with white sugar, is said to make an excellent and refreshing dish.

Children delight in making Cowslip Balls, or 'tosties,' from the flowers. The umbels are picked off close to the top of the main flowerstalk and about fifty to sixty are hung across a string which may be stretched for convenience between the backs of two chairs. The flowers are then pressed carefully together and the string tied tightly so as to collect them into a ball. Care must be taken to choose only such heads or umbels in which all the flowers are open, as otherwise the surface of the ball will be uneven.

Historical Medicinal Uses - For Entertainment ONLY

Part Used Medicinally: The yellow corolla is alone needed, no stalk or green part whatever is required, only the yellow part, plucked out of the green calyx.

Constituents: The roots and the flowers have somewhat of the odour of Anise, due to their containing some volatile oil identical with Mannite. Their acrid principle is Saponin.

Medicinal Action and Uses: Sedative, antispasmodic.

In olden days, Cowslip flowers were in great request for homely remedies, their special value lying in strengthening the nerves and the brain, and relieving restlessness and insomnia. The Cowslip was held good 'to ease paines in the head and is accounted next with Betony, the best for that purpose.'

Cowslip Wine made from the flowers, as above described, is an excellent sedative. Also, 1 lb. of the freshly gathered blossom infused in 1 1/2 pint of boiling water and simmered down with loaf sugar to a fine yellow syrup, taken with a little water is admirable for giddiness from nervous debility or from previous nervous excitement, and this syrup was formerly given against palsy.

In earlier times, the Cowslip was considered beneficial in all paralytic ailments, being, as we have seen, often called Palsy Wort or Herba paralysis. The root was also called in old Herbals Radix arthritica, from its use as a cure for muscular rheumatisrm.

In A Plain Plantain (Russell G. Alexander) we read:

'Cowslip water was considered to be good for the memory, and Cowslips of Jerusalem for mitigating "hectical fevers." Mrs. Raffald (English Housekeeper, 1778) gives a recipe for the wine. "For the future," says the poet Pope, in one of his letters, "I'll drown all high thoughts in the Lethe of Cowslip Wine" (which is pleasantly soporific). Our Lady's Cowslip is Gagea lutea.'

The old writers give a long list of ills that may be remedied by application of the roots or leaves of the plant; the juice of the flowers 'takes off spots and wrinkles from the face and other vices of the skin,' the water of the flowers being 'very proper medicine for weakly people.'

Turner says:

'Some weomen we find, sprinkle ye floures of cowslip wt whyte wine and after still it and wash their faces wt that water to drive wrinkles away and to make them fayre in the eyes of the worlde rather than in the eyes of God, Whom they are not afrayd to offend.'

Formerly an ointment was made from the flowers as a cosmetic. Culpepper says:

'Our city dames know well enough the ointment or distilled water of it adds to beauty or at least restores it when lost. The flowers are held to be more effectual than the leaves and the roots of little use. An ointment being made with them taketh away spots and wrinkles of the skin, sunburnings and freckles and promotes beauty; they remedy all infirmities of

the head coming of heat and wind, as vertigo, false apparitions, phrensies, falling sickess, palsies, convulsions, cramps, pains in the nerves, and the roots ease pains in the back and bladder. The leaves are good in wounds and the flowers take away trembling. Because they strengthen the brains and nerves and remedy palsies, the Greeks gave them the name Paralysio. The flowers preserved or conserved and a quantity the size of a nutmeg taken every morning is a sufficient dose for inward diseases, but for wounds, spots, wrinkles and sunburnings an ointment is made of the leaves and hog's lard.'

A later writer, Hill (1755), tells us that when boiled in ale, the powdered roots were taken with success by country folk for giddiness, wakefulness and similar nervous troubles for which the syrup made from the flowers was also taken.

The usual dose of the dried and powdered flowers is 15 to 20 grains.

From Hartman's Family Physitian, 1696:

'Another way to make Cowslip Wine

'Having boil'd your Water and Sugar together, pour it boiling hot upon your Cowslips beaten, stir them well together, and let them stand in a Vessel close cover'd till it be almost cold; then put into it the Yest beaten with the Juice of Lemons; let it stand for two days, then press it out with as much speed as you can, and put it up into a Cask, and leave a little hole open, for the working; when it hath quite done working stop it up close for a Month or Six Weeks, then Bottle it. Cowslip Wine is very Cordial, and a glass of it being drank at night Bedward, causes sleep and rest. . . .'

The Bird's-eye Primrose (*Primula farinosa*) is a plant of mountain slopes and pastures, and may be met with on the mountain ranges of Europe and Asia. It is not uncommon in the northern counties of England, though much less common in Scotland.

Gerard, in his Herball, says:

"These plants grow very plentifully in moist and squally grounds in the North parts of England, as in Harwood, neere to Blackburne in Lancashire, and ten miles from Preston in Aundernesse; also at Crosby, Ravensnaith, and Craig-close in Westmorland. They likewise grow in the meadows belonging to a village in Lancashire neere Maudsley called Harwood, and at Hasketh, not far from thence, and in many other places of Lancashire, but not on this side Trent' (Gerard writes as a Londoner) *'that I could ever have certain knowledge of. Lobel reporteth, That Doctor Penny, a famous Physition of our London Colledge, did find them in these Southerne Parts.'*

Specimens of the Bird's-eye Primrose growing in the North of Scotland, in Caithness and the Orkney Islands, and in other localities bordering on the sea, vary from the typical form of the plant in being of stouter habit and much smaller, in having leaves of broader proportions and flowers of a deeper purple; and some botanists are inclined to distinguish this variety by creating it an independent species, and calling it the ScotchBird's-eye (*P. Scotica*), while others are content to consider it but a variety from the type, and label it P. farinosa, var. Scotica.

All the hardy varieties of Primula, whether Primrose, Cowslip, Polyanthus or Auricula, may be easily propagated by dividing the roots of old plants in autumn. New varieties are raised from seed, which should be sown as soon as ripe, in leaf-mould, and pricked out into beds when large enough.

Among the many splendid flowers that are grown in our greenhouses none shows more improvement under the fostering hand of the British florist than the Chinese Primula which originally had small, inconspicuous flowers, but now bears trusses of magnificent blooms ranging from the purest white to the richest scarlet and crimson. The Star Primulas, which have attained an even greater popularity in late years, are considered perhaps even more elegant, being looser in growth and carrying their plentiful blossoms in more graceful, if not more beautiful trusses. Both varieties are among the most beautiful of our winter-flowering plants, the toothed and lobed, somewhat heart-shaped leaves being extremely handsome with their crimson tints.

Seeds of these greenhouse Primulas should be sown in the spring in gentle heat, the soil used being very fine and pleasantly moist. The seedlings must be pricked off and potted out as necessary, with a view to ensuring sturdy, healthy growth.

P. obconica is a slightly varying type of these greenhouse Primulas, the leaves approaching more the shape of those of the common Primrose, the plants are exceedingly floriferous and graceful, the full trusses of delicate lilac flowers are borne on tall slender stems and care must be used in the handling of it, as the leaves sometimes cause an eruption like eczema. Homoeopaths make a tincture from this species.

The broad, thick leaves of the Auricula (*P. auricula*), a frequent garden plant in this country, though not native to Great Britain, are used in the Alps as a remedy for coughs.

In its native state the Auricula is said to be either yellow or white. It is the skill of the gardener which has brought it to its present purple and brown. It was formerly known as Mountain Cowslip, or Bear's Ears.

Dandelion

Compositae.

Taraxacum officinale Web.

Quick Facts

Latin/Linnaen:	*Taraxacum officinale*
Family:	*Asteraceae*
Old English :	ægwyrt
Synonyms:	OE name means 'egg plant', other names include priest's crown, swine's snout, and the by-name 'piss-the-bed'
Action:	Choleretic, Diuretic, Appetite stimulant
Parts Used:	Herb and root
Indicated For:	Loss of appetite, disturbance in bile flow, dyspepsia, stimulation of diuresis
Dosage:	Herb only: Unless otherwise prescribed: 4-10g of herb 3 times daily, 4-10mg liquid extract 1:1 in 25% alcohol 3 times daily.
	Root with herb: Unless otherwise prescribed: as tea: 1 tablespoon of cut drug per cup of water, as decoction: 3-4g cut or powdered drug per cup of water, as tincture: 10-15 drops 3 times daily.
Preparation:	Liquid and solid preparations for oral use
Cautions:	Contraindications: Obstruction of bile ducts, gallbladder empyema, ileus. In cases of gallstones, use only after consultation with a physician
Other Uses:	**Beverages**: Flowers are used to make Dandelion wine, and ground roasted dandelion root can be used as a coffee substitute.
	"Dandelion and Burdock" is a soft drink that has long been popular in the United Kingdom with authentic recipes sold by health food shops. It has also been used in a saison ale called Pissenlit (literally "piss the bed" in French) made by Brasserie Fantôme in Belgium.
	Culinary: The greens are used in salads and in soups. Usually the young leaves and unopened buds are eaten raw in salads, while older leaves are cooked. Raw leaves have a slightly bitter taste. Dandelion salad is often accompanied with hard boiled eggs.
	Another recipe using the plant is dandelion flower jam.

In Silesia and also other parts of Poland and world, dandelion flowers are used to make a honey substitute syrup with added lemon (so-called May-honey). This "honey" is believed to have a medicinal value, in particular against liver problems.

Dye: Yellow or green dye colours can be obtained from the flowers

Description

Taraxacum officinale, the common dandelion (often simply called "dandelion"), is an herbaceous perennial plant of the family *Asteraceae* (*Compositae*). It can be found growing in temperate regions of the world, in lawns, on roadsides, on disturbed banks and shores of water ways, and other areas with moist soils. *T. officinale* is considered a weedy species, especially in lawns and along roadsides, but it is sometimes used as a medical herb and in food preparation. As a nearly cosmopolitan weed, common dandelion is best known for its yellow flower heads that turn into round balls of silver tufted fruits that blow away on the wind.

Taraxacum officinale grows from generally unbranched taproots and produces one to more than ten stems that are typically 5 to 40 cm tall but sometimes up to 70 cm tall. The stems can be tinted purplish, they are upright or lax, and produce flower heads that are held as tall or taller than the foliage. The foliage is upright growing or horizontally orientated, with leaves having narrowly winged petioles or being unwinged. The stems can be glabrous or are sparsely covered with short hairs. The 5–45 cm long and 1–10 cm wide leaves are oblanceolate, oblong, or obovate in shape with the bases gradually narrowing to the petiole. The leaf margins are typically shallowly lobed to deeply lobed and often lacerate or toothed with sharp or dull teeth. The calyculi (the cup like bracts that hold the florets) is composed of 12 to 18 segments: each segment is reflexed and sometimes glaucous. The lanceolate shaped bractlets are in 2 series with the apices acuminate in shape. The 14 to 25 mm wide involucres are green to dark green or brownish green with the tips dark gray or purplish. The florets number 40 to over 100 per head, having corollas that are yellow or orange-yellow in color. The fruits, which are called cypselae, range in color from olive-green or olive-brown to straw-colored to grayish, they are oblanceoloid in shape and 2 to 3 mm long with slender beaks. The fruits have 4 to 12 ribs that have sharp edges. The silky pappi, which form the parachutes, are white to silver-white in color and around 6 mm wide. Plants typically have 24 or 40 pairs of chromosomes but some plants have 16 or 32 chromosomes. Plants have milky sap and the leaves are all basal, each flowering stem lacks bracts and has one single flower head. The yellow flower heads lack receptacle bracts and all the flowers, which are called florets, are ligulate and bisexual. The fruits are mostly produced by apomixis. It blooms from March until October

Cultivation

Hardiness Zone:	3-10
Soil pH:	7.5 optimal, prefers alkaline soil
Soil type:	Moist-dry
Cultivation:	Readily self seed and regenerate from root pieces.
Sunlight:	Prefers full sun, but tolerant of shade
Habitat:	Can grow almost anywhere

Dandilion is a perennial plant which is extremely hardy. It can grow almost anywhere. It is considered a noxious weed and care should be taken not to promote its spread. Consult local laws before propagating dandelion.

Historical Notes

The Dandelion (*Taraxacum officinale*, Weber, T. Densleonis, Desf; Leontodon taraxacum, Linn.), though not occurring in the Southern Hemisphere, is at home in all parts of the north temperate zone, in pastures, meadows and on waste ground, and is so plentiful that farmers everywhere find it a troublesome weed, for though its flowers are more conspicuous in the earlier months of the summer, it may be found in bloom, and consequently also prolifically dispersing its seeds, almost throughout the year.

From its thick tap root, dark brown, almost black on the outside though white and milky within, the long jagged leaves rise directly, radiating from it to form a rosette lying close upon the ground, each leaf being grooved and constructed so that all the rain falling on it is conducted straight to the centre of the rosette and thus to the root which is, therefore, always kept well watered. The maximum amount of water is in this manner directed towards the proper region for utilization by the root, which but for this arrangement would not obtain sufficient moisture, the leaves being spread too close to the ground for the water to penetrate.

The leaves are shiny and without hairs, the margin of each leaf cut into great jagged teeth, either upright or pointing somewhat backwards, and these teeth are themselves cut here and there into lesser teeth. It is this somewhat fanciful resemblance to the canine teeth of a lion that (it is generally assumed) gives the plant its most familiar name of Dandelion, which is a corruption of the French Dent de Lion, an equivalent of this name being found not only in its former specific Latin name Dens leonis and in the Greek name for the genus to which Linnaeus assigned it, Leontodon, but also in nearly all the languages of Europe.

There is some doubt, however, as to whether it was really the shape of the leaves that provided the original notion, as there is really no similarity between them, but the leaves may perhaps be said to resemble the angular jaw of a lion fully supplied with teeth. Some authorities have suggested that the yellow flowers might be compared to the golden teeth of the heraldic lion, while others say that the whiteness of the root is the feature which provides the resemblance. Flückiger and Hanbury in Pharmacographia, say that the name was conferred by Wilhelm, a surgeon, who was so much impressed by the virtues of the plant that he likened it to Dens leonis. In the Ortus Sanitatis, 1485, under 'Dens Leonis,' there is a monograph of half a page (unaccompanied by any illustration) which concludes:

'The Herb was much employed by Master Wilhelmus, a surgeon, who on account of its virtues, likened it to "eynem lewen zan, genannt zu latin Dens leonis" (a lion's tooth, called in Latin Dens leonis).'

In the pictures of the old herbals, for instance, the one in Brunfels' Contrafayt Kreuterbuch, 1532, the leaves very much resemble a lion's tooth. The root is not illustrated at all in the old herbals, as only the herb was used at that time.

The name of the genus, *Taraxacum*, is derived from the Greek taraxos (disorder), and akos (remedy), on account of the curative action of the plant. A possible alternative derivation of *Taraxacum* is suggested in The Treasury of Botany:

'The generic name is possibly derived from the Greek taraxo ("I have excited" or "caused") and achos (pain), in allusion to the medicinal effects of the plant.'

There are many varieties of Dandelion leaves; some are deeply cut into segments, in others the segments or lobes form a much less conspicuous feature, and are sometimes almost entire.

The shining, purplish flower-stalks rise straight from the root, are leafless, smooth and hollow and bear single heads of flowers. On picking the flowers, a bitter, milky juice exudes from the broken edges of the stem, which is present throughout the plant, and which when it comes into contact with the hand, turns to a brown stain that is rather difficult to remove.

Each bloom is made up of numerous strapshaped florets of a bright golden yellow. This strap-shaped corolla is notched at the edge into five teeth, each tooth representing a petal, and lower down is narrowed into a claw-like tube, which rests on the singlechambered ovary containing a single ovule. In this tiny tube is a copious supply of nectar, which more than half fills it, and the presence of which provides the incentive for the visits of many insects, among whom the bee takes first rank. The Dandelion takes an important place among honey-producing plants, as it furnishes considerable quantities of both pollen and nectar in the early spring, when the bees' harvest from fruit trees is nearly over. It is also important from the beekeeper's point of view, because not only does it flower most in spring, no matter how cool the weather may be, but a small succession of bloom is also kept up until late autumn, so that it is a source of honey after the main flowers have ceased to bloom, thus delaying the need for feeding the colonies of bees with artificial food.

Many little flies also are to be found visiting the Dandelion to drink the lavishly-supplied nectar. By carefully watching, it has been ascertained that no less than ninety-three different kinds of insects are in the habit of frequenting it. The stigma grows up through the tube formed by the anthers, pushing the pollen before it, and insects smearing themselves with this pollen carry it to the stigmas of other flowers already expanded, thus ensuring cross-fertilization. At the base of each flower-head is a ring of narrow, green bracts the involucre. Some of these stand up to support the florets, others hang down to form a barricade against such small insects as might crawl up the stem and injure the bloom without taking a share in its fertilization, as the winged insects do.

The blooms are very sensitive to weather conditions: in fine weather, all the parts are outstretched, but directly rain threatens the whole head closes up at once. It closes against the dews of night, by five o'clock in the evening, being prepared for its night's sleep, opening again at seven in the morning though as this opening and closing is largely dependent upon the intensity of the light, the time differs somewhat in different latitudes and at different seasons.

When the whole head has matured, all the florets close up again within the green sheathing bracts that lie beneath, and the bloom returns very much to the appearance it had in the bud. Its shape being then somewhat reminiscent of the snout of a pig, it is termed in some districts 'Swine's Snout.' The withered, yellow petals are, however soon pushed off in a bunch, as the seeds, crowned with their tufts of hair, mature, and one day, under the influence of sun and wind the 'Swine's Snout' becomes a large gossamer ball, from its silky whiteness a very noticeable feature. It is made up of myriads of plumed seeds or pappus, ready to be blown off when quite ripe by the slightest breeze, and forms the 'clock' of the children, who by blowing at it till all the seeds are released, love to tell themselves the time of day by the number of puffs necessary to disperse every seed. When all the seeds have flown, the receptacle or disc on which they were placed remains bare, white, speckled and surrounded by merely the drooping remnants of the sheathing bracts, and we can see why the plant received another of its popular names, 'Priest's Crown,' common in the Middle Ages, when a priest's shorn head was a familiar object.

Small birds are very fond of the seeds of the Dandelion and pigs devour the whole plant greedily. Goats will eat it, but sheep and cattle do not care for it, though it is said to increase the milk of cows when eaten by them. Horses refuse to touch this plant, not appreciating its bitter juice. It is valuable food for rabbits and may be given them from April to September forming excellent food in spring and at breeding seasons in particular.

The young leaves of the Dandelion make an agreeable and wholesome addition to spring salads and are often eaten on the Continent, especially in France. The full-grown leaves should not be taken, being too bitter, but the young leaves, especially if blanched, make an excellent salad, either alone or in combination with other plants, lettuce, shallot tops or chives.

Young Dandelion leaves make delicious sandwiches, the tender leaves being laid between slices of bread and butter and sprinkled with salt. The addition of a little lemon-juice and pepper varies the flavour. The leaves should always be torn to pieces, rather than cut, in order to keep the flavour.

John Evelyn, in his Acetana, says: 'With thie homely salley, Hecate entertained Theseus.' In Wales, they grate or chop up Dandelion roots, two years old, and mix them with the leaves in salad. The seed of a special broad-leaved variety of Dandelion is sold by seedsmen for cultivation for salad purposes. Dandelion can be blanched in the same way as endive, and is then very delicate in flavour. If covered with an ordinary flower-pot during the winter, the pot being further buried under some rough stable litter, the young leaves sprout when there is a dearth of saladings and prove a welcome change in early spring. Cultivated thus, Dandelion is only pleasantly bitter, and if eaten while the leaves are quite young, the centre rib of the leaf is not at all unpleasant to the taste. When older the rib is tough and not nice to eat. If the flower-buds of plants reserved in a corner of the garden for salad purposes are removed at once and the leaves carefully cut, the plants will last through the whole winter.

The young leaves may also be boiled as a vegetable, spinach fashion, thoroughly drained, sprinkled with pepper and salt, moistened with soup or butter and served very hot. If considered a little too bitter, use half spinach, but the Dandelion must be partly cooked first in this case, as it takes longer than spinach. As a variation, some grated nutmeg or garlic, a teaspoonful of chopped onion or grated lemon peel can be added to the greens when they are cooked. A simple vegetable soup may also be made with Dandelions.

The dried Dandelion leaves are also employed as an ingredient in many digestive or diet drinks and herb beers. Dandelion Beer is a rustic fermented drink common in many parts of the country and made also in Canada. Workmen in the furnaces and potteries of the industrial towns of the Midlands have frequent resource to many of the tonic Herb Beers, finding them cheaper and less intoxicating than ordinary beer, and Dandelion stout ranks as a favourite. An agreeable and wholesome fermented drink is made from Dandelions, Nettles and Yellow Dock.

In Berkshire and Worcestershire, the flowers are used in the preparation of a beverage known as Dandelion Wine. This is made by pouring a gallon of boiling water over a gallon of the flowers. After being well stirred, it is covered with a blanket and allowed to stand for three days, being stirred again at intervals, after which it is strained and the liquor boiled for 30 minutes, with the addition of 3 1/2 lb. of loaf sugar, a little ginger sliced, the rind of 1 orange and 1 lemon sliced. When cold, a little yeast is placed in it on a piece of toast, producing fermentation. It is then covered over and allowed to stand two days until it has ceased 'working,' when it is placed in a cask, well bunged down for two months before bottling. This wine is suggestive of sherry slightly flat, and has the deserved reputation of being an excellent tonic, extremely good for the blood.

The roasted roots are largely used to form Dandelion Coffee, being first thoroughly cleaned, then dried by artificial heat, and slightly roasted till they are the tint of coffee, when they are ground ready for use. The roots are taken up in the autumn, being then most fitted for this purpose. The prepared powder is said to be almost indistinguishable from real coffee, and is claimed to be an improvement to inferior coffee, which is often an adulterated product. Of late years, Dandelion Coffee has come more into use in this country, being obtainable at most vegetarian restaurants and stores. Formerly it used occasionally to be given for medicinal purposes, generally mixed with true coffee to give it a better flavour. The ground root was sometimes mixed with chocolate for a similar purpose. Dandelion Coffee is a natural beverage without any of the injurious effects that ordinary tea and coffee have on the nerves and digestive organs. It exercises a stimulating influence over the whole system, helping the liver and kidneys to do their work and keeping the bowels in a healthy condition, so that it offers great advantages to dyspeptics and does not cause wakefulness.

History

The first mention of the Dandelion as a medicine is in the works of the Arabian physicians of the tenth and eleventh centuries, who speak of it as a sort of wild Endive, under the name of Taraxcacon. In this country, we find allusion to it in the Welsh medicines of the thirteenth century. Dandelion was much valued as a medicine in the times of Gerard and Parkinson, and is still extensively employed.

Dandelion roots have long been largely used on the Continent, and the plant is cultivated largely in India as a remedy for liver complaints.

The root is perennial and tapering, simple or more or less branched, attaining in a good soil a length of a foot or more and 1/2 inch to an inch in diameter. Old roots divide at the crown into several heads. The root is fleshy and brittle, externally of a dark brown, internally white and abounding in an inodorous milky juice of bitter, but not disagreeable taste.

Only large, fleshy and well-formed roots should be collected, from plants two years old, not slender, forked ones. Roots produced in good soil are easier to dig up without breaking, and are thicker and less forked than those growing on waste places and by the roadside. Collectors should, therefore only dig in good, free soil, in moisture and shade, from meadow-land. Dig up in wet weather, but not during frost, which materially lessens the activity of the roots. Avoid breaking the roots, using a long trowel or a fork, lifting steadily and carefully. Shake off as much of the earth as possible and then cleanse the roots, the easiest way being to leave them in a basket in a running stream so that the water covers them, for about an hour, or shake them, bunched, in a tank of clean water. Cut off the crowns of leaves, but be careful in so doing not to leave any scales on the top. Do not cut or slice the roots or the valuable milky juice on which their medicinal value depends will be wasted by bleeding.

As only large, well-formed roots are worth collecting, some people prefer to grow Dandelions as a crop, as by this means large roots are insured and they are more easily dug, generally being ploughed up. About 4 lb. of seed to the acre should be allowed, sown in drills, 1 foot apart. The crops should be kept clean by hoeing, and all flower-heads should be picked off as soon as they appear, as otherwise the grower's own land and that of his neighbours will be smothered with the weed when the seeds ripen. The yield should be 4 or 5 tons of fresh roots to the acre in the second year. Dandelion roots shrink very much in drying, losing about 76 per cent of their weight, so that 100 parts of fresh roots yield only about 22 parts of dry material. Under favourable conditions, yields at the rate of 1,000 to 1,500 lb. of dry roots per acre have been obtained from second-year plants cultivated.

Dandelion root can only be economically collected when a meadow in which it is abundant is ploughed up. Under such circumstances the roots are necessarily of different ages and sizes, the seeds sowing themselves in successive years. The roots then collected after washing and drying, have to be sorted into different grades.

The largest, from the size of a lead pencil upwards, are cut into straight pieces 2 to 3 inches long, the smaller side roots being removed, these are sold at a higher price as the finest roots. The smaller roots fetch a less price, and the trimmings are generally cut small, sold at a lower price and used for making Dandelion Coffee. Every part of the root is thus used. The root before being dried should have every trace of the leaf-bases removed as their presence lessens the value of the root.

In collecting cultivated Dandelion advantage is obtained if the seeds are all sown at one time, as greater uniformity in the size of the root is obtainable, and in deep soil free from stones, the seedlings will produce elongated, straight roots with few branches, especially if allowed to be somewhat crowded on the same principles that coppice trees produce straight trunks. Time is also saved in digging up the roots which can thus be sold at prices competing with those obtained as the result of cheaper labour on the Continent. The edges of fields when room is allowed for the plough-horses to turn, could easily be utilized if the soil is good and free from stones for both Dandelion and Burdock, as the roots are usually much branched in stony ground, and the roots are not generally collected until October when the harvest is over. The roots gathered in this month have stored up their food reserve of Inulin, and when dried present a firm appearance, whilst if collected in spring, when the food reserve in the root is used up for the leaves and flowers, the dried root then presents a shrivelled and porous appearance which renders it unsaleable. The medicinal properties of the root are, therefore, necessarily greater in proportion in the spring. Inulin being soluble in hot water, the solid extract if made by boiling the root, often contains a large quantity of it, which is deposited in the extract as it cools.

The roots are generally dried whole, but the largest ones may sometimes be cut transversely into pieces 3 to 6 inches long. Collected wild roots are, however, seldom large enough to necessitate cutting. Drying will probably take about a fortnight. When finished, the roots should be hard and brittle enough to snap, and the inside of the roots white, not grey

The roots should be kept in a dry place after drying, to avoid mould, preferably in tins to prevent the attacks of moths and beetles. Dried Dandelion is exceedingly liable to the attacks of maggots and should not be kept beyond one season.

Dried Dandelion root is 1/2 inch or less in thickness, dark brown, shrivelled, with wrinkles running lengthwise, often in a spiral direction; when quite dry, it breaks easily with a short, corky fracture, showing a very thick, white bark, surrounding a wooden column. The latter is yellowish, very porous, without pith or rays. A rather broad but indistinct cambium zone separates the wood from the bark, which latter exhibits numerous well-defined, concentric layers, due to the milk vessels. This structure is quite characteristic and serves to distinguish Dandelion roots from other roots like it. There are several flowers easily mistaken for the Dandelion when in blossom, but these have either hairy leaves or branched flower-stems, and the roots differ either in structure or shape.

Dried Dandelion root somewhat resembles Pellitory and Liquorice roots, but Pellitory differs in having oil glands and also a large radiate wood, and Liquorice has also a large radiate wood and a sweet taste.

The root of Hawkbit (*Leontodon hispidus*) is sometimes substituted for Dandelion root. It is a plant with hairy, not smooth leaves, and the fresh root is tough, breaking with difficulty and rarely exuding much milky juice. Some kinds of Dock have also been substituted, and also Chicory root. The latter is of a paler colour, more bitter and has the laticiferous vessels in radiating lines. In the United States it is often substituted for Dandelion. Dock roots have a prevailing yellowish colour and an astringent taste.

During recent years, a small form of a Dandelion root has been offered by Russian firms, who state that it is sold and used as Dandelion in that country. This root is always smaller than the root of T. officinale, has smaller flowers, and the crown of the root has often a tuft of brown woolly hairs between the leaf bases at the crown of the root, which are never seen in the Dandelion plant in this country (UK), and form a characteristic distinction, for the root shows similar concentric, horny rings in the thick white bark as well as a yellow porous woody centre. These woolly hairs are mentioned in Greenish's Materia Medica, and also in the British Pharmaceutical Codex, as a feature of Dandelion root, but no mention is made of them in the Pharmacographia, nor in the British Pharmacopceia or United States Pharmacopceia, and it is probable, therefore, that Russian specimens have been used for describing the root, and that the root with brown woolly hairs belongs to some other species of *Taraxacum*.

Chemical Constituents

The chief constituents of Dandelion root are Taraxacin, acrystalline, bitter substance, of which the yield varies in roots collected at different seasons, and

Taraxacerin, an acrid resin, with Inulin (a sort of sugar which replaces starch in many of the Dandelion family, Compositae), gluten, gum and potash. The root contains no starch, but early in the year contains much uncrystallizable sugar and laevulin, which differs from Inulin in being soluble in cold water. This diminishes in quantity during the summer and becomes Inulin in the autumn. The root may contain as much as 24 per cent. In the fresh root, the Inulin is present in the cell-sap, but in the dry root it occurs as an amorphodus, transparent solid, which is only slightly soluble in cold water, but soluble in hot water.

There is a difference of opinion as to the best time for collecting the roots. The British Pharmacopceia considers the autumn dug root more bitter than the spring root, and that as it contains about 25 per cent insoluble Inulin, it is to be preferred on this account to the spring root, and it is, therefore, directed that in England the root should be collected between September and February, it being considered to be in perfection for Extract making in the month of November.

Bentley, on the other hand, contended that it is more bitter in March and most of all in July, but that as in the latter month it would generally be inconvenient for digging it, it should be dug in the spring, when the yield of Taraxacin, the bitter soluble principle, is greatest.

On account of the variability of the constituents of the plant according to the time of year when gathered, the yield and composition of the extract are very variable. If gathered from roots collected in autumn, the resulting product yields a turbid solution with water; if from spring-collected roots, the aqueous solution will be clear and yield but very little sediment on standing, because of the conversion of the Inulin into Laevulose and sugar at this active period of the plant's life.

In former days, Dandelion Juice was the favourite preparation both in official and domestic medicine. Provincial druggists sent their collectors for the roots and expressed the juice while these were quite fresh. Many country druggists prided themselves on their Dandelion Juice. The most active preparations of Dandelion, the Juice (*Succus Taraxaci*) and the Extract (*Extractum Taraxaci*), are made from the bruised fresh root. The Extract prepared from the fresh root is sometimes almost devoid of bitterness. The dried root alone was official in the United States Pharmacopoeia.

The leaves are not often used, except for making Herb-Beer, but a medicinal tincture is sometimes made from the entire plant gathered in the early summer. It is made with proof spirit.

When collecting the seeds care should be taken when drying them in the sun, to cover them with coarse muslin, as otherwise the down will carry them away. They are best collected in the evening, towards sunset, or when the damp air has caused the heads to close up.

The tops should be cut on a dry day, when quite free of rain or dew, and all insect-eaten or stained leaves rejected.

Historical Medicinal Uses - For Entertainment ONLY

Parts Used Medicinally

The root, fresh and dried, the young tops. All parts of the plant contain a somewhat bitter, milky juice (latex), but the juice of the root being still more powerful is the part of the plant most used for medicinal purposes.

Medicinal Action and Uses: Diuretic, tonic and slightly aperient. It is a general stimulant to the system, but especially to the urinary organs, and is chiefly used in kidney and liver disorders.

Dandelion is not only official but is used in many patent medicines. Its beneficial action is best obtained when combined with other agents.

The tincture made from the tops may be taken in doses of 10 to 15 drops in a spoonful of water, three times daily.

It is said that its use for liver complaints was assigned to the plant largely on the doctrine of signatures, because of its bright yellow flowers of a bilious hue.

In the hepatic complaints of persons long resident in warm climates, Dandelion is said to afford very marked relief. A broth of Dandelion roots, sliced and stewed in boiling water with some leaves of Sorrel and the yolk of an egg, taken daily for some months, has been known to cure seemingly intractable cases of chronic liver congestion.

A strong decoction is found serviceable in stone and gravel: the decoction may be made by boiling 1 pint of the sliced root in 20 parts of water for 15 minutes, straining this when cold and sweetening with brown sugar or honey. A small teacupful may be taken once or twice a day.

Dandelion is used as a bitter tonic in atonic dyspepsia, and as a mild laxative in habitual constipation. When the stomach is irritated and where active treatment would be injurious, the decoction or extract of Dandelion administered three or four times a day, will often prove a valuable remedy. It has a good effect in increasing the appetite and promoting digestion.

Dandelion combined with other active remedies has been used in cases of dropsy and for induration of the liver, and also on the Continent for phthisis and some cutaneous diseases. A decoction of 2 OZ. of the herb or root in 1 quart of water, boiled down to a pint, is taken in doses of one wineglassful every three hours for scurvy, scrofula, eczema and all eruptions on the surface of the body.

Preparations and Dosages

Fluid extract, B.P., 1/2 to 2 drachms. Solid extract, B.P. 5 to 15 grains. Juice, B.P., 1 to 2 drachms. Leontodin, 2 to 4 grains.

Dandelion Tea

Infuse 1 OZ. of Dandelion in a pint of boiling water for 10 minutes; decant, sweeten with honey, and drink several glasses in the course of the day. The use of this tea is efficacious in bilious affections, and is also much approved of in the treatment of dropsy.

Or take 2 OZ. of freshly-sliced Dandelion root, and boil in 2 pints of water until it comes to 1 pint; then add 1 OZ. of compound tincture of Horseradish. Dose, from 2 to 4 OZ. Use in a sluggish state of the liver.

Or 1 OZ. Dandelion root, 1 OZ. Black Horehound herb, 1/2 OZ. Sweet Flag root, 1/4 OZ. Mountain Flax. Simmer the whole in 3 pints of water down to 1 1/2 pint, strain and take a wineglassful after meals for biliousness and dizziness.

For Gall Stones

1 OZ. Dandelion root, 1 OZ. Parsley root, 1 OZ. Balm herb, 1/2 OZ. Ginger root, 1/2 OZ. Liquorice root. Place in 2 quarts of water and gently simmer down to 1 quart, strain and take a wineglassful every two hours.

For a young child suffering from jaundice: 1 OZ. Dandelion root, 1/2 oz. Ginger root, 1/2 oz. Caraway seed, 1/2 oz. Cinnamon bark, 1/4 oz. Senna leaves. Gently boil in 3 pints of water down to 1 1/2 pint, strain, dissolve 1/2 lb. sugar in hot liquid, bring to a boil again, skim all impurities that come to the surface when clear, put on one side to cool, and give frequently in teaspoonful doses.

A Liver and Kidney Mixture

1 OZ. Broom tops, 1/2 oz. Juniper berries, 1/2 oz. Dandelion root, 1 1/2 pint water. Boil in gredients for 10 minutes, then strain and adda small quantity of cayenne. Dose, 1 tablespoonful, three times a day.

A Medicine for Piles

1 OZ. Long-leaved Plantain, 1 OZ. Dandelion root, 1/2 oz. Polypody root, 1 OZ. Shepherd's Purse. Add 3 pints of water, boil down to half the quantity, strain, and add 1 OZ. of tincture of Rhubarb. Dose, a wineglassful three times a day. Celandine ointment to be applied at same time.

In Derbyshire, the juice of the stalk is applied to remove warts.

Dill

Quick Facts

Latin/Linnaen:	*Anethum Graveolens*
Family:	*Apiaceae*
Old English :	Dyle, Dile
Synonyms:	None
Action:	Antispasmodic, Bacteriostatic
Parts Used:	Seed
Indicated For:	Dyspepsia
Dosage:	Unless otherwise prescribed: Avrage daily dosage: Seed, 3 g; essential oil, 0.1 - 0.3; Equivalent preparations.
Preparation:	Whole seeds for teas and other galenical preparations for internal application.
Cautions:	
Other Uses:	**Culinary**: In Manipur, India Dill locally known as "Pakhon" is an essential ingredient of Chagem Pomba – a traditional Manipuri dish with fermented soya bean, and rice.

Description

Dill (*Anethum graveolens*) is a perennial herb. It is the sole species of the genus *Anethum*, though classified by some botanists in a related genus as *Peucedanum graveolens* (L.) C.B.Clarke.

40–60 cm (16–24 in), with slender stems and alternate, finely divided, softly delicate leaves 10–20 cm (3.9–7.9 in) long. The ultimate leaf divisions are 1–2 mm (0.039–0.079 in) broad, slightly broader than the similar leaves of fennel, which are threadlike, less than 1 mm (0.039 in) broad, but harder in texture. The flowers are white to yellow, in small umbels 2–9 cm (0.79–3.5 in) diameter. The seeds are 4–5 mm (0.16–0.20 in) long and 1 mm (0.039 in) thick, and straight to slightly curved with a longitudinally ridged surface.

Dill originated within an area around the Mediterranean and the South of Russia. Zohary and Hopf remark that "wild and weedy types of dill are widespread in the Mediterranean basin and in West Asia. Although several twigs of dill were found in the tomb of Amenhotep II, they report that the earliest archeological evidence for its cultivation comes from late Neolithic lake shore settlements in Switzerland. Traces have been found in Roman ruins in Great Britain.

In Semitic languages it is known by the name of Shubit. The Talmud requires that tithes shall be paid on the seeds, leaves, and stem of dill.

The name dill comes from Old English dile, thought to have originated from a Norse or Anglo-Saxon word dylle meaning to soothe or lull, the plant having the carminative property of relieving gas. In Romania it is called Mărar and is used for preparing Borscht or Pickles.

Fresh and dried dill leaves (sometimes called "dill weed" to distinguish it from dill seed) are used as herbs, mainly in Finland, Sweden, the Baltic, in Russia, and in central Asia.

Like caraway, its fernlike leaves are aromatic and are used to flavor many foods, such as gravlax (cured salmon), borscht and other soups, and pickles (where the dill flower is sometimes used). Dill is best when used fresh, as it loses its flavor rapidly if dried; however, freeze-dried dill leaves preserve their flavor relatively well for a few months.

Dill seed is used as a spice, with a flavor somewhat similar to caraway but also resembling that of fresh or dried dill weed. Dill seeds were traditionally used to soothe the stomach after meals. Dill oil can be extracted from the leaves, stems and seeds of the plant.

Dill is the eponymous ingredient in Dill Pickles; cucumbers preserved in salty brine and/or vinegar.

In Arabic, dill seed is called ain jaradeh (means cricket eye) used as a spice in cold dishes like fattoush and pickles.

In Arab coutries of the Persian Gulf, dill is called "shibint" and is used mostly in fish dishes; dill is also used in Iranian "Aash" recipes, and is called "sheved" (also "shevid") in Persian. Very rarely it is used in chicken dishes.

In Lao cuisine and parts of northern Thailand, dill is known in English as Laotian coriander and Lao cilantro. In the Lao language, it is called Phak See, and in Thai, it is known as Phak Chee Lao. In Lao cuisine, the herb is typically used in mok pa (steamed fish in banana leaf) and several coconut milk-based curries that contain fish or prawns.

In Romania dill is used on a national scale as an ingredient for soups and other dishes; it is often mixed with salted cheese and used as a filling for the langos. Another popular dish with dill as a base ingredient is the dill sauce.

In Vietnam, the use of dill in cooking is regional, specifically northern Vietnamese cuisine.

In Iran, dill is known as "Shevid" and is sometimes used with rice and called "Shevid-Polo".

In India, dill is known as "SHEPU" or "SHAPU" in Marathi, 'Savaa' in Hindi or 'Soa' not related to Soy, in Punjabi. In Telugu it is called soya and soya-kura (for herb greens). It is also called 'sapsige soppu' in Kannada. In Tamil it is known as Sada kuppi. In Sanskrit, this herb is called Shatapushpa. In Gujrati it is known as hariz. In India, dill is prepared in the manner of yellow Moong dal as a main-course dish. It is considered to have very good anti-gas properties, and hence it is used as mukhwas, or an after-meal digestive. It is also traditionally given to mothers immediately after childbirth.

In Serbia, dill is known as "Mirodjija" and used in addition to soups and dishes, also in potato salads and French fries.

In Canada, dill is a favourite herb to accompany poached salmon.

In Santa Maria, Azores, dill (Endro) is the most important ingredient of the traditional Holy Ghost soup (Sopas do Espírito Santo). Dill is found practically anywhere in Santa Maria, and curiously rare in the other Azorean Islands.

In Anglo-Saxon England, as prescribed in Leechdoms, Wortcunning, and Starcraft of Early England (also called Læceboc) (many of whose recipes were borrowed from Greek medicinal texts), dill was used in many medicines, including medicines against jaundice, headache, boils, lack of appetite, stomach problems, nausea, liver problems, and much more.

Cultivation

Hardiness Zone:	Not applicable/annual plant
Soil pH:	5.5-6.5 preferred, can tolerate up to 7.5
Soil type:	Well drained rich loose soil
Cultivation:	Started in early spring by seed
Sunlight:	Full sun
Habitat:	Native to the Middle East and Europe

Cultivate dill frequently, lay seed on cotton sheet to dry naturally and store in cotton sacks in a dry place. The leaves of the dill plant are best harvested in the early morning after the dew has dried. They can be used fresh or dried for later use in seasoning food.

When used as a companion planting, dill draws in many beneficial insects as the umbrella flower heads go to seed. Fittingly, it makes a good companion plant for cucumbers. It is a poor companion for carrots and tomatoes.

Historical Notes

Dill is a hardy annual, a native of the Mediterranean region and Southern Russia. It grows wild among the corn in Spain and Portugal and upon the coast of Italy, but rarely occurs as a cornfield weed in Northern Europe.

The plant is referred to in St. Matthew XXiii., 23, though the original Greek name Anethon, was erroneously rendered Anise by English translators, from Wicklif (1380) downwards.

Dill is commonly regarded as the Anethon of Dioscorides. It was well known in Pliny's days and is often mentioned by writers in the Middle Ages. As a drug it has been in use from very early times. It occurs in the tenth-century vocabulary of Alfric, Archbishop of Canterbury.

The name is derived, according to Prior's Popular Names of English Plants, from the old Norse word, dilla (to lull), in allusion to the carminative properties of the drug.

Lyte (Dodoens, 1578) says Dill was sown in all gardens amongst worts and pot-herbs.

In the Middle Ages, Dill was also one of the herbs used by magicians in their spells, and charms against witchcraft.

In Drayton's Nymphidia are the lines:

'Therewith her Vervain and her Dill,

That hindereth Witches of their Will.'

Culpepper tells us that:

'Mercury has the dominion of this plant, and therefore to be sure it strengthens the brain.... It stays the hiccough, being boiled in wine, and but smelled unto being tied in a cloth. The seed is of more use than the leaves, and more effectual to digest raw and vicious humours, and is used in medicines that serve to expel wind, and the pains proceeding therefrom....'

The plant grows ordinarily from 2 to 2 1/2 feet high and is very like fennel, though smaller, having the same feathery leaves, which stand on sheathing foot-stalks, with linear and pointed leaflets. Unlike fennel, however, it has seldom more than one stalk and its long, spindle-shaped root is only annual. It is of very upright growth, its stems smooth, shiny and hollow, and in midsummer bearing flat terminal umbels with numerous yellow flowers, whose small petals are rolled inwards. The flat fruits, the so-called seeds, are produced in great quantities. They are very pungent and bitter in taste and very light, an ounce containing over 25,000 seeds. Their germinating capacity lasts for three years. The whole plant is aromatic.

The plant was placed by Linnaeus in a separate genus, *Anethum*, whence the name Fructus Anethi, by which Dill fruit goes in medicine. It is now included in the genus *Peucedanum*.

Cultivation

This annual is of very easy culture. When grown on a large scale for the sake of its fruits, it may be sown in drills 10 inches apart, in March or April, 10 lb. of the seed being drilled to the acre, and thinned out to leave 8 to 10 inches room each way Sometimes the seed is sown in autumn as soon as ripe, but it is not so advisable as spring sowing. Careful attention must be given to the destruction of weeds. The crop is considered somewhat exhaustive of soil fertility.

Harvesting

Mowing starts as the lower seeds begin, the others ripening on the straw. In dry periods, cutting is best done in early morning or late evening, care being taken to handle with the least possible shaking to prevent loss. The loose sheaves are built into stacks of about twenty sheaves, tied together. In hot weather, threshing may be done in the field, spreading the sheaves on a large canvas sheet and beating out. The average yield is about 7 cwt. of Dill fruits per acre.

The seeds are finally dried by spreading out on trays in the sun, or for a short time over the moderate heat of a stove, shaking occasionally.

Dill fruits are oval, compressed, winged about one-tenth inch wide, with three longitudinal ridges on the back and three dark lines or oil cells (vittae) between them and two on the flat surface. The taste of the fruits somewhat resembles caraway. The seeds are smaller, flatter and lighter than caraway and have a pleasant aromatic odour. They contain a volatile oil (obtained by distillation) on which the action of the fruit depends. The bruised seeds impart their virtues to alcohol and to boiling water.

Constituents

Oil of Dill is of a pale yellow colour, darkening on keeping, with the odour of the fruit and a hot, acrid taste. Its specific gravity varies between 0.895 and 0.915. The fruit yields about 3.5 per cent of the oil, which is a mixture of a paraffin hydrocarbon and 40 to 60 per cent of d-carvone, with d-limonene. Phellandrine is present in the English and Spanish oils, but not to any appreciable extent in the German oil.

In spite of the difference in odour between Dill and Caraway oils, the composition of the two is almost identical, both consisting nearly entirely of limonene and carvone. Dill oil, however, contains less carvone than caraway oil.

English-distilled oils usually have the highest specific gravity, from 0.910 to 0.916, and are consequently held in the highest esteem.

Uses

As a sweet herb, Dill is not much used in this country (UK). When employed, it is for flavouring soups, sauces, etc., for which purpose the young leaves only are required. The leaves added to fish, or mixed with pickled cucumbers give them a spicy taste.

Dill vinegar, however, forms a popular household condiment. It is made by soaking the seeds in vinegar for a few days before using.

The French use Dill seeds for flavouring cakes and pastry, as well as for flavouring sauces.

Perhaps the chief culinary use of Dill seeds is in pickling cucumbers: they are employed in this way chiefly in Germany where pickled cucumbers are largely eaten.

SOME OLD-FASHIONED FENNEL AND DILL RECIPES

Dill and Collyflower Pickle

'*Boil the Collyflowers till they fall inpieces; then with some of the stalk and worst of the flower boil it in a part of the liquer till pretty strong. Then being taken off strain it- and when settled, clean it from the bottom. Then with Dill, gross pepper, a pretty quantity of salt, when cold add as much vinegar as will make it sharp and pour all upon the Collyflower.' (From Acetaria, a book about Sallets, 1680, by John Evelyn.)*

To Pickle Cucumbers in Dill

'*Gather the tops of the ripest dill and cover the bottom of the vessel, and lay a layer of Cucumbers and another of Dill till you have filled the vessel within a handful of the top. Then take as much water as you think will fill the vessel and mix it with salt and a quarter of a pound of allom to a gallon of water and poure it on them and press them down with a stone on them and keep them covered close. For that use I think the water will be best boyl'd and cold, which will keep longer sweet, or if you like not this pickle, doe it with water, salt and white wine vinegar, or (if you please) pour the water and salt on them scalding hot which will make them ready to use the sooner.' (From Receipt Book of Joseph Cooper, Cook to Charles I, 1640.)*

Historical Medicinal Uses - For Entertainment ONLY

Medicinal Action and Uses

Like the other umbelliferous fruits and volatile oils, both Dill fruit and oil of Dill possess stimulant, aromatic, carminative and stomachic properties, making them of considerable medicinal value.

Oil of Dill is used in mixtures, or administered in doses of 5 drops on sugar, but its most common use is in the preparation of Dill Water, which is a common domestic remedy for the flatulence of infants, and is a useful vehicle for children's medicine generally.

Preparations

Dill water, 1 to 8 drachms. Oil, 1 to 5 drops.

Oil of Dill is also employed for perfuming soaps.

The British Pharmacopoeia directs that only the fruits from English-grown plants shall be employed pharmaceutically, and it is grown in East Anglia for that purpose. The Dill fruits of commerce are imported from central and southern Europe, the plant being largely cultivated in Germany and Roumania.

Considerable quantities of Dill fruit are imported from India and Japan - they are the fruits of a species of *Peucedanum* that has been considered by some botanists entitled to rank as a distinct species, P. Sowa (Kurz), but is included by others in the species, *P. graveolens*. Indian dill is widely grown in the Indies under the name of 'Soyah,' its fruit and leaves being used for flavouring pickles. Its fruits are narrower and more convex than European dill, with paler, more distinct ridges and narrower wings.

The oils from both Japanese and Indian dill differ from European dill oil, in having a higher specific gravity (0.948 to 0.968), which is ascribed to the presence of dill apiol, and in containing much less carvone than the European oil. It should not be substituted for the official oil.

African dill oil is produced from plants grown from English imported seed. The fruits are slightly larger than the English fruits and a little paler in colour, their odour closely resembling the English. The yield of oil is slightly larger than that of

English fruits, and it is considered that if the fruits can be produced in Cape Colony, they should form a most useful source of supply.

Elder

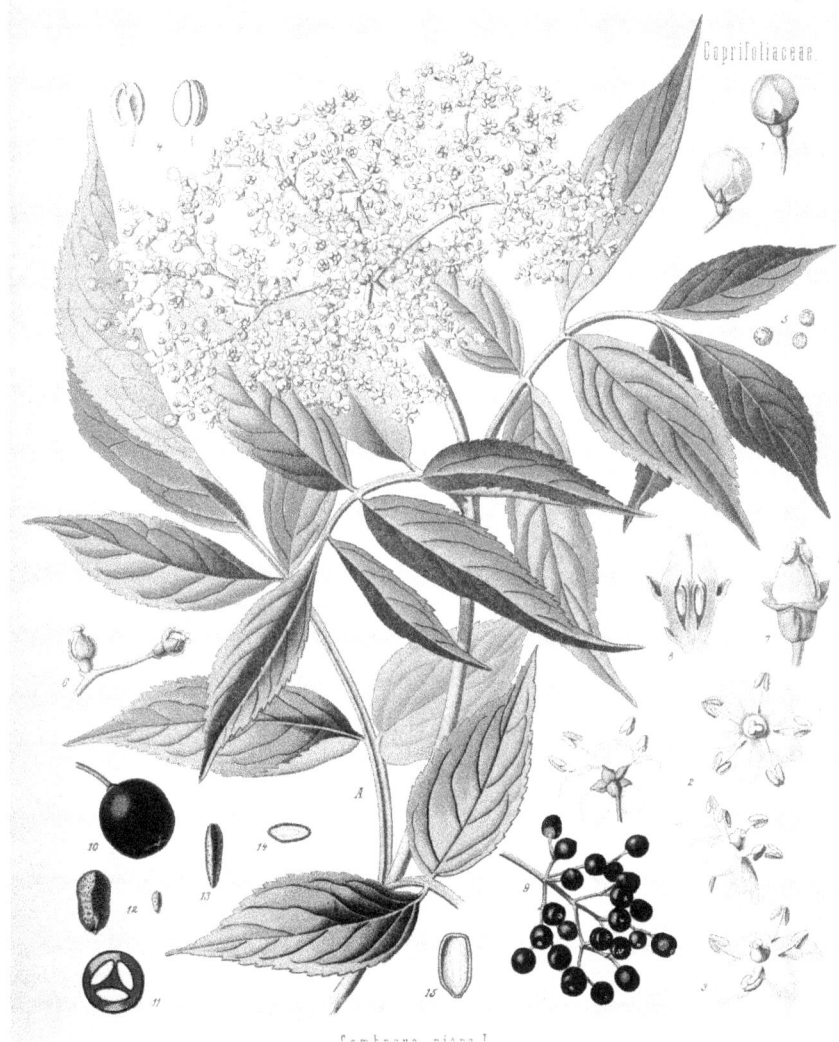

Quick Facts

Latin/Linnaen: *Sambucus nigra*

Family: *Adoxaceae*

Old English :   Ellen

Synonyms: Dwarf Elder, Danewort (different species), Elderberry, Black Elder, European Elder, European Elderberry, European Black Elderberry, Common Elder, or Elder Bush, Pipe Tree, Bore Tree, Bour Tree, (Fourteenth Century) Hylder, Hylantree, (Anglo-Saxon) Eldrum, (Low Saxon) Ellhorn, (German) Hollunder, (French) Sureau.

Action: Diaphoretic, Increase bronchial secretion

Parts Used: Flower

Indicated For: Colds

Dosage: Unless otherwise prescribed: Average daily dosage: 10 -15g drug; 1.5 - 3g fluidextract (according to Erg. B. 6); 2.5 - 7.5g tincture (according to Erg. B. 6); equivalent preparations.

Preparation: Whole herb and other galenical preparations for teas, 1-2 cups of tea sipped several times daily, as hot as possible.

Cautions:

Other Uses: The dark blue/purple berries can be eaten when fully ripe but are mildly poisonous in their unripe state. All green parts of the plant are poisonous, containing cyanogenic glycosides (Vedel & Lange 1960). The berries are edible after cooking and can be used to make jam, jelly, chutney and Pontack sauce. Also when cooked they go well with blackberries and with apples in pies.

The flowerheads are commonly used in infusions, giving a very common refreshing drink in Northern Europe and Balkans. Commercially these are sold as elderflower cordial, etc. In Europe, the flowers are made into a syrup or cordial (in Romanian: Socată, in Swedish: fläder(blom)saft), which is diluted with water before drinking. The popularity of this traditional drink has recently encouraged some commercial soft drink producers to introduce elderflower-flavoured drinks (Fanta Shokata, Freaky Fläder). The flowers can also be dipped into a light batter and then fried to make elderflower fritters. In Scandinavia and Germany, soup made from the elder berry (e.g. the German Fliederbeersuppe) is a traditional meal.

Both flowers and berries can be made into elderberry wine, and in Hungary an elderberry brandy is made that requires 50 kg of fruit to produce 1 litre of brandy. In south-western Sweden, it is traditional to make a snaps liqueur flavored with elderflower. Elderflowers are also used in liqueurs such as St. Germain and a mildly alcoholic sparkling elderflower 'champagne'.

In Beerse, Belgium, a variety of Jenever called Beers Vlierke is made from the berries.

Description

Sambucus nigra is a species complex of elder native to most of Europe.

It is most commonly called Elder, Elderberry, Black Elder, European Elder, European Elderberry, European Black Elderberry, Common Elder, or Elder Bush when distinction from other species of Sambucus is needed. It grows in a variety of conditions including both wet and dry fertile soils, primarily in sunny locations.

It is a deciduous shrub or small tree growing to 4–6 m (rarely to 10 m) tall. The bark, light grey when young, changes to a coarse grey outer bark with lengthwise furrowing. The leaves are arranged in opposite pairs, 10–30 cm long, pinnate with five to seven (rarely nine) leaflets, the leaflets 5–12 cm long and 3–5 cm broad, with a serrated margin.

The hermaphrodite flowers are borne in large corymbs 10–25 cm diameter in mid summer, the individual flowers white, 5–6 mm diameter, with five petals; they are pollinated by flies.

The fruit is a dark purple to black berry 3–5 mm diameter, produced in drooping clusters in the late autumn; they are an important food for many fruit-eating birds, notably Blackcaps.

This plant is traditionally used as a medicinal plant by many native peoples and herbalists alike.

Stembark, leaves, flowers, fruits, root extracts are used to treat bronchitis, cough, upper respiratory cold infections, fever. A small double blind clinical trial published in 2004 showed reduction in both duration and severity of flu-like symptoms for patients receiving elderberry syrup versus placebo.

In a placebo-controlled, double-blind study, black elderberry (*Sambucus nigra*) was shown to be effective for treating Influenza B. People using the elderberry extract recovered much faster than those only on a placebo. The study was published in the Journal of Alternative Complementary Medicine.

A small study published in 2004 showed that 93% of flu patients given extract were completely symptom-free within two days; those taking a placebo recovered in about six days. This current study shows that, indeed, it works for type A flu, reports lead researcher Erling Thom, with the University of Oslo in Norway. However, the study that showed these results was sponsored by an Israeli company that produces various black elderberry extracts.

Elderberry flowers are sold in Ukrainian and Russian drugstores for relief of congestion, specifically as an expectorant to relieve dry cough and make it productive. The dried flowers are simmered for 15 minutes; the resulting flavorful and aromatic tea is poured through a coffee filter. Some individuals find it better hot, others cold, and some may experience an allergic reaction.

The flowers can be used to make an herbal tea as a remedy for inflammation caused by colds and fever.

Cultivation

Hardiness Zone:	4-10
Soil pH:	5.5-6.5, tolerant of a wider range
Soil type:	Fertile moist soil, tolerant to some standing water.
Cultivation:	Hard or softwood cuttings, root cuttings or suckers.
Sunlight:	Full sun to part sun
Habitat:	Native to Europe, grows in ditches, grasslands and near water.

Historical Notes

The Elder, with its flat-topped masses of creamy-white, fragrant blossoms, followed by large drooping bunches of purplish-black, juicy berries, is a familiar object in English countryside and gardens. It has been said, with some truth, that English summer is not here until the Elder is fully in flower, and that it ends when the berries are ripe.

The word 'Elder' comes from the Anglo-Saxon word aeld. In Anglo-Saxon days we find the tree called Eldrun, which becomes Hyldor and Hyllantree in the fourteenth century. One of its names in modern German - Hollunder - is clearly derived from the same origin. In Low-Saxon, the name appears as Ellhorn. Æld meant 'fire,' the hollow stems of the young branches having been used for blowing up a fire: the soft pith pushes out easily and the tubes thus formed were used as pipes - hence it was often called Pipe-Tree, or Bore-tree and Bour-tree, the latter name remaining in Scotland and being traceable to the Anglo-Saxon form, Burtre.

The generic name Sambucus occurs in the writings of Pliny and other ancient writers and is evidently adapted from the Greek word Sambuca, the Sackbut, an ancient musical instrument in much use among the Romans, in the construction of which, it is surmised, the wood of this tree, on account of its hardness, was used. The difficulty, however, of accepting this is that the Sambuca was a stringed instrument, while anything made from the Elder would doubtless be a wind instrument, something of the nature of a Pan-pipe or flute. Pliny records the belief held by country folk that the shrillest pipes and the most sonorous horns were made of Elder trees which were grown out of reach of the sound of cock-crow. At the present day, Italian peasants construct a simple pipe, which they call sampogna, from the branches of this plant.

The popular pop-gun of small boys in the country has often been made of Elder stems from which the pith has been removed, which moved Culpepper to declare: 'It is needless to write any description of this (Elder), since every boy that plays with a pop-gun will not mistake another tree for the Elder.' Pliny's writings also testify that pop-guns and whistles are manufactures (products) many centuries old!

A wealth of folk-lore, romance and superstition centre round this English tree. Shakespeare, in Cymbeline, referring to it as a symbol of grief, speaks slightingly of it as 'the stinking Elder,' yet, although many people profess a strong dislike to the scent of its blossom, the shrub is generally beloved by all who see it. In countrysides where the Elder flourishes it is certainly one of the most attractive features of the hedgerow, while its old-world associations have created for it a place in the hearts of English people.

In Love's Labour Lost reference is made to the common medieval belief that 'Judas was hanged on an Elder.' We meet with this tradition as far back in English literature as Langland's Vision of Piers Plowman (middle of the fourteenth century, before Chaucer):

'Judas he japed with Jewen silver

And sithen an eller hanged hymselve.'

Why the Elder should have been selected as a gallows for the traitor Apostle is, considering the usual size of the tree, puzzling; but Sir John Mandeville in his travels, written about the same time, tells us that he was shown 'faste by' the Pool of Siloam, the identical 'Tree of Eldre that Judas henge himself upon, for despeyr that he hadde, when he solde and betrayed oure Lord.' Gerard scouts the tradition and says that the Judas-tree (Cercis siliquastrum) is 'the tree whereon Judas did hange himselfe.'

Another old tradition was that the Cross of Calvary was made of it, and an old couplet runs:

'Bour tree - Bour tree: crooked rong

Never straight and never strong;

Ever bush and never tree

Since our Lord was nailed on thee.'

In consequence of these old traditions, the Elder became the emblem of sorrow and death, and out of the legends which linger round the tree there grew up a host of superstitious fancies which still remain in the minds of simple country folk. Even in these prosaic days, one sometimes comes across a hedge-cutter who cannot bring himself to molest the rampant growth of its spreading branches for fear of being pursued by ill-luck. An old custom among gypsies forbade them using the wood to kindle their camp fires and gleaners of firewood formerly would look carefully through the faggots lest a stick of Elder should have found its way into the bundle, perhaps because the Holy Cross was believed to have been fashioned out of a giant elder tree, though probably the superstitious awe of harming the Elder descended from old heathen myths of northern Europe. In most countries, especially in Denmark, the Elder was intimately connected with magic. In its branches was supposed to dwell a dryad, Hylde-Moer, the Elder-tree Mother, who lived in the tree and watched over it. Should the tree be cut down and furniture be made of the wood, Hylde-Moer was believed to follow her property and haunt the owners. Lady Northcote, in The Book of Herbs, relates:

'There is a tradition that once when a child was put in a cradle of Elder-wood, HyldeMoer came and pulled it by the legs and would give it no peace till it was lifted out Permission to cut Elder wood must always be asked first and not until Hylde-Moer has given consent by keeping silence, may the chopping begin.'

Arnkiel relates:

'Our forefathers also held the Ellhorn holy wherefore whoever need to hew it down (or cut its branches) has first to make request "Lady Ellhorn, give me some of thy wood and I will give thee some of mine when it grows in the forest" - the which, with partly bended knees, bare head and folded arms was ordinarily done, as I myself have often seen and heard in my younger years.'

Mr. Jones (quoted in The Treasury of Botany), in his Notes on Certain Superstitions in the Vale of Gloucester, cites the following, said to be no unusual case:

'Some men were employed in removing an old hedgerow, partially formed of Eldertrees. They had bound up all the other wood into faggots for burning, but had set apart the elder and enquired of their master how it was to be disposed of. Upon his saying that he should of course burn it with the rest, one of the men said with an air of undisguised alarm, that he had never heard of such a thing as burning Ellan Wood, and in fact, so strongly did he feel upon the subject, that he refused to participate in the act of tying it up. The word Ellan (still common with us) indicates the origin of the superstition.'

In earlier days, the Elder Tree was supposed to ward off evil influence and give protection from witches, a popular belief held in widely-distant countries. **Lady Northcote says**:

'The Russians believe that Elder-trees drive away evil spirits, and the Bohemians go to it with a spell to take away fever. The Sicilians think that sticks of its wood will kill serpents and drive away robbers, and the Serbs introduce a stick of Elder into their wedding ceremonies to bring good luck. In England it was thought that the Elder was never struck by lightning, and a twig of it tied into three or four knots and carried in the pocket was a charm against rheumatism. A cross made of Elder and fastened to cowhouses and stables was supposed to keep all evil from the animals.'

In Cole's Art of Simpling (1656) we may read how in the later part of the seventeenth century:

'in order to prevent witches from entering their houses, the common people used to gather Elder leaves on the last day of April and affix them to their doors and windows,'

and the tree was formerly much cultivated near English cottages for protection against witches .

The use of the Elder for funeral purposes was an old English custom referred to by Spenser,

'The Muses that were wont green Baies to weave,

Now bringen bittre Eldre braunches seare.'

- Shepheard's Calendar - November.

And Canon Ellacombe says that in the Tyrol:

'An Elder bush, trimmed into the form of a cross, is planted on a new-made grave, and if it blossoms, the soul of the person lying beneath it is happy.'

Green Elder branches were also buried in a grave to protect the dead from witches and evil spirits, and in some parts it was a custom for the driver of the hearse to carry a whip made of Elder wood.

In some of the rural Midlands, it is believed that if a child is chastised with an Elder switch, it will cease to grow, owing, in this instance, to some supposed malign influence of the tree. On the other hand, Lord Bacon commended the rubbing of warts with a green Elder stick and then burying the stick to rot in the mud, and for erysipelas, it was recommended to wear about the neck an amulet made of Elder 'on which the sun had never shined.'

In Denmark we come across the old belief that he who stood under an Elder tree on Midsummer Eve would see the King of Fairyland ride by, attended by all his retinue. Folkard, in Plant-Lore, Legends and Lyrics, relates:

'The pith of the branches when cut in round, flat shapes, is dipped in oil, lighted, and then put to float in a glass of water; its light on Christmas Eve is thought to reveal to the owner all the witches and sorcerers in the neighbourhood'; and again,

'On Bertha Night (6th January), the devil goes about with special virulence. As a safeguard, persons are recommended to make a magic circle, in the centre of which they should stand, with Elderberries gathered on St. John's night. By doing this, the mystic Fern-seed may be obtained, which possesses the strength of thirty or forty men.'

This is a Styrian tradition.

The whole tree has a narcotic smell, and it is not considered wise to sleep under its shade. Perhaps the visions of fairyland were the result of the drugged sleep! No plant will grow under the shadow of it, being affected by its exhalations.

Apart from all these traditions, the Elder has had from the earliest days a firm claim on the popular affection for its many sterling virtues.

Its uses are manifold and important. The wood of old trees is white and of a fine, close grain, easily cut, and polishes well, hence it was used for making skewers for butchers, shoemakers' pegs, and various turned articles, such as tops for angling rods and needles for weaving nets, also for making combs, mathematical instruments and several different musical instruments, and the pith of the younger stems, which is exceedingly light, is cut into balls and is used for electrical experiments and for making small toys. It is also considerably used for holding small objects for sectioning for microscopical purposes.

In a cutting of Worlidge's Mystery of Husbandry (dated 1675) the Elder is included in the 'trees necessary and proper for fencing and enclosing of Lands.'

'A considerable Fence,' he writes, 'may be made of Elder, set of reasonable hasty Truncheons, like the Willow and may be laid with great curiosity: this makes a speedy shelter for a garden from Winds, Beasts and suchlike injuries,' though he adds and emphasizes with italics, 'rather than from rude Michers.'

The word 'micher' is now obsolete, but it means a lurking thief, a skulking vagabond. By clipping two or three times a year, an Elder hedge may, however, be made close and compact in growth. There is an old tradition that an Elder stake will last in the ground longer than an iron bar of the same size, hence the old couplet:

'An eldern stake and a black thorn ether (hedge)

Will make a hedge to last for ever.'

The leaves have an unpleasant odour when bruised, which is supposed to be offensive to most insects, and a decoction of the young leaves is sometimes employed by gardeners to sprinkle over delicate plants and the buds of the flowers to keep off the attacks of aphis and minute caterpillars. Moths are fond of the blossoms, but it was stated by Christopher Gullet (Phil. Trans., 1772, LXII) that if turnips, cabbages, fruit trees or corn be whipped with bunches of the green leaves, they gain immunity from blight. Though this does not sound a very practical procedure, there is evidently some foundation for this statement, as the following note which appeared in the Chemist and Druggist, January 6, 1923, would seem to prove:

'A liquid preparation for preventing, and also curing, blight in fruit trees, wherein the base is a liquid obtained by boiling the young shoots of the Elder tree or bush, mixed with suitable proportions of copper sulphate, iron sulphate, nicotine, soft soap, methylated spirit and slaked lime.'

The leaves, bruised, if worn in the hat or rubbed on the face, prevent flies settling on the person. In order to safeguard the skin from the attacks of mosquitoes, midges and other troublesome flies, an infusion of the leaves may be dabbed on with advantage. Gather a few fresh leaves from the elder, tear them from their stalks and place them in a jug, pouring boiling water on them and covering them at once, leaving for a few hours. When the infusion is cold, it is fit for use and should be at once poured off into a bottle and kept tightly corked. It is desirable to make a fresh infusion often. The leaves are said to be valued by the farmer for driving mice away from granaries and moles from their usual haunts.

The bark of the older branches has been used in the Scotch Highlands as an ingredient in dyeing black, also the root. The leaves yield, with alum, a green dye and the berries dye blue and purple, the Juice yielding with alum, violet; with alum and salt, a lilac colour.

The botanist finds in this plant an object of considerable interest, for if a twig is partially cut, then cautiously broken and the divided portions are carefully drawn asunder, the spiral air-vessels, resembling a screw, may be distinctly seen.

Linnaeus observed that sheep eat the leaves, also cows, but that horses and goats refuse it. If sheep that have the foot-rot can get at the bark and young shoots, they will cure themselves. Elderberries are eaten greedily by young birds and pigeons, but are said to have serious effects on chickens: the flowers are reported to be fatal to turkeys, and according to Linnaeus, also to peacocks.

Elder Flowers and Elder Berries have long been used in the English countryside for making many home-made drinks and preserves that are almost as great favourites now as in the time of our great-grandmothers. The berries make an excellent home-made wine and winter cordial, which improves with age, and taken hot with sugar, just before going to bed, is an old-fashioned and well established cure for a cold.

In Kent, there are entire orchards of Elder trees cultivated solely for the sake of their fruit, which is brought regularly to market and sold for the purpose of making wine. The berries are not only used legitimately for making Elderberry Wine, but largely in the manufacture of so-called British wines - they give a red colour to raisin wine - and in the adulteration of foreign wines. Judiciously flavoured with vinegar and sugar and small quantities of port wine, Elder is often the basis of spurious 'clarets' and 'Bordeaux.' 'Men of nice palates,' says Berkeley (Querist, 1735), 'have been imposed on by Elder Wine for French Claret.' Cheap port is often faked to resemble tawny port by the addition of Elderberry juice, which forms one of the least injurious ingredients of factitious port wines. Doctoring port wine with Elderberry juice seems to have assumed such dimensions that in 1747 this practice was forbidden in Portugal, even the cultivation of the Elder tree was forbidden on this account. The practice proving so lucrative, however, is by no means obsolete, but as the berries possess valuable medicinal properties, this adulteration has no harmful results. The circumstances under which this was proved are somewhat curious. In 1899 an American sailor informed a physician of Prague that getting drunk on genuine, old, dark-red port was a sure remedy for rheumatic pains. This unedifying observation started a long series of investigations ending in the discovery that while genuine port wine has practically no anti-neuralgic properties, the cheap stuff faked to resemble tawny port by the addition of elderberry juice often banishes the pain of sciatica and other forms of neuralgia, though of no avail in genuine neuritis. Cases of cure have been instanced after many tests carried out by leading doctors in Prague and other centres abroad, the dose recommended being 30 grams of Elderberry juice mixed with 10 grams of port wine.

The Romans, as Pliny records, made use of it in medicine, as well as of the Dwarf Elder (*Sambucus Ebulus*). Both kinds were employed in Britain by the ancient English and Welsh leeches and in Italy in the medicine of the School of Salernum. Elder still keeps its place in the British Pharmacopoeia, the cooling effects of Elder flowers being well known. In many parts of the country, Elder leaves and buds are used in drinks, poultices and ointments.

It has been termed 'the medicine chest of the country people' (Ettmueller) and 'a whole magazine of physic to rustic practitioners,' and it is said the great physician Boerhaave never passed an Elder without raising his hat, so great an opinion had he of its curative properties. How great was the popular estimation of it in Shakespeare's time may be gauged by the line in the Merry Wives of Windsor, Act II, Sc. 3:

'What says my Æsculapius? my Galen? my heart of Elder?'

John Evelyn, writing in praise of the Elder, says:

'If the medicinal properties of its leaves, bark and berries were fully known, I cannot tell what our countryman could ail for which he might not fetch a remedy from every hedge, either for sickness, or wounds.'

'The buds boiled in water gruel have effected wonders in a fever, the spring buds are excellently wholesome in pattages; and small ale in which Elder flowers have been infused is esteemed by many so salubrious that this is to be had in most of the eatinghouses about our town.'

He also, as we have seen, recommends Elder flowers infused in vinegar as an ingredient of a salad, 'though the leaves are somewhat rank of smell and so not commendable in sallet they are of the most sovereign virtue,' and goes so far as to say, 'an extract composed of the berries greatly assists longevity. Indeed this is a catholicum against all infirmities whatever.'

Some twenty years before Evelyn's eulogy there had appeared in 1644 a book entirely devoted to its praise: The Anatomie of the Elder, translated from the Latin of Dr. Martin Blockwich by C. de Iryngio (who seems to have been an army doctor), a treatise of some 230 pages, that in Latin and English went through several editions. It deals very learnedly with the medicinal virtues of the tree - its flowers, berries, leaves, 'middle bark,' pith, roots and 'Jew's ears,' a large fungus often to be found on the Elder (*Hirneola auricula Judae*), the name a corruption of 'Judas's ear,' from the tradition, referred to above, that Judas hanged himself on the Elder. It is of a purplish tint, resembling in shape and softness the human ear, and though it occurs also on the Elm, it grows almost exclusively on Elder trunks in damp, shady places. It is curious that on account of this connexion with Judas, the fungus should have (as Sir Thomas Browne says) 'become a famous medicine in quinses, sore-throats, and strangulation ever since.' Gerard says, 'the jelly of the Elder otherwise called Jew's ear, taketh away inflammations of the mouth and throat if they be washed therewith and doth in like manner help the uvula,' and Salmon, writing in the early part of the eighteenth century, recommends an oil of Jew's ears for throat affections. The fungus is edible and allied species are eaten in China.

Evelyn refers to this work (or rather to the original by 'Blockwitzius,' as he calls him!) for the comprehensive statement in praise of the Elder quoted above. It sets forth that as every part of the tree was medicinal, so virtually every ailment of the body was curable by it, from toothache to the plague. It was used externally and internally, and in amulets (these were especially good for epilepsy, and in popular belief also for rheumatism), and in every kind of form - in rob and syrup, tincture, mixture, oil, spirit, water, liniment, extract, salt, conserve, vinegar, oxymel, sugar, decoction, bath, cataplasm and powder. Some of these were prepared from one part of the plant only, others from several or from all. Their properties are summed up as 'desiccating, conglutinating, and digesting,' but are extended to include everything necessary to a universal remedy. The book prescribes in more or less detail for some seventy or more distinct diseases or classes of diseases, and the writer is never at a loss for an authority - from Dioscorides to the Pharmacopoeias of his own day-while the examples of cures he adduces are drawn from all classes of people, from Emylia, Countess of Isinburg, to the tradesmen of Heyna and their dependants.

The interest in the Elder evinced about this period is also demonstrated by a tract on 'Elder and Juniper Berries, showing how useful they may be in our Coffee Houses,' which was published with The Natural History of Coffee, in 1682.

SOME ELDER WINE RECIPES

An old recipe for Elder Wine

'To every quart of berries put 2 quarts of water; boil half an hour, run the liquor and break the fruit through a hair sieve; then to every quart of juice, put 3/4 of a pound of Lisbon sugar, coarse, but not the very coarsest. Boil the whole a quarter of an hour with some Jamaica peppers, ginger, and a few cloves. Pour it into a tub, and when of a proper warmth, into the barrel, with toast and yeast to work, which there is more difficulty to make it do than most other liquors. When it ceases to hiss, put a quart of brandy to eight gallons and stop up. Bottle in the spring, or at Christmas. The liquor must be in a warm place to make it work.'

The following recipe for making Elder Wine is given by Mrs. Hewlett in a work entitled Cottage Comforts:

'If two gallons of wine are to be made, get one gallon of Elderberries, and a quart of damsons, or sloes; boil them together in six quarts of water, for half an hour, breaking the fruit with a stick, flat at one end; run off the liquor, and squeeze the pulp through a sieve, or straining cloth; boil the liquor up again with six pounds of coarse sugar, two ounces of ginger, two ounces of bruised allspice, and one ounce of hops; (the spice had better be loosely tied in a bit of muslin); let this boil above half an hour; then pour it off, when quite cool, stir in a teacupful of yeast, and cover it up to work. After two days, skim off the yeast, and put the wine into the barrel, and when it ceases to hiss, which will be in about a fortnight, paste a stiff brown paper over the bung-hole. After this, it will be fit for use in about 8 weeks, but will keep 8 years, if required. The bag of spice may be dropped in at the bung-hole, having a string fastened outside, which shall keep it from reaching the bottom of the barrel.'

Another Recipe

'Strip the berries, which must be quite ripe, into a dry pan and pour 2 gallons of boiling water over 3 gallons of berries. Cover and leave in a warm place for 24 hours; then strain, pressing the juice well out. Measure it and allow 3 pounds of sugar, half an ounce of ginger and 1/4 ounce of cloves to each gallon. Boil for 20 minutes slowly, then strain it into a cask and ferment when lukewarm. Let it remain until still, before bunging, and bottle in six months.

'If a weaker wine is preferred, use 4 gallons of water to 3 gallons of berries and leave for two days before straining.

'If a cask be not available, large stone jars will answer: then the wine need not be bottled.'

Parkinson tells us that fresh Elder Flowers hung in a vessel of new wine and pressed every evening for seven nights together, *'giveth to the wine a very good relish and a smell like Muscadine.'* Ale was also infused with Elder flowers.

The berries make good pies, if blended with spices, and formerly used to be preserved with spice and kept for winter use in pies when fruit was scarce. Quite a delicious jam can also be made of them, mixed with apples, which has much the flavour of Blackberry jam. They mix to very great advantage with Crab Apple, or with the hard Catillac cooking Pear, or with Vegetable Marrow, and also with Blackberries or Rhubarb.

The Fruit Preserving Section of the Food Ministry issued during the War (WWI) the following recipe for Elderberry and Apple Jam: 6 lb. Elderberries, 6 lb. sliced apples, 12 lb. sugar. Make a pulp of the apples by boiling in water till soft and passing through a coarse sieve to remove any seeds or cores. The Elderberries should also be stewed for half an hour to soften them. Combine the Apple pulp, berries and sugar and return to the fire to boil till thick.

Another Recipe

Equal quantities of Elderberries and Apples, 3/4 lb. sugar and one lemon to each pound of fruit. Strip the berries from the stalks, peel, core and cut up the apples and weigh both fruits. Put the Elderberries into a pan over low heat and bruise them with a wooden spoon. When the juice begins to flow, add the Apples and one-third of the sugar and bring slowly to the boil. When quite soft, rub all through a hair sieve. Return the pulp to the pan, add the rest of the sugar, the grated lemon rind and juice and boil for half an hour, or until the jam sets when tested. Remove all scum, put into pots and cover.

Elderberry Jam without Apples

To every pound of berries add 1/4 pint of water, the juice of 2 lemons and 1 lb. of sugar. Boil from 30 to 45 minutes, until it sets when tested. Put into jars and tie down when cold.

The Elderberry will, of course, also make a jelly. As it is a juicy fruit, it will not need the addition of any more liquid than, perhaps, a squeeze of lemon. Equal quantities of Elderberry juice and apple juice, and apple juice from peeling, will require 3/4 lb. of sugar to a pint. Elderberry Jelly is firm and flavorous, with a racy tang.

When the fruit is not quite ripe, it may be preserved in brine and used as a substitute for capers.

The juice from Elder Berries, too, was formerly distilled and mixed with vinegar for salad dressings and flavouring sauces. Vinegars used in former times frequently to be aromatized by steeping in them barberries, rosemary, rose leaves, gilliflowers, lavender, violets - in short, any scented flower or plant though tarragon is now practically the only herb used in this manner to any large extent. **Elderflower Vinegar** is made thus:

Take 2 lb. of dried flowers of Elder. If you use your own flowers, pluck carefully their stalks from them and dry them carefully and thoroughly. This done, place in a large vessel and pour over them 2 pints of good vinegar. Close the vessel hermetically, keep it in a very warm place and shake them from time to time. After 8 days, strain the vinegar through a paper filter. Keep in well-stoppered bottles.

This is an old-world simple, but rarely met with nowadays, but worth the slight trouble of making. It was well-known and appreciated in former days and often mentioned in old books; Steele, in The Tatler, says: 'They had dissented about the preference of Elder to Wine vinegar.'

One seldom has the chance of now tasting the old country pickle made from the tender young shoots and flowers. John Evelyn, writing in 1664, recommends Elder flowers infused in vinegar as an ingredient of a salad. The pickled blossoms are said by those who have tried them to be a welcome relish with boiled mutton, as a substitute for capers. Clusters of the flowers are gathered in their unripened green state, put into a stone jar and covered with boiling vinegar. Spices are unnecessary. The jar is tied down directly the pickle is cold. This pickle is very good and has the advantage of costing next to nothing.

The pickle made from the tender young shoots - sometimes known as 'English Bamboo' - is more elaborate. During May, in the middle of the Elder bushes in the hedges, large young green shoots may be observed. Cut these, selecting the greenest, peel off every vestige of the outer skin and lay them in salt and water overnight. Each individual length must be carefully chosen, for while they must not be too immature, if the shoots are at all woody, they will not be worth eating, The following morning, prepare the pickle for the Mock Bamboo. To a quart of vinegar, add an ounce of white pepper, an ounce of ginger, half a saltspoonful of mace and boil all well together. Remove the Elder shoots from the salt and water, dry in a cloth and slice up into suitable pieces, laying them in a stone jar. Pour the boiling mixture over them and either place them in an oven for 2 hours, or in a pan of boiling water on the stove. When cold, the pickle should be green in colour. If not, strain the liquor, boil it up again, pour over the shoots and repeat the process. The great art of obtaining and retaining the essence of the plant lies in excluding air from the tied-down jar as much as possible.

The young shoots can also be boiled in salted water with a pinch of soda to preserve the colour, they prove beautifully tender, resembling spinach, and form quite a welcome addition to the dinner table.

Good use can be made of the berries for Ketchup and Chutney, and the following recipes will be found excellent.

Elderberry Chutney

2 lb. Elderberries, 1 large Onion, 1 pint vinegar, 1 teaspoonful salt, 1 teaspoonful ground ginger, 2 tablespoonsful sugar, 1 saltspoonful cayenne and mixed spices, 1 teaspoonful mustard seed.

Stalk, weigh and wash the berries; put them into a pan and bruise with a wooden spoon; chop the onion and add with the rest of the ingredients and vinegar. Bring to the boil and simmer till it becomes thick. Stir well, being careful not to let it burn as it thickens. Put into jars and cover.

Another Recipe

Rub 1 1/2 lb. of berries through a wire sieve, pound 1 onion, 6 cloves, 1/4 oz. ground ginger, 2 oz. Demerara sugar, 3 oz. stoned raisins, a dust of cayenne and mace, 1 teaspoonful salt and 1 pint vinegar. Put all in an enamelled saucepan and boil with the pulp of the berries for 10 minutes. Take the pan from the fire and let it stand till cold. Put the chutney into jars and cork securely.

Elderberry Ketchup

1 pint Elderberries, 1 oz. shallots, 1 blade mace, 1/2 oz. peppercorns, 1 1/2 oz. whole ginger, 1 pint vinegar.

Pick the berries (which must be ripe) from the stalks, weigh and wash them. Put them into an unglazed crock or jar, pour over the boiling vinegar and leave all night in a cool oven. Next day, strain the liquor from the berries through a cloth tied on to the legs of an inverted chair and put it into a pan, with the peeled and minced shallots, the ginger peeled and cut up small, the mace and peppercorns. Boil for 10 minutes, then put into bottles, dividing the spices among the bottles. Cork well.

All parts of the tree - bark, leaves, flowers and berries - have long enjoyed a high reputation in domestic medicine. From the days of Hippocrates, it has been famous for its medicinal properties.

Historical Medicinal Uses - For Entertainment ONLY

Parts Used Medicinally: The bark, leaves, flowers and berries.

Bark: The Inner Bark should be collected in autumn, from young trees. It is best dried in a moderate sun-heat, being taken indoors at night. When ready for use, it is a light grey, soft and corky externally, with broad fissures; white and smooth on the inner surface. The taste of the bark is sweetish at first, then slightly bitter and nauseous. It is without odour.

Chemical Constituents: The active principle of the bark is a soft resin, and Viburnic acid, which has been proved identical with Valeric acid. Other constituents are traces of a volatile oil, albumen, resin, fat, wax, chlorophyll, tannic acid, grape sugar, gum, extractive, starch, pectin and various alkaline and earthy salts. (According to an analysis by Kramer in 1881.)

Medicinal Action and Uses: The bark is a strong purgative which may be employed with advantage, an infusion of 1 oz. in a pint of water being taken in wineglassful doses; in large doses it is an emetic. Its use as a purgative dates back to Hippocrates. It has been much employed as a diuretic, an aqueous solution having been found very useful in cardiac and renal dropsies. It has also been successfully employed in epilepsy.

An emollient ointment is made of the green inner bark, and a homoeopathic tincture made from the fresh inner bark of the young branches, in diluted form, relieves asthmatic symptoms and spurious croup of children - dose, 4 or 5 drops in water.

Culpepper states:

'The first shoots of the common Elder, boiled like Asparagus, and the young leaves and stalks boiled in fat broth, doth mightily carry forth phlegm and choler. The middle or inward bark boiled in water and given in drink wortheth much more violently; and the berries, either green or dry, expel the same humour, and are often given with good success in dropsy; the bark of the root boiled in wine, or the juice thereof drunk, worketh the same effects, but more powerfully than either the leaves or fruit. The juice of the root taken, causes vomitings and purgeth the watery humours of the dropsy.'

Though the use of the root is now obsolete, its juice was used from very ancient times to promote both vomiting and purging, and taken, as another old writer recommends, in doses of 1 to 2 tablespoonsful, fasting, once in the week, was held to be 'the most excellent purge of water humours in the world and very singular against dropsy.' A tea was also made from the roots of Elder, which was considered an effective preventative for incipient dropsy, in fact the very best remedy for such cases.

Leaves: Elder leaves are used both fresh and dry.

Collect the leaves in June and July. Gather only in fine weather, in the morning, after the dew has been dried by the sun. Strip the leaves off singly, rejecting any that are stained or insect-eaten. Drying is then done in the usual manner.

Constituents: Elder leaves contain an alkaloid Sambucine, a purgative resin and the glucoside Sambunigrin, which crystallizes in white, felted needles. Fresh Elder leaves yield about 0.16 per cent of hydrocyanic acid. They also contain cane sugar, invertin, a considerable quantity of potassium nitrate and a crystalline substance, Eldrin, which has also been found in other white flowering plants.

De Sanctis claims to have isolated the alkaloid Coniine from the branches and leaves of *Sambucus nigra*. Alpes (Proc. Amer. Pharm. Assoc., 1900) found undoubted evidence of an alkaloid in the roots of the American Elder (*S. Canadensis*), its odour being somewhat similar to that of coniine and also suggesting nicotine. This alkaloid was evidently volatile. It appeared to be much less abundant in the dried roots after some months keeping. The fresh root of *S. Canadensis* has been found extremely poisonous, producing death in children within a short time after being eaten with symptoms very similar to those of poisoning by Hemlock (Conium).

Elder leaves are used in the preparation of an ointment, *Unguentum Sambuci Viride*, Green Elder Ointment, which is a domestic remedy for bruises, sprains, chilblains, for use as an emollient, and for applying to wounds. It can be compounded as follows: Take 3 parts of fresh Elder leaves, 4 parts of lard and 2 of prepared suet, heat the Elder leaves with the melted lard and suet until the colour is extracted, then strain through a linen cloth with pressure and allow to cool.

Sir Thomas Browne (1655) stated: 'The common people keep as a good secret in curing wounds the leaves of the Elder, which they have gathered the last day of April.' The leaves, boiled soft with a little linseed oil, were used as a healing application to piles. An ointment concocted from the green Elderberries, with camphor and lard, was formerly ordered by the London College of Surgeons to relieve the same complaint. The leaves are an ingredient of many cooling ointments: Here is another recipe, not made from Elder leaves alone, and very much recommended by modern herbalists as being very cooling and softening and excellent for all kinds of tumours, swellings and wounds: Take the Elder leaves 1/2 lb., Plantain leaves 1/4 lb., Ground Ivy 2 oz., Wormwood 4 oz. (all green); cut them small, and boil in 4 lb. of lard, in the oven, or over a slow fire; stir them continually until the leaves become crisp, then strain, and press out the ointment for use.

Oil of Elder Leaves (*Oleum Viride*), Green Oil, or Oil of Swallows, is prepared by digesting 1 part of bruised fresh Elder leaves in 3 parts of linseed oil. In commerce, it is said to be generally coloured with verdigris.

Like the bark, the leaves are also purgative, but more nauseous than the bark. Their action is likewise expectorant, diuretic and diaphoretic. They are said to be very efficacious in dropsy. The juice of Elder leaves is stated by the old herbalists to be good for inflammation of the eyes, and 'snuffed up the nostrils,' Culpepper declares, 'purgeth the brain.' Another old notion was that if the green leaves were warmed between two hot tiles and applied to the forehead, they would promptly relieve nervous headache.

The use of the leaves, bruised and in decoction to drive away flies and kill aphides and other insect pests has already been referred to.

Flowers: Elder Flowers are chiefly used in pharmacy in the fresh state for the distillation of Elder Flower Water, but as the flowering season only lasts for about three weeks in June, the flowers are often salted, so as to be available for distillation at a later season, 10 per cent of common salt being added, the flowers being them termed 'pickled.' They are also dried, for making infusions.

The flowers are collected when just in full bloom and thrown into heaps, and after a few hours, during which they become slightly heated the corollas become loosened and can then be removed by sifting. The Elder 'flowers' of pharmacy consist of the small white wheel-shaped, five-lobed, monopetalous corollas only, in the short tube of which the five stamens with very short filaments and yellow anthers are inserted. When fresh, the flowers have a slightly bitter taste and an odour scarcely pleasant. The pickled flowers, however, gradually acquire an agreeable fragrance and are therefore generally used for the preparation of Elder Flower Water. A similar change also takes place in the water distilled from the fresh flowers.

In domestic herbal medicines, the dried flowers are largely used in country districts and are sold by herbalists either in dried bunches of flowers, or sifted free from flower stalks. The flowers are not easily dried of good colour. If left too late exposed to the sun before gathering, the flowers assume a brownish colour when dried, and if the flower bunches are left too long in heaps, to cause the flowers to fall off, these heaps turn black. If the inflorescence is only partly open when gathered, the flower-heads have to be sifted more than once, as the flowers do not open all at the same time. The best and lightest coloured flowers are obtained at the first sifting, when the flowers that have matured and fallen naturally are free from stalks, and dried quickly in a heated atmosphere. They may be very quickly dried in a heated copper pan, being stirred about for a few minutes. They can also be dried almost as quickly in a cool oven, with the door open. Quickness in drying is essential.

The dried flowers, which are so shrivelled that their details are quite obscured, have a dingy, brownish-yellow colour and a faint, but characteristic odour and mucilaginous taste. As a rule, imported flowers have a duller yellow colour and inferior odour and are sold at a cheaper rate. When the microscope does not reveal tufts of short hairs in the sinuses of the calyx, the drug is not of this species. Most pharmacopoeias specify that dark brown or blackish flowers should be rejected. This appearance may be due to their having been collected some time after opening, to carelessness in drying, or to having been preserved too long.

The flowers of the Dwarf Elder, a comparatively uncommon plant in this country are distinguished from those of the Common Elder by having dark red anthers.

The flowers of the Yarrow (*Achillea millefolium*), and other composite plants, which have been used as adulterants of Elder flowers differ still more markedly in appearance and their presence in the drug is readily detected.

Constituents: The most important constituent of Elder flowers is a trace of semisolid volatile oil, present to the extent only of 0.32, per cent possessing the odour of the flowers in a high degree. It is obtained by distilling the fresh flowers with water, saturating the distillate with salt and shaking it with ether. On evaporating the ethereal solution, the oil is obtained as a yellowish, buttery mass. Without ether, fresh Elder flowers yield 0.037 per cent of the volatile oil and the dried flowers 0.0027 per cent only.

Elder Flower Water (*Aqua Sambuci*) is an official preparation of the British Pharmacopoeia, which directs that it be made from 100 parts of Elder flowers distilled with 500 parts of water (about 10 lb. to the gallon), and that if fresh Elder flowers are not obtainable, an equivalent quantity of the flowers preserved with common salt be used. The product has at first a distinctly unpleasant odour, but gradually acquires an agreeably aromatic odour, and it is preferable not to use it until this change has taken place.

Elder Flower Water is employed in mixing medicines and chiefly as a vehicle for eye and skin lotions. It is mildly astringent and a gentle stimulant. It is the Eau de Sureau of the Continent, Sureau being the French name of the Eider.

Here is a recipe that can be carried out at home: Fill a large jar with Elder blossoms, pressing them down, the stalks of course having been removed previously. Pour on them 2 quarts of boiling water and when slightly cooled, add 1 1/2 oz. of rectified spirits. Cover with a folded cloth, and stand the jar in a warm place for some hours. Then allow it to get quite cold and strain through muslin. Put into bottles and cork securely.

Elderflower Water in our great-grandmothers' days was a household word for clearing the complexion of freckles and sunburn, and keeping it in a good condition. Every lady's toilet table possessed a bottle of the liquid, and she relied on this to keep her skin fair and white and free from blemishes, and it has not lost its reputation. Its use after sea-bathing has been recommended, and if any eruption should appear on the face as the effect of salt water, it is a good plan to use a mixture composed of Elder Flower Water with glycerine and borax, and apply it night and morning.

Elder flowers, if placed in the water used for washing the hands and face, will both whiten and soften the skin-a convenient way being to place them in a small muslin bag. Such a bag steeped in the bathwater makes a most refreshing bath and a well known French doctor has stated that he considers it a fine aid in the bath in cases of irritability of the skin and nerves.

The flowers were used by our forefathers in bronchial and pulmonary affections, and in scarlet fever, measles and other eruptive diseases. An infusion of the dried flowers, Elder Flower Tea, is said to promote expectoration in pleurisy; it is gently laxative and aperient and is considered excellent for inducing free perspiration. It is a good old fashioned remedy for colds and throat trouble, taken hot on going to bed. An almost infallible cure for an attack of influenza in its first stage is a strong infusion of dried Elder Blossoms and Peppermint. Put a handful of each in a jug, pour over them a pint and a half of boiling water, allow to steep, on the stove, for half an hour then strain and sweeten and drink in bed as hot as possible. Heavy perspiration and refreshing sleep will follow, and the patient will wake up well on the way to recovery and the cold or influenza will probably be banished within thirty-six hours. Yarrow may also be added.

Elder Flower Tea, cold, was also considered almost as good for inflammation of the eyes as the distilled Elder Flower Water.

Tea made from Elder Flowers has also been recommended as a splendid spring medicine, to be taken every morning before breakfast for some weeks, being considered an excellent blood purifier.

Externally, Elder Flowers are used in fomentations, to ease pain and abate inflammation. An old writer tells us:

'There be nothing more excellent to ease the pains of the haemorrhoids than a fomentation made of the flowers of the Elder and Verbusie, or Honeysuckle in water or milk for a short time. It easeth the greatest pain. '

A lotion, too, can be made by pouring boiling water on the dried blossoms, which is healing, cooling and soothing. Add 2 1/2 drachms of Elder flowers to 1 quart of boiling water, infuse for an hour and then strain. The liquor can be applied as a lotion by means of a linen rag, for tumours boils, and affections of the skin, and is said to be effective put on the temples against headache and also for warding off the attacks of flies.

A salad of young Elder buds, macerated a little in hot water and dressed with oil, vinegar and salt, has been used as a remedy against skin eruptions.

Elder Vinegar made from the flowers is an old remedy for sore throat.

A good ointment is also prepared from the flowers by infusion in warm lard, useful for dressing wounds, burns and scalds, which is used, also, as a basis for pomades and cosmetic ointments, Elder Flower Ointment (*Unguentum Sambuci*) was largely used for wounded horses in the War (WWI)- the Blue Cross made a special appeal for supplies - but it is also good for human use and is an old remedy for chapped hands and chilblains. Equal quantities of the fresh flowers and of lard are taken, the flowers are heated with the lard until they become crisp, then strained through a linen cloth with pressure and allowed to cool. For use as a Face Cream, (This preparation is hardly suitable as a cosmetic, as lard induces the growth of hair.) the directions are a little more elaborate, but it is essentially the same: Melt lard in a pan then add a small cup of cold water and stir well. Simmer with the lid on for about an hour and finally let the mixture boil with the lid off until all the water has evaporated; this will have happened when, on stirring, no steam arises. Place on one side to cool a little and then pass the liquid fat through a piece of muslin so that it may be well strained and free from impurities. Take a quantity of Elder Flowers equal in weight to the lard and place these in the lard. Then boil up the mixture again, keeping it simmering for a good hour. At the end of that time, strain the whole through a coarse cloth and when cool, the ointment will be ready for use.

Elder Flowers, with their subtle sweet scent, entered into much delicate cookery, in olden days. Formerly the creamy blossoms were beaten up in the batter of flannel cakes and muffins, to which they gave a more delicate texture. They were also boiled in gruel as a fever-drink, and were added to the posset of the Christening feast.

Berries: All the other parts of the Elder plant, except the wood and pith, are more active than either the flowers or the fruit. Fresh Elder Berries are found to contain sudorific properties similar to those of the flowers, but weaker. Chemically, the berries furnish Viburnic acid, with an odorous oil, combined with malates of potash and lime. The fresh, ripe fruits contain Tyrosin.

The blue colouring matter extracted from them has been considerably used as an indication for alkalis, with which it gives a green colour, being red with acids. (Alkalis redden some vegetable yellows and change some vegetable blues to green.) According to Cowie this colouring matter is best extracted in the form of a 20 per cent tincture from the refuse remaining after the expression of the first juice. The colouring matter is precipitated blue by lead acetate (National Standard Dispensatory, 1909.)

The Romans made use of Elderberry juice as a hair-dye, and Culpepper tells us that 'the hair of the head washed with the berries boiled in wine is made black.'

English Elder Berries, as we have seen, are extensively used for the preparation of Elder Wine. French and other Continental Elder berries, when dried, are not liked for this purpose, as they have a more unpleasant odour and flavour, and English berries are preferred. Possibly this may be due to the conditions of growth, or variety, or to the presence of the berries of the Dwarf Elder. Aubrey (1626-97) tells us that:

'the apothecaries well know the use of the berries, and so do the vintners, who buy vast quantities of them in London, and some do make no inconsiderable profit by the sale of them.'

They were held by our forefathers to be efficacious in rheumatism and erysipelas. They have aperient, diuretic and emetic properties, and the inspissated juice of the berries has been used as an alterative in rheumatism and syphilis in doses of from one to two drachms, also as a laxative in doses of half an ounce or more. It promotes all fluid secretions and natural evacuations.

For colic and diarrhoea, a tea made of the dried berries is said to be a good remedy.

In The Anatomie of the Elder, it is stated that the berries of the Elder and Herb Paris are useful in epilepsy. Green Elderberry Ointment has already been mentioned as curative of piles.

After enumerating many uses of the Elder, Gerard says:

'The seeds contained within the berries, dried, are good for such as have the dropsie, and such as are too fat, and would faine be leaner, if they be taken in a morning to the quantity of a dram with wine for a certain space. The green leaves, pounded with Deeres suet or Bulls tallow are good to be laid to hot swellings and tumors, and doth assuage the paine of the gout.'

Parkinson, physician to James I, also tells us of the same use of the seeds, which he recommends to be taken powdered, in vinegar.

Elderberry Wine has a curative power of established repute as a remedy, taken hot, at night, for promoting perspiration in the early stages of severe catarrh, accompanied by shivering, sore throat, etc. Like Elderflower Tea, it is one of the best preventives known against the advance of influenza and the ill effects of a chill. A little cinnamon may be added. It has also a reputation as an excellent remedy for asthma.

Almost from time immemorial, a 'Rob' (a vegetable juice thickened by heat) has been made from the juice of Elderberries simmered and thickened with sugar, forming an invaluable cordial for colds and coughs, but only of late years has science proved that Elderberries furnish Viburnic acid, which induces perspiration, and is especially useful in cases of bronchitis and similar troubles.

To make **Elderberry Rob**, 5 lb. of fresh ripe, crushed berries are simmered with 1 lb. of loaf sugar and the juice evaporated to the thickness of honey. It is cordial, aperient and diuretic. One or two tablespoonsful mixed with a tumblerful of hot water, taken at night, promotes perspiration and is demulcent to the chest.

The Rob when made can be bottled and stored for the winter. Herbalists sell it ready for use.

'Syrup of Elderberries' is made as follows: Pick the berries when throughly ripe from the stalks and stew with a little water in a jar in the oven or pan. After straining, allow 1/2 oz. of whole ginger and 18 cloves to each gallon. Boil the ingredients an hour, strain again and bottle. The syrup is an excellent cure for a cold. To about a wineglassful of Elderberry syrup, add hot water, and if liked, sugar.

Both Syrup of Elderberries and the Rob were once official in this country (as they are still in Holland), the rob being the older of of the two, and the one that retained its place longer in our Pharmacopoeia. In 1788, its name was changed to Succus Sambuci spissatus, and in 1809 it disappeared altogether. Brookes in 1773 strongly recommended it as a 'saponaceous Resolvent' promoting 'the natural secretions by stool, urine and sweat,' and, diluted with water, for common colds. John Wesley, in his Primitive Physick, directs it to be taken in broth, and in Germany it is used as an ingredient in soups.

There were six or seven robs in the old London Pharmacopceia, to most of which sugar was added. They were thicker than syrups, but did not differ materially from them; among them was a rob of Elderberries, and both Quincy and Bates had a syrup of Elder.

An old prescription for sciatica (called the Duke of Monmouth's recipe) was compounded of ripe haws and fennel roots, distilled in white wine and taken with syrup of Elder.

The use of the juicy berries, not as medicine, but as a pleasant article of food, in jam, jelly, chutney and ketchup has already been described.

Medicinal Preparations: Fluid extract of bark, 1/2 to 1 drachm. Water, B.P.

Fennel

Foeniculum officinale All. Gebräuchlicher Fenchel.

Quick Facts

Latin/Linnaen:	*Foeniculum Vulgare*
Family:	*Apiaceae (formerly Umbelliferae)*
Old English :	Finol, Finule, Fenel, Fenyl
Synonyms:	Fenkel, Sweet Fennel, Wild Fennel
Action:	Promoted gastrointestinal motility, in higher concentrations acts as an antispasmodic. Experimentally, anethole and fenchone have been shown to have a secretolytic action in the respiratory tract.
Parts Used:	Oil and seed
Indicated For:	Peptic discomforts, such as mild, spastic disorders of the gastrointestinal tract, feeling of fullness, flatulence. Catarrhs of the upper respiratory tract. Fennel honey: catarrhs of the upper respiratory tract in children.
Dosage:	**Oil**: Unless otherwise prescribed: Daily dosage: 0.1-0.6 ml, equivalent to 0.1-0.6g of herb; equivalent preparations. Fennel honey syrup with 0.5g fennel oil/kg: 10-20g; equivalent preparations. **Seed**: Unless otherwise prescribed: 5-7g of herb; 10-20 g fennel syrup or honey; 5-7.5g compound fennel tincture; equivalent preparations.
Preparation:	**Oil**: Essential oil and galenical preparations for internal use. Seed: Crushed or ground seeds for teas, tea like products, as well as other galenical preparations.
Cautions:	Contraindications: pregnancy and infants and toddlers.
Other Uses:	**Culinary:** Fennel features prominently in Mediterranean cuisine, where bulbs and fronds are used, both raw and cooked, in side dishes, salads, pastas, vegetable dishes and risottos. Fennel seed is a common ingredient in Italian sausages and meatballs and northern European rye breads. Fennel is one of the most important spices in Kashmiri Pandit and Gujarati cooking.[citation needed] It is an essential ingredient of the Assamese/Bengali/Oriya spice mixture panch phoron and in Chinese five-spice powders. In many parts of India and Pakistan, roasted fennel seeds are consumed as mukhwas, an after-meal digestive and breath freshener. Fennel leaves are used as leafy green vegetables either by themselves or

mixed with other vegetables, cooked to be served and consumed as part of a meal, in some parts of India. In Lebanon, it is used to make a special kind of egg omelette (along with onions, and flour) called ijjeh.

Many egg, fish, and other dishes employ fresh or dried fennel leaves. Florence fennel is a key ingredient in some Italian and German salads, often tossed with chicory and avocado, or it can be braised and served as a warm side dish. It may be blanched or marinated, or cooked in risotto.

Beverages: Florence fennel was one of the three main herbs used in the preparation of absinthe, an alcoholic mixture which originated as a medicinal elixir in Switzerland and became, by the late 19th century, a popular alcoholic drink in France and other countries.

Toothpaste: Fennel is also used as a flavouring in some natural toothpastes.

Description

Fennel (*Foeniculum vulgare*) is a plant species in the genus *Foeniculum* (treated as the sole species in the genus by most botanists). It is a member of the family *Apiaceae* (formerly the *Umbelliferae*). It is a hardy, perennial, umbelliferous herb, with yellow flowers and feathery leaves. It is indigenous to the shores of the Mediterranean, but has become widely naturalised in many parts of the world, especially on dry soils near the sea-coast and on riverbanks.

It is a highly aromatic and flavourful herb with culinary and medicinal uses, and, along with the similar-tasting anise, is one of the primary ingredients of absinthe. Florence fennel or finocchio is a selection with a swollen, bulb-like stem base that is used as a vegetable.

Fennel is used as a food plant by the larvae of some Lepidoptera species including the mouse moth and the anise swallowtail.

The word fennel developed from the Middle English fenel or fenyl. This came from the Old English fenol or finol, which in turn came from the Latin feniculum or foeniculum, the diminutive of fenum or faenum, meaning "hay". The Latin word for the plant was ferula, which is now used as the genus name of a related plant. As

Old English finule it is one of the nine plants invoked in the pagan Anglo-Saxon Nine Herbs Charm, recorded in the 10th century.

In Greek mythology, Prometheus used the stalk of a fennel plant to steal fire from the gods. Also, it was from the giant fennel, Ferula communis, that the Bacchanalian wands of the god Dionysus and his followers were said to have come.

Fennel, Foeniculum vulgare, is a perennial herb. It is erect, glaucous green, and grows to heights of up to 2.5 m, with hollow stems. The leaves grow up to 40 cm long; they are finely dissected, with the ultimate segments filiform (threadlike), about 0.5 mm wide. (Its leaves are similar to those of dill, but thinner.) The flowers are produced in terminal compound umbels 5–15 cm wide, each umbel section having 20–50 tiny yellow flowers on short pedicels. The fruit is a dry seed from 4–10 mm long, half as wide or less, and grooved.

Cultivation

Hardiness Zone:	5-10
Soil pH:	6.5
Soil type:	Average well drained soil.
Cultivation:	Sow seeds directly in the garden.
Sunlight:	Full sun
Habitat:	Native to the Mediterranean, but naturalized in many parts of the world.

Do not plant fennel near coriander, caraway, or wormwood as they don't do well together. Fennel seeds can be harvested when the flower starts to brown. They are best kept in a paper bag in a cool dry place.

Fennel will thrive anywhere, and a plantation will last for years. It is easily propagated by seeds, sown early in April in ordinary soil. It likes plenty of sun and is adapted to dry and sunny situations, not needing heavily manured ground, though it will yield more on rich stiff soil. From 4 1/2 to 5 lb. of seed are sown per acre, either in drills, 15 inches apart, lightly, just covered with soil and the plants afterwards thinned to a similar distance, or sewn thinly in a bed and transplanted when large enough. The fruit is heavy and a crop of 15 cwt. per acre is an average yield.

Historical Notes

Parts Used: Seeds, leaves, roots.

Habitat: Fennel, a hardy, perennial, umbelliferous herb, with yellow flowers and feathery leaves, grows wild in most parts of temperate Europe, but is generally considered indigenous to the shores of the Mediterranean, whence it spreads eastwards to India. It has followed civilization, especially where Italians have colonized, and may be found growing wild in many parts of the world upon dry soils near the sea-coast and upon river-banks. It flourishes particularly on limestone soils and is now naturalized in some parts of this country, being found from North Wales southward and eastward to Kent, being most frequent in Devon and Cornwall and on chalk cliffs near the sea. It is often found in chalky districts inland in a semi-wild state.

For the medicinal use of its fruits, commonly called seeds, Fennel is largely cultivated in the south of France, Saxony, Galicia, and Russia, as well as in India and Persia.

This plant was attached by Linnaeus to the genus Anethum, but was separated from it by De Candolle and placed with three or four others in a new genus styled Foeniculum, which has been generally adopted by botanists. (Foeniculum was the name given to this plant by the Romans, and is derived from the Latin word, foenum = hay).

This was corrupted in the Middle Ages into Fanculum, and this gave birth to its alternative popular name, 'fenkel.'

The Anethum Foeniculum of Linnaeus embraced two varieties, the Common or Wild Fennel and the Sweet Fennel. These are considered by De Candolle as distinct species named respectively F. vulgare (Gaertn.) - the garden form of which is often named F. Capillaceum (Gilibert) - and F. dulce.

History: Fennel was well known to the Ancients and was cultivated by the ancient Romans for its aromatic fruits and succulent, edible shoots. Pliny had much faith in its medicinal properties, according no less than twenty-two remedies to it, observing also that serpents eat it 'when they cast their old skins, and they sharpen their sight with the juice by rubbing against the plant.' A very old English rhyming Herbal, preserved at Stockholm, gives the following description of the virtue of the plant:

'Whaune the heddere (adder) is hurt in eye

Ye red fenel is hys prey,

And yif he mowe it fynde

Wonderly he doth hys kynde.

He schall it chow wonderly,

And leyn it to hys eye kindlely,

Ye jows shall sang and hely ye eye

Yat beforn was sicke et feye.'

Many of the older herbalists uphold this theory of the peculiarly strengthening effect of this herb on the sight.

Longfellow alludes to this virtue in the plant:

'Above the lower plants it towers,

The Fennel with its yellow flowers;

And in an earlier age than ours

Was gifted with the wondrous powers

Lost vision to restore.'

In mediaeval times, Fennel was employed, together with St. John's Wort and other herbs, as a preventative of witchcraft and other evil influences, being hung over doors on Midsummer's Eve to warn off evil spirits. It was likewise eaten as a condiment to the salt fish so much consumed by our forefathers during Lent. Like several other umbelliferae, it is carminative.

Though the Romans valued the young shoots as a vegetable, it is not certain whether it was cultivated in northern Europe at that time, but it is frequently mentioned in Anglo-Saxon cookery and medical recipes prior to the Norman Conquest. Fennel shoots, Fennel water and Fennel seed are all mentioned in an ancient record of Spanish agriculture dating A.D. 961. The diffusion of the plant in Central Europe was stimulated by Charlemagne, who enjoined its cultivation on the imperial farms.

It is mentioned in Gerard (1597), and Parkinson (Theatricum Botanicum, 1640) tells us that its culinary use was derived from Italy, for he says:

'The leaves, seede and rootes are both for meate and medicine; the Italians especially doe much delight in the use thereof, and therefore transplant and whiten it, to make it more tender to please the taste, which being sweete and somewhat hot helpeth to digest the crude qualitie of fish and other viscous meats. We use it to lay upon fish or to boyle it therewith and with divers other things, as also the seeds in bread and other things.'

William Coles, in Nature's Paradise (1650) affirms that -

'both the seeds, leaves and root of our Garden Fennel are much used in drinks and broths for those that are grown fat, to abate their unwieldiness and cause them to grow more gaunt and lank.'

The ancient Greek name of the herb, Marathron, from maraino, to grow thin, probably refers to this property.

It was said to convey longevity, and to give strength and courage.

There are many references to Fennel in poetry. Milton, in Paradise Lost alludes to the aroma of the plant:

'A savoury odour blown,

Grateful to appetite, more pleased my sense

Than smell of sweetest Fennel.'

Description: Fennel is a beautiful plant. It has a thick, perennial root-stock, stout stems, 4 to 5 feet or more in height, erect and cylindrical, bright green and so smooth as to seem polished, much branched bearing leaves cut into the very finest of segments. The bright golden flowers, produced in large, flat terminal umbels, with from thirteen to twenty rays, are in bloom in July and August.

In the kitchen garden this naturally ornamental, graceful plant, generally has its stems cut down to secure a constant crop of green leaves for flavouring and garnishing, so that the plant is seldom seen in the same perfection as in the wild state. In the original wild condition, it is variable as to size, habit, shape and colour of leaf, number of rays in the flower-head or umbel, and shape of fruit, but it has been under cultivation for so long that there are now several well-marked species. The Common Garden Fennel (*F. Capillaceum* or *officinale*) is distinguished from its wild relative (*F. vulgare*) by having much stouter, taller, tubular and larger stems, and less divided leaves, but the chief distinction is that the leaf-stalks form a curved sheath around the stem, often even as far as the base of the leaf above. The flower-stalks, or pedicels, of the umbels are also sturdier, and the fruits, 1/4 to 1/2 inch long, are double the size of the wild ones.

The roots of Fennel were formerly employed in medicine, but are generally inferior in virtues to the fruit, which is now the only portion recognized by any of the Pharmacopoeias.

The cessation of the supply of Fennel fruits from the Continent during the War (WWI) led to its being grown more extensively here, any crop produced being almost certain to sell well.

There are several varieties of Fennel fruit known in commerce - sweet or Roman Fennel, German or Saxon Fennel, wild or bitter Fennel, Galician Russian and Roumanian Fennel, Indian, Persian and Japanese. The fruits vary very much in length, breadth, taste and other characters, and are of very different commercial value.

The most esteemed Fennel fruit vary from three to five lines in length, are elliptical, slightly curved, somewhat obtuse at the ends and pale greyish green in colour. Wild fruits are short, dark coloured and blunt at their ends, and have a less agreeable flavour and odour than those of sweet Fennel - they are not official.

Fennel fruits are frequently distinguished into 'shorts' and 'longs' in commerce, the latter being the most valued.

The odour of Fennel seed is fragrant, its taste, warm, sweet and agreeably aromatic. It yields its virtues to hot water, but more freely to alcohol. The essential oil may be separated by distillation with water.

For medicinal use, the fruits of the cultivated Fennel, especially those grown in Saxony, are alone official, as they yield the most volatile oil. Saxon fruits are greenish to yellowish-brown in colour, oblong, smaller and straighter than the French or Sweet Fennel (*F. dulce*). This French Fennel, known also as Roman Fennel, is distinguished by its greater length, more oblong form, yellowish-green colour and sweet taste; its anise-like odour is also stronger. It is cultivated in the neighbourhood of Nimes, in the south of France, but yields comparatively little oil, which has no value medicinally.

Indian Fennel is brownish, usually smaller, straighter and not quite so rounded at the ends with a sweet anise taste. Persian and Japanese fennel, pale greenish brown in colour, are the smallest and have a sweeter, still more strongly anise taste and an odour intermediate between that of French and Saxon.

The Saxon, Galician, Roumanian and Russian varieties all yield 4 to 5 per cent of volatile oil, and these varieties are alone suitable for pharmaceutical use. In the ordinary way they furnish some of the best Fennel crops, and from their fruit a large portion of the oil of commerce is derived.

For family use, 1/2 oz. of seed will produce an ample supply of plants and for several years, either from the established roots, or by re-seeding. Unless seed is needed for household or sowing purposes, the flower stems should be cut as soon as they appear.

Adulteration: Commercial Fennel varies greatly in quality, this being either due to lack of care in harvesting, or deliberate adulteration. It may contain so much sand, dirt, stem tissues, weed seeds or other material, that it amounts to adulteration and is unfit for medicinal use, or it may have had some of its oil removed by distillation.

Fruits exhausted by water or steam are darker, contain less oil and sink at once in water, but those exhausted by alcohol still retain 1 to 2 per cent, and are but little altered in appearance, they acquire, however, a peculiar fusel oil odour.

Exhausted, or otherwise inferior fennel is occasionally improved in appearance by the use of a factitious colouring, but old exhausted fruits that have been re-coloured may be detected by rubbing the fruit between the hands, when the colour will come off.

Constituents: As found in commerce, oil Fennel is not uniform.

The best varieties of Fennel yield from 4 to 5 per cent of volatile oil (sp. gr. 0.960 to 0.930), the principal constituents of which are Anethol (50 to 60 per cent) and Fenchone (18 to 22 per cent). Anethol is also the chief constituent of Anise oil.

Fenchone is a colourless liquid possessing a pungent, camphoraceous odour and taste, and when present gives the disagreeable bitter taste to many of the commercial oils. It probably contributes materially to the medicinal properties of the oil, hence only such varieties of Fennel as contain a good proportion of fenchone are suitable for medicinal use.

There are also present in oil of Fennel, d-pinene, phellandrine, anisic acid and anisic aldehyde. Schimmel mentions limonene as also at times present as a constituent.

There is reason to believe that much of the commercial oil is adulterated with oil from which the anethol or crystalline constituent has been separated. Good oil will contain as much as 60 per cent.

Saxon Fennel yields 4.7 per cent of volatile oil, containing 22 per cent of fenchone.

Russian, Galician and Roumanian, which closely resembles one another, yield 4 to 5 per cent of volatile oil, of which about 18 per cent is fenchone. They have a camphoraceous taste.

French sweet or Roman Fennel yields only 2.1 per cent. of oil, containing much less anethol and with a milder and sweeter taste, probably due to the entire absence of the bitter fenchone.

French bitter Fennel oil differs considerably, anethol being only present in traces. The oil (Essence de Fenouil amer) is distilled from the entire herb, collected in the south of France, where the plant grows without cultivation.

Indian Fennel yields only 0.72 per cent of oil, containing only 6.7 per cent of fenchone.

Japanese Fennel yields 2.7 per cent of oil, containing 10.2 of fenchone and 75 per cent of anethol.

Sicilian Fennel oil is yielded from F. *piperitum*.

It was formerly the practice to boil Fennel with all fish, and it was mainly cultivated in kitchen gardens for this purpose. Its leaves are served nowadays with salmon, to correct its oily indigestibility, and are also put into sauce, in the same way as parsley, to be eaten with boiled mackerel.

The seeds are also used for flavouring and the carminative oil that is distilled from them, which has a sweetish aromatic odour and flavour, is employed in the making of cordials and liqueurs, and is also used in perfumery and for scenting soaps. A pound of oil is the usual yield of 500 lb. of the seed.

Historical Medicinal Uses - For Entertainment ONLY

Medicinal Action and Uses: On account of its aromatic and carminative properties, Fennel fruit is chiefly used medicinally with purgatives to allay their tendency to griping and for this purpose forms one of the ingredients of the well-known compound Liquorice Powder. Fennel water has properties similar to those of anise and dill water: mixed with sodium bicarbonate and syrup, these waters constitute the domestic 'Gripe Water,' used to correct the flatulence of infants. Volatile oil of Fennel has these properties in concentration.

Fennel tea, formerly also employed as a carminative, is made by pouring half a pint of boiling water on a teaspoonful of bruised Fennel seeds.

Syrup prepared from Fennel juice was formerly given for chronic coughs.

Fennel is also largely used for cattle condiments.

It is one of the plants which is said to be disliked by fleas, and powdered Fennel has the effect of driving away fleas from kennels and stables. The plant gives off ozone most readily.

Culpepper says:

'One good old custom is not yet left off, viz., to boil fennel with fish, for it consumes the phlegmatic humour which fish most plentifully afford and annoy the body with, though few that use it know wherefore they do it. It benefits this way, because it is a herb of Mercury, and under Virgo, and therefore bears antipathy to Pisces. Fennel expels wind, provokes urine, and eases the pains of the stone, and helps to break it. The leaves or seed boiled in barley water and drunk, are good for nurses, to increase their milk and make it more wholesome for the child. The leaves, or rather the seeds, boiled in water, stayeth the hiccup and taketh away nausea or inclination to sickness. The seed and the roots much more help to open obstructions of the liver, spleen, and gall, and thereby relieve the painful and windy swellings of the spleen, and the yellow jaundice, as also the gout and cramp. The seed is of good use in medicines for shortness of breath and wheezing, by stoppings of the lungs. The roots are of most use in physic, drinks and broths, that are taken to cleanse the blood, to open obstructions of the liver, to provoke urine, and amend the ill colour of the face after sickness, and to cause a good habit through the body; both leaves, seeds, and

roots thereof, are much used in drink, or broth, to make people more lean that are too fat. A decoction of the leaves and root is good for serpent bites, and to neutralize vegetable poison, as mushrooms, etc.' 'In warm climates,' says Mattiolus, 'the stems are cut and there exudes a resinous liquid, which is collected under the name of Fennel Gum.'

In Italy and France, the tender leaves are often used for garnishes and to add flavour to salads, and are also added, finely chopped, to sauces served with puddings. Roman bakers are said to put the herb under their loaves in the oven to make the bread taste agreeably.

The tender stems are employed in soups in Italy, though are more frequently eaten raw as a salad. John Evelyn, in his Acetaria (1680), held that the peeled stalks, soft and white, of the cultivated garden Fennel, when dressed like celery exercised a pleasant action conducive to sleep. The Italians eat these peeled stems, which they call 'Cartucci' as a salad, cutting them when the plant is about to bloom and serving with a dressing of vinegar and pepper.

Formerly poor people used to eat Fennel to satisfy the cravings of hunger on fast days and make unsavoury food palatable; it was also used in large quantities in the households of the rich, as may be seen by the record in the accounts of Edward I.'s household, 8 1/2 lb. of Fennel were bought for one month's supply.

Preparations: Fluid extract, 5 to 30 drops. Oil, 1 to 5 drops. Water, B.P. and U.S.P., 4 drachms.

SOME OLD-FASHIONED FENNEL AND DILL RECIPES

A Sallet of Fennel

'Take young Fennel, about a span long in the spring, tye it up in bunches as you do Sparragrass; when your Skillet boyle, put in enough to make a dish; when it is boyled and drained, dish it up as you do Sparragrass, pour on butter and vinegar and send it up.' (From The Whole Body of Cookery Dissected, 1675, by William Tabisha.)

Fennel and Gooseberry Sauce

'Brown some butter in a saucepan with a pinch of flour, then put in a few cives shred small, add a little Irish broth to moisten it, season with salt and pepper; make these boil, then put in two or three sprigs of Fennel and some Gooseberries. Let all simmer together till the Gooseberries are soft and then put in some Cullis.' (From Receipt Book of Henry Howard, Cook to the Duke of Ormond, 1710.)

Fenugreek

XVII. 3.   106. Leguminosae.

433. Trigonella Foenum graecum L.   Griechisches Heu.

Quick Facts

Latin/Linnaen:	*Trigonella foenum-graecum*
Family:	*Fabaceae*
Old English :	Wyllecerse
Synonyms:	Well cress, Bird's Foot, Greek Hay-seed
Action:	Secretolytic, Hyperemic, Mild Antiseptic
Parts Used:	Seed
Indicated For:	Internal: Loss of appetite, External: As a poultice for local inflammation
Dosage:	Unless otherwise prescribed: Internal: 6g drug; equivalent preparations, External: 50g powdered drug with ¼ liter of water.
Preparation:	Liniments in the form of alcoholic solutions, ointments, gels, emulsions, oils. Also bath additive and as an inhalant.
Cautions:	Repeated external applications can result in undesirable skin reactions.
Other Uses:	**Culinary:** Fenugreek is used both as an herb (the leaves) and as a spice (the seed, often called methi in Urdu/Hindi/Nepali). The leaves and sprouts are also eaten as vegetables.

Descripton

Fenugreek (*Trigonella foenum-graecum*) is a plant in the family *Fabaceae*. Fenugreek is used both as an herb (the leaves) and as a spice (the seed, often called methi in Urdu/Hindi/Nepali). The leaves and sprouts are also eaten as vegetables. The plant is cultivated worldwide as a semi-arid crop and is a common ingredient in many curries.

The name fenugreek or foenum-graecum is from Latin for "Greek hay". The plant's similarity to wild clover has likely spawned its Swedish name:

"bockhornsklöver" as well as the German: "Bockshornklee", both literally meaning: "ram's horn clover".

The cuboid yellow to amber coloured fenugreek seeds are frequently used in the preparation of pickles, curry powders, and curry paste, and the spice is often encountered in the cuisine of the Indian subcontinent. The dried leaves – also called kasuri methi (or kasoori methi in North India and Pakistan), after the region of Kasur in Punjab, Pakistan province, where it grows abundantly – have a bitter taste and a characteristically strong smell. When harvested as microgreens, it also known as Samudra Methi, in Maharashtra, especially in and around Mumbai, where it is often grown near the sea in the sandy tracts, hence the name (Samudra means "ocean" in Sanskrit). Fenugreek is used in Eritrean and Ethiopian cuisine. The word for fenugreek in Amharic is abesh (or abish), and the seed is used in Ethiopia as a natural herbal medicine in the treatment of diabetes.

Cultivation

Hardiness Zone:	Annual herb
Soil pH:	5.3-8.2
Soil type:	Rich, well drained soil.
Cultivation:	Sow seeds in spring and harvest dry seedpods in early-mid fall.
Sunlight:	Full sun
Habitat:	Native to the Mediterranean and Asia, now grown in many different countries.

Fenugreek seeds can lose some flavor if overly fertilized, so go lightly on the fertilizer. Fenugreek will not do well in cold wet environments.

Historical Notes

The name comes from *Foenum-graecum*, meaning Greek Hay, the plant being used to scent inferior hay. The name of the genus, *Trigonella*, is derived from the old Greek name, denoting 'three-angled,' from the form of its corolla. The seeds of

Fenugreek have been used medicinally all through the ages and were held in high repute among the Egyptians, Greeks and Romans for medicinal and culinary purposes.

Fenugreek is an erect annual herb, growing about 2 feet high, similar in habit to Lucerne. The seeds are brownish, about 1/8 inch long, oblong, rhomboidal, with a deep furrow dividing them into two unequal lobes. They are contained, ten to twenty together, in long, narrow, sickle-like pods.

Taste - bitter and peculiar, not unlike lovage or celery. Odour, similar.

Charred fenugreek seeds have been recovered from Tell Halal, Iraq, (radiocarbon dating to 4000 BC) and Bronze Age levels of Lachish, as well as desiccated seeds from the tomb of Tutankhamen. Cato the Elder lists fenugreek with clover and vetch as crops grown to feed cattle.

Constituents: About 28 per cent mucilage; 5 per cent of a stronger-smelling, bitter fixed oil, which can be extracted by ether; 22 per cent proteids; a volatile oil; two alkaloids, Trigonelline and Choline, and a yellow colouring substance. The chemical composition resembles that of cod-liver oil, as it is rich in phosphates, lecithin and nucleoalbumin, containing also considerable quantities of iron in an organic form, which can be readily absorbed. Reutter has noted the presence of trimethylamine, neurin and betain; like the alkaloids in cod-liver oil, these substances stimulate the appetite by their action on the nervous system, or produce a diuretic or ureo-poietic effect.

Historical Medicinal Uses - For Entertainment ONLY

Medicinal Action and Uses: In Cairo it is used under the name of Helba. This is an Egyptian preparation, made by soaking the seeds in water till they swell into a thick paste. Said to be equal to quinine in preventing fevers; is comforting to the stomach and has been utilized for diabetes. The seeds are soaked in water, then allowed to sprout, and when grown about 2 or 3 inches high, the green eaten raw with the seeds.

The seeds yield the whole of their odour and taste to alcohol and are employed in the preparation of emollient cataplasms, ointments and plasters.

They give a strong mucilage, which is emollient and a decoction of 1 oz. seeds to 1 pint water is used internally in inflamed conditions of the stomach and intestines. Externally it is used as a poultice for abscesses, boils, carbuncles, etc. It can be employed as a substitute for cod-liver oil in scrofula, rickets, anaemia, debility following infectious diseases. For neurasthenia, gout and diabetes it can be combined with insulin. It possesses the advantage of being cheap and readily taken by children, if its bitter taste is disguised: 1 or 2 teaspoonful of the powder is taken daily in jam, etc.

The ground seeds are used also to give a maple-flavouring to confectionery and nearly all cattle like the flavour of Fenugreek in their forage. The powder is also employed as a spice in curry. At the present day, the ground seeds are utilized to an enormous extent in the manufactures of condition powders for horses and cattle; Funugreek is the principal ingredient in most of the quack nostrums which find so much favour among grooms and horsekeepers. It has a powerful odour of coumarin and is largely used for flavouring cattle foods and to make damaged hay palatable.

In India the fresh plant is employed as an esculent.

Arthritis has a low incidence rate in India where a lot of fenugreek is consumed. Drinking 1 cup of fenugreek tea per day, made from the leaves, is said to relieve the discomfort of arthritis.

A June 2011 study at the Australian Centre for Integrative Clinical and Molecular Medicine found that men aged 25 to 52 who took a fenugreek extract twice daily for six weeks scored 25% higher on tests gauging libido levels than those who took a placebo.

Fenugreek seeds are a rich source of the polysaccharide galactomannan. They are also a source of saponins such as diosgenin, yamogenin, gitogenin, tigogenin, and neotigogens. Other bioactive constituents of fenugreek include mucilage, volatile oils, and alkaloids such as choline and trigonelline.

Fenugreek seeds are used as a medicinal in Traditional Chinese Medicine under the name Hu Lu Ba, where they are considered to warm and tonify kidneys, disperse cold and alleviate pain. Main indications are hernia, pain in the groin. They are used raw or toasted. In India about 2-3g of raw fenugreek seeds (called Methi in India) are swallowed raw early in the morning with warm water, before brushing the teeth and before drinking tea or coffee, where they are supposed to have a therapeutic and healing effect on joint pains, without any side effects.

In Persian cuisine Fenugreek leaves are used and called shambalile. In Arabic traditional medicine, it is known as Helba or Hulba. Tea made from the seeds is used in the Near East to treat various kidney, heart, abdominal illnesses and Diabetes. Seeds are used by Bedouin women to strengthen pregnant and breastfeeding women.

Fenugreek is frequently used in the production of flavoring for artificial maple syrups. The taste of toasted fenugreek, like cumin, is additionally based on substituted pyrazines. By itself, fenugreek has a bitter taste.

Fenugreek seed is widely used as a galactagogue (milk producing agent) by nursing mothers to increase inadequate breast milk supply. Studies have shown that fenugreek is a potent stimulator of breast milk production and its use was associated with increases in milk production. It can be found in capsule form in many health food stores.

Several human intervention trials demonstrated that the antidiabetic effects of fenugreek seeds ameliorate most metabolic symptoms associated with type-1 and type-2 diabetes in both humans and relevant animal models by reducing serum glucose and improving glucose tolerance. Fenugreek is currently available commercially in encapsulated forms and is being prescribed as dietary supplements for the control of hypercholesterolemia and diabetes by practitioners of complementary and alternative medicine. Fenugreek contains high dietary fiber, so a few seeds taken with warm water before going to sleep helps avoiding constipation.

Flax

Linum usitatissimum L.

Quick Facts

Latin/Linnaen:	*Linum Usitatissimum*
Family:	*Linaceae*
Old English :	Linwyrt, Lynsaed
Synonyms:	Common flax, Linseed
Action:	Laxative effects due to increase in volume and consequent initiation of intestinal peristalsis due to stretching reflexes. Protective effect on the mucosa because of coating action.
Parts Used:	Seed
Indicated For:	Internal: Chronic constipation, for colons damaged by abuse of laxatives, irritable colon, diverticulitis, as mucilage for gastritis and enteritis. External: As cataplasm for local inflammation.
Dosage:	Unless otherwise prescribed: Internal: 1 tablespoon of whole or "bruised" seed (not ground) with 150ml of liquid 2-3 times daily, 2-3 tablespoons of milled flaxseed for the preparation of flaxseed mucilage (gruel). External: 30-50g flaxseed flour for a moist-heat cataplasm for compress.
Preparation:	Internal: As seed, as cracked or coarsely ground seed, in which only the cuticle and mucilage epidermis are damaged; as flaxseed mucilage (gruel) and other galenical preparations. External: As flaxseed flour or flaxseed expellant.
Cautions:	Ileus (intestinal obstruction or lack of motor activity in the GI tract, for any reason. As with any mucilage, the absorption of other drugs may be impacted.
Other Uses:	**Culinary:** Flax seed sprouts are edible, with a slightly spicy flavor. Flaxseed is called 'Tisi' in northern India, particularly in the Bihar region. Roasted 'Tisi' is powdered and eaten with boiled rice, a little water, and a little salt since ancient times in the villages.
	Oil: Flax seeds produce a vegetable oil known as flaxseed or linseed oil, which is one of the oldest commercial oils, and solvent-processed flax seed oil has been used for centuries as a drying oil in painting and varnishing.

Clothing: Flax fibers can be spun into linen.

Descripton

Flax (also known as common flax or linseed) (binomial name: *Linum usitatissimum*) is a member of the genus *Linum* in the family *Linaceae*. It is native to the region extending from the eastern Mediterranean to India and was probably first domesticated in the Fertile Crescent. Flax was extensively cultivated in ancient Ethiopia and ancient Egypt. In a prehistoric cave in the Republic of Georgia, dyed flax fibers have been found that date to 30,000 BC, implicating it as the first domesticated species in human history. New Zealand flax is not related to flax but was named after it, as both plants are used to produce fibers.

(It is known as Linari in Greek, Aalas in Nepali, Agasi/Akshi in Kannada, Aazhi Vidhai in Tamil, Jawas/Javas) or Alashi in Marathi and Alsi in Urdu and Hindi, Tisi in Bengali and Avisalu in Telugu.)

Flax is an erect annual plant growing to 1.2 m (3 ft 11 in) tall, with slender stems. The leaves are glaucous green, slender lanceolate, 20–40 mm long and 3 mm broad. The flowers are pure pale blue, 15–25 mm diameter, with five petals; they can also be bright red. The fruit is a round, dry capsule 5–9 mm diameter, containing several glossy brown seeds shaped like an apple pip, 4–7 mm long.

In addition to referring to the plant itself, the word "flax" may refer to the unspun fibers of the flax plant.

Flax is grown both for its seeds and for its fiber. Various parts of the plant have been used to make fabric, dye, paper, medicines, fishing nets, hair gels, and soap. Flax seed is the source of linseed oil, which is used as an edible oil, as a nutritional supplement and as an ingredient in many wood finishing products. Flax is also grown as an ornamental plant in gardens.

Flax seeds come in two basic varieties: (1) brown; and (2) yellow or golden. Most types have similar nutritional characteristics and equal numbers of short-chain omega-3 fatty acids. The exception is a type of yellow flax called solin (trade name Linola), which has a completely different oil profile and is very low in omega-3 FAs. Although brown flax can be consumed as readily as yellow, and has been for thousands of years, it is better known as an ingredient in paints, fiber and cattle feed.

One hundred grams of ground flax seed supplies about 450 kilocalories, 41 grams of fat, 28 grams of fiber, and 20 grams of protein.

Flax seed sprouts are edible, with a slightly spicy flavor. Excessive consumption of flax seeds with inadequate water can cause bowel obstruction.

Flax seeds contain high levels of dietary fiber as well as lignans, an abundance of micronutrients and omega-3 fatty acids. Flax seeds may lower cholesterol levels, especially in women. Initial studies suggest that flax seeds taken in the diet may benefit individuals with certain types of breast and prostate cancers. A study done at Duke university suggests that flaxseed may stunt the growth of prostate tumors, although a meta-analysis found the evidence on this point to be inconclusive. Flax may also lessen the severity of diabetes by stabilizing blood-sugar levels. There is some support for the use of flax seed as a laxative due to its dietary fiber content though excessive consumption without liquid can result in intestinal blockage. Consuming large amounts of flax seed may impair the effectiveness of certain oral medications, due to its fiber content, and may have adverse effects due to its content of neurotoxic cyanogen glycosides and immunosuppressive cyclic nonapeptides.

One of the main components of flax is lignan, which has plant estrogen as well as antioxidants (flax contains up to 800 times more lignans than other plant foods contain).

Cultivation

Hardiness Zone:	Annual plant
Soil pH:	6.0-6.5
Soil type:	Rich loamy soil with lots of organic matter.
Cultivation:	Seed propagation, harvest when seed heads turn yellow and start to open.
Sunlight:	Full sun

Habitat:	Native to the Mediterranean and India.

Historical Notes

Flax is one of the English-grown medicinal herbs, the products of which are included in the British Pharmacopoeia, its seed known as Linseed, being much employed in medicine.

Flax fibers are amongst the oldest fiber crops in the world. The use of flax for the production of linen goes back at least to ancient Egyptian times. Dyed flax fibers found in a cave in Dzudzuana (prehistoric Georgia) have been dated to 30,000 years ago. Pictures on tombs and temple walls at Thebes depict flowering flax plants. The use of flax fiber in the manufacturing of cloth in northern Europe dates back to Neolithic times. In North America, flax was introduced by the Puritans.

Flax fiber is extracted from the bast or skin of the stem of the flax plant. Flax fiber is soft, lustrous and flexible; bundles of fiber have the appearance of blonde hair, hence the description "flaxen". It is stronger than cotton fiber but less elastic. The best grades are used for linen fabrics such as damasks, lace and sheeting. Coarser grades are used for the manufacturing of twine and rope. Flax fiber is also a raw material for the high-quality paper industry for the use of printed banknotes and rolling paper for cigarettes and tea bags. Flax mills for spinning flaxen yarn were invented by John Kendrew and Thomas Porthouse of Darlington in 1787. This process was improved in the early 1800's by Ross M. Brown. New methods of processing flax and the rising price of cotton have led to renewed interest in the use of flax as an industrial fiber. Naturally Advanced's Crailar technology is one proprietary method that is increasing the industrial adoption of this plant.

The 'fine linen' mentioned in the Bible has been satisfactorily proved to have been spun from Flax; it was the plant to which the plague of hail proved so disastrous (Exodus ix. 31). Joseph was arrayed in this product (Genesis xii. 42), and it also furnished the garments of the Jewish High-Priests (Exodus xxviii.) as well as the curtains of the Tabernacle (Exodus xxvi. 1). We learn that the knowledge of spinning this linen was known to the Canaanites (see Joshua ii. 6), and in New

Testament times it formed the clothing of the Saviour (Jesus) in the tomb where Joseph of Arimathaea laid Him.

It was used for cord and sail-cloth ('white sails' are mentioned by Homer in the Odyssey), and it was used for lamp-wicks (Isaiah xlii. 3).

The seed-vessels with their five-celled capsules are referred to in the Bible as 'bolls,' and the expression 'the flax was bolled' (Exodus ix. 31) means that it had arrived at a state of maturity. When the bolls are ripe, the Flax is pulled and tied in bundles, and in order to assist the separation of the fibre from the stalks, the bundles are placed in water for several weeks, and then spread out to dry. This custom is alluded to in Joshua ii. 6. (The Bible)

Pliny writes:

'What department is there to be found of active life in which flax is not employed? And in what production of the Earth are there greater marvels to us than in this? To think that here is a plant which brings Egypt to close proximity to Italy! - so much so, in fact, that Galerius and Balbillus, both of them prefects of Egypt, made the passage to Alexandria from the Straits of Sicily, the one in six days, the other in five! . . . What audacity in man! What criminal perverseness! Thus to sow a thing in the ground for the purpose of catching the winds and tempests; it being not enough for him, forsooth, to be borne upon the waves alone!'

Bartholomew the mediaeval herbalist, refers to the making of linen from the soaking of Flax in water till it is dried and turned in the sun and then bound in 'praty bundels' and afterwards 'knockyd, beten and brayd and carflyd, rodded and gnodded; ribbyd and heklyd, and at the last sponne'; of the bleaching, and finally of its many uses for making clothing, and for sails, and fish-nets, and thread and ropes, and strings ('for bows'), and measuring lines, and sheets ('to reste in'), and 'sackes and bagges, and purses (to put and to kepe thynges in').

Of the making of tow 'uneven and full of knobs' used for stuffing into the cracks in ships, and 'for bonds and byndynges and matches for candelles, for it is full drye and taketh sone fyre and brenneth.' 'And so,' he concludes somewhat breathlessly, 'none herbe is so needfull to so many dyurrse uses to mankynde as is the flexe.'

Darwin studied several species of Linum, and found that some like the primrose had flowers with two forms of stamens and pistil. His object was to test the relative degrees of fertility of the long and short-styled pistils. L. perenne, for instance, is dimorphic:

'Of the flowers on the long-styled plants he found that twelve were fertilized with their own form pollen, but from a different plant. A seed capsule was only set when pollinated from anthers of the same height as the stigmas.'

So Darwin concluded:

'We have the clearest evidence that the stigmas of each form require for full fertility that pollen from the stamens of a corresponding height, belonging to the opposite form, should be brought to them.' (Forms of Flowers, p. 92.)

This plant is visited by bees, who perform the function Darwin describes.

Many traditions are associated with this useful plant. Flax flowers were believed in the Middle Ages to be a protection against sorcery. The Bohemians have a belief that if seven-year-old children dance among Flax, they will become beautiful, and the whole plant was supposed to be under the protection of the goddess Hulda, who, in Teuton mythology, was held to have first taught mortals the art of growing Flax, of spinning, and of weaving it.

Cultivation and Preparation for Market:

Its cultivation in this country (UK) could only pay on a large scale. The very exhausting nature of the crop has prevented its extensive cultivation in England, and the area under cultivation has declined in consequence. This peculiarity was well known to the Ancients, and Pliny asserted that it scorched the ground. Its culture requires care and suitable soil to secure a good crop. It has been grown in large quantities in the alluvial soils of Lincolnshire and in the eastern counties, and flourishes well in Ireland. It succeeds best in deep, moist loams such as contain a large proportion of vegetable matter, in good condition, firm, not loose. Strong clays do not answer well, nor poor soils, nor such as are of a gravelly or sandy nature, nor should the soil be freshly manured.

It is best treated as a farm crop. Being quickly grown and quickly harvested, it can be grown after a winter root crop, being over and reaped in time to secure a catch crop for the following season. The seed, which must be kept dry, as damp injures it, is sown in March or April, in drills, 70 lb. to the acre, on land carefully prepared and freed from weeds by ploughing. The crop itself must be handweeded, or the roots, being surface rooted, will be injured. It should be reaped in August, before the seed is fully ripe. The fibres of the plant, when grown for Flax, are found to be softer and stronger when the blossom has just fallen and the stalk begins to turn yellow before the leaves fall, than if left standing till the seeds are quite mature. The seeds, however, will ripen after the plant is gathered, if they be allowed to remain on the plant for a time. The Dutch avail themselves of this fact with regard to their Flax crops. After pulling the plants they stack them. The seeds by this means ripen, while the fibres are collected at the most favourable period of their growth. They thus obtain both of the valuable products of the plant.

Historical Medicinal Uses - For Entertainment ONLY

Parts Used Medicinally: The fruit is a globular capsule, about the size of a small pea, containing in separate cells ten seeds, which are brown (white within), oval-oblong and flattened, pointed at one end, shining and polished on the surface, 1/6 to 1/4 inch long. They are inodorous except when powdered, but the taste is mucilaginous and slightly unpleasant.

Linseed varies much in size and tint - a yellowish variety occurring in India. Holland, Russia, the United States, Canada, the Argentine and India furnish the principal supplies. The Russian seed or Dutch-grown of Russian origin, though small, is preferred for Flax-growing, as it is hardier than the large southern seed from the Mediterranean and India. For medicinal purposes, English and Dutch seeds are preferred, on account of their freedom from weed-seeds and dirt. If containing more than 4 per cent of weedseeds, linseed may be said to be adulterated. Of English and Dutch seeds about twelve weigh 1 grain, but some of the Indian and Mediterranean varieties are twice as large and heavy.

Constituents: The envelope or testa of the seed contains about 15 per cent of mucilage. The seeds themselves contain in the cotyledons and endosperm from 30 to 40 per cent of a fixed oil, of a light yellow colour, and about 25 per cent proteids, together with wax, resin, sugar, phosphates, acetic acid, and a small quantity of the glucoside Linamarin. On incineration, linseed should not yield more than 5 per cent of ash.

The oil is obtained by expression, with little or no heat. The cake which remains after expressing the oil, and which contains the farinaceous and mucilaginous part of the seed, is familiarly known as oil-cake, and is largely used as a fattening food for cattle. It is also used as a manure. When ground up, it is known as linseed meal, which is employed for making poultices. The meal is sold in two forms, crushed linseed and linseed meal. Formerly linseed meal was always obtained by grinding English oil-cake to powder and contained little oil, but now the crushed seeds, containing all the oil, are official. Crushed linseed of good quality usually contains from 30 to 35 per cent of oil.

Linseed oil rapidly absorbs oxygen from the air and forms, when laid on in thin layers, a hard, transparent varnish. It is largely used in the arts for its properties as a drying oil. It is a viscid, yellow liquid, its chief constituent being Linolein. It also contains palmitin, stearin and myristin, with glyceride of linoleic acid. Boiled oil, produced by heating raw linseed oil to a temperature of 150 degrees C., together with a small proportion of a metallic drier, possesses the drying properties of linseed oil to an enhanced degree. It becomes of a brown colour and dries much more rapidly, and in this state is used in the manufacture of printer's ink.

Medicinal Action and Uses: Emollient, demulcent, pectoral. The crushed seeds or linseed meal make a very useful poultice, either alone or with mustard. In ulceration and superficial or deep-seated inflammation a linseed poultice allays irritation and pain and promotes suppuration. The addition of a little lobelia seed makes it of greater value in cases of boils. It is commonly used for abscesses and other local affections.

Linseed is largely employed as an addition to cough medicines. As a domestic remedy for colds, coughs and irritation of the urinary organs, linseed tea is most valuable. A little honey and lemon juice makes it very agreeable and more efficacious. This demulcent infusion contains a large quantity of mucilage, and is made from 1 oz. of the ground or entire seeds to 1 pint of boiling water. It is taken in wineglassful doses, which may be repeated ad libitum.

Linseed oil, mixed with an equal quantity of lime water, known then as Carron Oil, is an excellent application for burns and scalds.

Internally, the oil is sometimes given as a laxative; in cases of gravel and stone it is excellent, and has been administered in pleurisy with great success. It may also be used as an injection in constipation. Mixed with honey, linseed oil has been used as a cosmetic for removing spots from the face.

The oil enters into veterinary pharmacy as a purgative for sheep and horses, and a jelly formed by boiling the seeds is often given to calves.

Linseed is often employed, with other seeds, as food for small birds.

Plantain seeds, also a favourite food of small birds, can, it is said, be used instead of linseed in making poultices, as they contain much mucilage, though not so much oil.

Linseed has occasionally been employed as human food - we hear of the seeds being mixed with corn by the ancient Greeks and Romans for making bread - but it affords little actual nourishment and is apparently unwholesome, being difficult of digestion and provoking flatulence.

The meal has sometimes been used fraudulently for adulterating pepper.

Garlic

Quick Facts

Latin/Linnaen:	*Alium Sativum*
Family:	*Amaryllidaceae*
Old English :	Garleac
Synonyms:	Poor Man's Treacle
Action:	Antibacterial, Antimycotic, Lipid-lowering, Inhibition of platelet aggregation, Prolongation of bleeding and clotting time, enhancement of fibrinolytic activity.
Parts Used:	Root
Indicated For:	Supportive to dietary measures at elevated levels of lipids in blood. Preventative measures for age-dependent vascular changes.
Dosage:	Unless otherwise prescribed: Average daily dosage: 4g fresh garlic; equivalent preparations.
Preparation:	Minced bulb and preparations thereof for internal use.
Cautions:	Rare occasions: gastrointestinal symptoms, changes to the flora of the intestine, or allergic reactions. Note: the odor of garlic can pervade the breath and skin.
Other Uses:	**Culinary**: Commonly used in cooking

Description

Allium sativum, commonly known as garlic, is a species in the onion genus, *Allium*. Its close relatives include the onion, shallot, leek, chive, and rakkyo. Dating back over 6,000 years, garlic is native to central Asia, and has long been a staple in the Mediterranean region, as well as a frequent seasoning in Asia, Africa, and Europe. It was known to Ancient Egyptians, and has been used throughout its history for both culinary and medicinal purposes.

The ancestry of cultivated garlic is not definitively established. According to Zohary and Hopf, "A difficulty in the identification of its wild progenitor is the sterility of the cultivars", though it is thought to be descendent from the species Allium longicuspis, which grows wild in central and southwestern Asia. *Allium sativum* grows in the wild in areas where it has become naturalised. The "wild garlic", "crow garlic", and "field garlic" of Britain are members of the species *Allium ursinum*, *Allium vineale*, and *Allium oleraceum*, respectively. In North America, *Allium vineale* (known as "wild garlic" or "crow garlic") and *Allium canadense*, known as "meadow garlic" or "wild garlic" and "wild onion", are common weeds in fields. One of the best-known "garlics", the so-called elephant garlic, is actually a wild leek (*Allium ampeloprasum*), and not a true garlic. Single clove garlic (also called pearl or solo garlic) originated in the Yunnan province of China.

Cultivation

Hardiness Zone:	3-8
Soil pH:	6.0-7.5
Soil type:	Soil rich in organic matter, well drained.
Cultivation:	Grown from bulbs or bulblets (produced from the flower of the garlic plant) planted in fall after a good frost. For best bulbs, remove scapes (the flower tops) before they flower. Ready to harvest when the top of the plant dries up and starts to bend.
Sunlight:	Full sun is best, but can tolerate partial sun
Habitat:	Native to central Asia, but is now grown all over the world

Weeding is crucial for garlic to thrive. Clove size is a more reliable determinant than bulb size for the future bulb. Garlic scapes can be used in place of garlic in cooking before the bulb is ready. Do not store garlic in the refrigerator as the cold will set it to sprouting. Once the bulbs are harvested, they need to cure. This should be done in a shady dry area. They are ready to be stored when the root crowns are hard, the skin is papery and the cloves separate easily. They can be braided and stored in a cool dry place for many months. Do not store in oil, as there is a risk of botulism.

Historical Notes

Garlic has been used as both food and medicine in many cultures for thousands of years, dating at least as far back as when the Giza pyramids were built. Garlic is mentioned in the Bible and the Talmud. Hippocrates, Galen, Pliny the Elder, and Dioscorides all mention the use of garlic for many conditions, including parasites, respiratory problems, poor digestion, and low energy. Its use in China was first mentioned in AD 510.

It was consumed by ancient Greek and Roman soldiers, sailors, and rural classes, and, according to Pliny the Elder, by the African peasantry. Galen eulogizes it as the "rustic's theriac" (cure-all), and Alexander Neckam, a writer of the 12th century, recommends it as a palliative for the heat of the sun in field labor.

In the account of Korea's establishment as a nation, gods were said to have given mortal women with bear and tiger temperaments an immortal's black garlic before mating with them. This is a genetically unique, six-clove garlic that was to have given the women supernatural powers and immortality. This garlic is still cultivated in a few mountain areas today.

In his Natural History, Pliny gives an exceedingly long list of scenarios in which it was considered beneficial. Dr. T. Sydenham valued it as an application in confluent smallpox, and, says Cullen, found some dropsies cured by it alone. Early in the 20th century, it was sometimes used in the treatment of pulmonary tuberculosis or phthisis.

Garlic was rare in traditional English cuisine (though it is said to have been grown in England before 1548) and has been a much more common ingredient in Mediterranean Europe. Garlic was placed by the ancient Greeks on the piles of stones at crossroads, as a supper for Hecate (Theophrastus, Characters, The Superstitious Man). A similar practice of hanging garlic, lemon and red chilli at the door or in a shop to ward off potential evil, is still very common in India. According to Pliny, garlic and onions were invoked as deities by the Egyptians at the taking of oaths. (Pliny also stated garlic demagnetizes lodestones, which is not factual.)The inhabitants of Pelusium, in lower Egypt (who worshiped the onion), are said to have had an aversion to both onions and garlic as food.

To prevent the plant from running to leaf, Pliny advised bending the stalk downward and covering with earth; seeding, he observes, may be prevented by twisting the stalk (by "seeding", he most likely meant the development of small, less potent bulbs).The Common Garlic a member of the same group of plants as the Onion, is of such antiquity as a cultivated plant, that it is difficult with any certainty to trace the country of its origin. De Candolle, in his treatise on the Origin of Cultivated Plants, considered that it was apparently indigenous to the southwest of Siberia, whence it spread to southern Europe, where it has become naturalized, and is said to be found wild in Sicily. It is widely cultivated in the Latin countries bordering on the Mediterranean. Dumas has described the air of Provence as being 'particularly perfumed by the refined essence of this mystically attractive bulb.'

The leaves are long, narrow and flat like grass. The bulb (the only part eaten) is of a compound nature, consisting of numerous bulblets, known technically as 'cloves,' grouped together between the membraneous scales and enclosed within a whitish skin, which holds them as in a sac.

The flowers are placed at the end of a stalk rising direct from the bulb and are whitish, grouped together in a globular head, or umbel, with an enclosing kind of leaf or spathae, and among them are small bulbils.

It was largely consumed by the ancient Greeks and Romans, as we may read in Virgil's Eclogues. Horace, however, records his detestation of Garlic, the smell of which, even in his days (as much later in Shakespeare's time), was accounted a sign of vulgarity. He calls it 'more poisonous than hemlock,' and relates how he was made ill by eating it at the table of Maecenas. Among the ancient Greeks, persons who partook of it were not allowed to enter the temples of Cybele. Homer, however, tells us that it was to the virtues of the 'Yellow Garlic' that Ulysses owed his escape from being changed by Circe into a pig, like each of his companions.

Homer also makes Garlic part of the entertainment which Nestor served up to his guest Machaon.

There is a Mohammedan legend that:

'when Satan stepped out from the Garden of Eden after the fall of man, Garlick sprang up from the spot where he placed his left foot, and Onion from that where his right foot touched.'

There is a curious superstition in some parts of Europe, that if a morsel of the bulb be chewed by a man running a race it will prevent his competitors from getting ahead of him, and Hungarian jockeys will sometimes fasten a clove of Garlic to the bits of their horses in the belief that any other racers running close to those thus baited, will fall back the instant they smell the offensive odour.

Many of the old writers praise Garlic as a medicine, though others, including Gerard, are sceptical as to its powers. Pliny gives an exceedingly long list of complaints, in which it was considered beneficial, and Galen eulogizes it as the rustics' Theriac, or Heal-All. One of its older popular names in this country was 'Poor Man's Treacle,' meaning theriac, in which sense we find it in Chaucer and many old writers.

A writer in the twelfth century - Alexander Neckam - recommends it as a palliative for the heat of the sun in field labour, and in a book of travel, written by Mountstuart Elphinstone about 100 years ago, he says that-

'the people in places where the Simoon is frequent eat Garlic and rub their lips and noses with it when they go out in the heat of the summer to prevent their suffering from the Simoon.'

Garlic is mentioned in several Old English vocabularies of plants from the tenth to the fifteenth centuries, and is described by the herbalists of the sixteenth century from Turner (1548) onwards. It is stated to have been grown in England before the year 1540. In Cole's Art of Simpling we are told that cocks which have been fed on Garlic are *'most stout to fight, and 50 are Horses'*: and that if a garden is infested with moles, Garlic or leeks will make them *'leap out of the ground presently.'*

The name is of Anglo-Saxon origin, being derived from gar (a spear) and lac (a plant), in reference to the shape of its leaves.

Cultivation: The ground should be prepared in a similar manner as for the closely allied onion.

The soil may be sandy, loam or clay, though Garlic flourishes best in a rich, moist, sandy soil. Dig over well, freeing the ground from all lumps and dig some lime into it. Tread firmly. Divide the bulbs into their component 'cloves' - each fair-sized bulb will divide into ten or twelve cloves - and with a dibber put in the cloves separately, about 2 inches deep and about 6 inches apart, leaving about 1 foot between the rows. It is well to give a dressing of soot.

Garlic beds should be in a sunny spot. They must be kept thoroughly free from weeds and the soil gathered up round the roots with a Dutch hoe from time to time.

When planted early in the spring, in February or March, the bulbs should be ready for lifting in August, when the leaves will be beginning to wither. Should the summer have been wet and cold, they may probably not be ready till nearly the middle of September.

The use of Garlic as an antiseptic was in great demand during the past war (WWI). In 1916 the Government asked for tons of the bulbs, offering 1s. per lb. for as much as could be produced. Each pound generally represents about 20 bulbs, and 5 lb. divided up into cloves and planted, will yield about 38 lb. at the end of the growing season, so it will prove a remunerative crop.

The following appeared in the Morning Post of December 12, 1922:

'A Dog's Recovery

'*Mr. W. H. Butlin, Tiptree, records the following experience: A fox-terrier, aged 14 years, appeared to be developing rapidly a pitiable condition, with a swollen neck and an ugly intractable sore at the root of the tail, and dull, coarse coat shedding abundantly. I administered "Yadil Antiseptic" in his drinking water and in less than a month the dog became perfectly sound and well, a mirabile dictu, his coat became firm, soft, and glossy.*' *(Yadil is a patent medicine said to contain Garlic.)*

'In cases of arterial tension, MM. Chailley-Bert, Cooper, and Debrey, at the Society of Biology, recommended about 30 drops of alcoholic extract as a remedy. To be administered by the mouth or intravenously.'

The crow garlic (*A. vineale*) is widely distributed and fairly common in many districts, but the bulbs are very small and the labour of digging them would be great. It is frequent in pastures and communicates its rank taste to milk and butter, when eaten by cows.

NOTE.--Professor Henslow calls *A. vineale* the Field Garlic, and *A. oleraceum* the Crow Garlic.

Ramsons (*A. ursinum*) grows in woods and has a very acrid taste and smell, but it also has very small bulbs, which would hardly render it of practical use.

Ransoms is also very generally known as 'Broad-leaved Garlic.'

The field garlic (*A. oleraceum*) is rather a rare plant. Both this and the Crow Garlic have, however, occasionally been employed as potherbs or for flavouring. It is an old country notion that if crows eat Crow Garlic, it stupefies them.

Ramsons, the wild Wood Garlic, but for its evil smell would rank among the most beautiful of British plants. Its broad leaves are very similar to those of the Lily-of-the-Valley, and its star-like flowers are a dazzling white, but its odour is too strong to admit of it being picked for its beauty, and many woods, especially in the Cotswold Hills, are spots to be avoided when it is in flower, being so closely carpeted with the plants that every step taken brings out the offensive odour.

There are many species of Allium grown in the garden, the flowers of some of which are even sweet-smelling (as *A. odorum* and *A. fragrans*), but they are the exceptions, and even these have the Garlic scent in their leaves and roots.

Constituents: The active properties of Garlic depend on a pungent, volatile, essential oil, which may readily be obtained by distillation with water. It is a sulphide of the radical Allyl, present in all the onion family. This oil is rich in sulphur, but contains no oxygen. The pecular penetrating odour of Garlic is due to this intensely smelling sulphuret of allyl, and is so diffusive that even when the bulb is applied to the soles of the feet, its odour is exhaled by the lungs.

Historical Medicinal Uses - For Entertainment ONLY

Medicinal Action and Uses: Diaphoretic, diuretic, expectorant, stimulant. Many marvellous effects and healing powers have been ascribed to Garlic. It possesses stimulant and stomachic properties in addition to its other virtues.

As an antiseptic, its use has long been recognized. In the late war it was widely employed in the control of suppuration in wounds. The raw juice is expressed, diluted with water, and put on swabs of sterilized Sphagnum moss, which are applied to the wound. Where this treatment has been given, it has been proved that there have been no septic results, and the lives of thousands of men have been saved by its use.

It is sometimes externally applied in ointments and lotions, and as an antiseptic, to disperse hard swellings, also pounded and employed as a poultice for scrofulous sores. It is said to prevent anthrax in cattle, being largely used for the purpose.

In olden days, Garlic was employed as a specific for leprosy. It was also believed that it had most beneficial results in cases of smallpox, if cut small and applied to the soles of the feet in a linen cloth, renewed daily.

It formed the principal ingredient in the 'Four Thieves' Vinegar,' which was adapted so successfully at Marseilles for protection against the plague when it prevailed there in 1722. This originated, it is said, with four thieves who confessed, that whilst protected by the liberal use of aromatic vinegar during the plague, they plundered the dead bodies of its victims with complete security.

It is stated that during an outbreak of infectious fever in certain poor quarters of London, early last century (1800's), the French priests who constantly used Garlic in all their dishes, visited the worst cases with impunity, whilst the English clergy caught the infection, and in many instances fell victims to the disease.

Syrup of Garlic is an invaluable medicine for asthma, hoarseness, coughs, difficulty of breathing, and most other disorders of the lungs, being of particular virtue in chronic bronchitis, on account of its powers of promoting expectoration. It is made by pouring a quart of water, boiled hot, upon a pound of the fresh root, cut into slices, and allowed to stand in a closed vessel for twelve hours, sugar then being added to make it of the consistency of syrup. Vinegar and honey greatly improve this syrup as a medicine. A little caraway and sweet fennel seed bruised and boiled for a short time in the vinegar before it is added to the Garlic, will cover the pungent smell of the latter.

A remedy for asthma, that was formerly most popular, is a syrup of Garlic, made by boiling the bulbs till soft and adding an equal quantity of vinegar to the water in which they have been boiled, and then sugared and boiled down to a syrup. The syrup is then poured over the boiled bulbs, which have been allowed to dry meanwhile, and kept in a jar. Each morning a bulb or two is to be taken, with a spoonful of the syrup.

Syrup made by melting 1 1/2 oz. of lump sugar in 1 oz. of the raw expressed juice may be given to children in cases of coughs without inflammation.

The successful treatment of tubercular consumption by Garlic has been recorded, the freshly expressed juice, diluted with equal quantities of water, or dilute spirit of wine, being inhaled antiseptically.

Bruised and mixed with lard, it has been proved to relieve whooping-cough if rubbed on the chest and between the shoulder-blades.

An infusion of the bruised bulbs, given before and after every meal, has been considered of good effect in epilepsy.

A clove or two of Garlic, pounded with honey and taken two or three nights successively, is good in rheumatism.

Garlic has also been employed with advantage in dropsy, removing the water which may already have collected and preventing its future accumulation. It is stated that some dropsies have been cured by it alone.

If sniffed into the nostrils, it will revive a hysterical sufferer. Amongst physiological results, it is reported that Garlic makes the eye retina more sensitive and less able to bear strong light.

The juice of Garlic, and milk of Garlic made by boiling the bruised bulbs in milk is used as a vermifuge.

Preparations: Juice, 10 to 30 drops. Syrup, 1 drachm. Tincture, 1/2 to 1 drachm.

Wine of Garlic - made by macerating three or four bulbs in a quart of proof spirit is a good stimulant lotion for baldness of the head.

Used in cookery it is a great aid to digestion, and keeps the coats of the stomach healthy. For this reason, essential oil is made from it and is used in the form of pills.

If a very small piece is chopped fine and put into chicken's food daily, it is a sure preventative of the gapes. Pullets will lay finer eggs by having garlic in their food before they start laying, but when they commence to lay it must be stopped, otherwise it will flavour the eggs.

Mrs. Beeton (in an old edition of her Household Management, 1866) gives the following recipe for making 'Bengal Mango Chutney,' which she states was given by a native to an English lady who had long been a resident in India, and who since her return to England had become quite celebrated amongst her friends for the excellence of this Eastern relish.

Ingredients. 1 1/2 lb. moist sugar, 3/4 lb. salt, 1/4 lb. Garlic, 1/4 lb. onions, 3/4 lb. powdered ginger, 1/4 lb. dried chillies, 3/4 lb. dried mustard-seed, 3/4 lb. stoned raisins, 2 bottles of best vinegar, 30 large, unripe, sour apples.

Mode. The sugar must be made into syrup; the Garlic, onions and ginger be finely pounded in a mortar; the mustard-seed be washed in cold vinegar and dried in the sun; the apples be peeled, cored and sliced, and boiled in a bottle and a half of the vinegar. When all this is done, and the apples are quite cold, put them into a large pan and gradually mix the whole of the rest of the ingredients, including the remaining half-bottle of vinegar. It must be well stirred until the whole is thoroughly blended, and then put into bottles for use. Tie a piece of wet bladder over the mouths of the bottles, after which they are well corked. This chutney is very superior to any which can be bought, and one trial will prove it to be delicious.

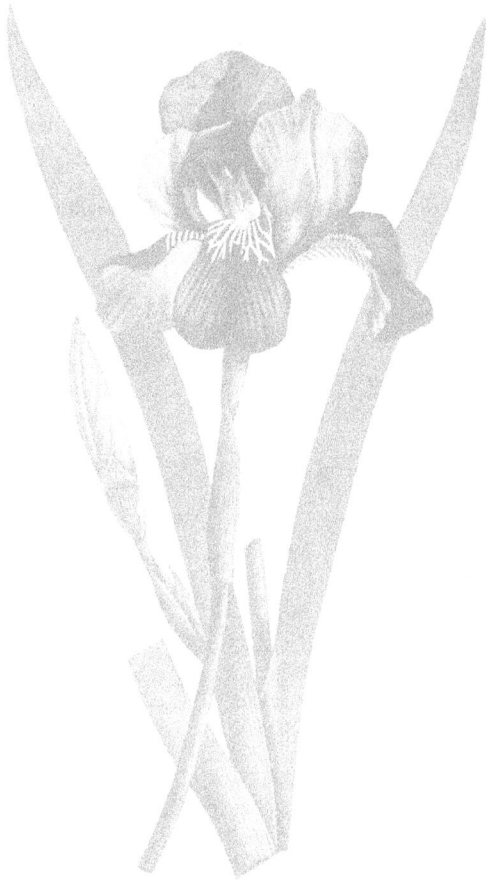

Heartsease

Violaceae

Viola tricolor L.

Quick Facts

Latin/Linnaen:	*Viola tricolor*
Family:	*Violaceae*
Old English :	Banwyrt, Banwort, Banewort
Synonyms:	Bonewort, Bullweed, Wild pansy', Viola, Johnny Jump-up, Wild Pansy. Love-Lies-Bleeding. Love-in-Idleness. Live-in-Idleness. Loving Idol, Cull Me, Cuddle Me, Call-me-to-you, Jackjump-up-and-kiss-me, Meet-me-in-the-Entry, Kiss-her-in-the-Buttery, Three-Faces-under-a-Hood, Kit-run-in-the-Fields, Pink-o'-the-Eye, Kit-run-about, Godfathers and Godmothers, Stepmother, Herb Trinitatis, Herb Constancy, Pink-eyed-John, Bouncing Bet, Flower o'luce, Bird's Eye, (French) Pensée. Heartsease has up to two hundred colloquial names!
Action:	Unknown
Parts Used:	Above ground parts.
Indicated For:	External: mild seborrheic skin diseases, milk scall (crust) in children.
Dosage:	Unless otherwise prescribed: 1.5g of drug per cup of water as tea, 3 times daily, equivalent preparations.
Preparation:	Chopped herb for teas and decoctions and for other galenical preparations for external use.
Cautions:	
Other Uses:	**Dye:** The flowers have been used to make yellow, green and blue-green dyes, **Misc:** The leaves can be used to make a chemical indicator.

Description

Viola tricolor, known as Heartsease, is a common European wild flower, growing as an annual or short-lived perennial. It has been introduced into North

America, where it has spread widely, and is known as the Johnny Jump Up (though this name is also applied to similar species such as the Yellow Pansy). It is the progenitor of the cultivated Pansy, and is therefore sometimes called Wild Pansy; before the cultivated Pansies were developed, "Pansy" was an alternative name for the wild form.

Heartsease is a small plant of creeping and ramping habit, reaching at most 15 cm in height, with flowers about 1.5 cm in diameter. It grows in short grassland on farms and wasteland, chiefly on acid or neutral soils. It is usually found in partial shade. It flowers from April to September. The flowers can be purple, blue, yellow or white. They are hermaphrodite and self-fertile, pollinated by bees.

As its name implies, Heartsease has a long history of use in herbalism. It has been recommended, among other uses, for epilepsy, asthma, skin diseases and eczema. *V. tricolor* has a history in folk medicine of helping respiratory problems such as bronchitis, asthma, and cold symptoms. It has expectorant properties, and so has been used in the treatment of chest complaints such as bronchitis and whooping cough. It is also a diuretic, leading to its use in treating rheumatism and cystitis.

Cultivation

Hardiness Zone:	4-10 (annual/short lived perennial)
Soil pH:	6.0-6.5
Soil type:	Prefers cool moist well drained soil.
Cultivation:	Sow by seed, in fall or spring.
Sunlight:	Full sun-part shade
Habitat:	Native to Europe, north Africa and Asia. Lawns and meadows

Heartsease freely self seeds and does well in a cool environment. They often appear early in spring and fade during the heat of summer to reappear once the temperature cools. The flowers make a colorful addition to salads.

Historical Notes

Long before cultivated pansies were released into the trade in 1839, Heartsease was associated with thought in the "language of flowers", often by its alternative name of pansy (from the French "pensée" - thought) hence Ophelia's often quoted line in Shakespeare's Hamlet, "There's pansies, that's for thoughts". What Shakespeare had in mind was Heartsease, not a modern garden pansy.

Shakespeare makes a more direct reference, probably to Heartsease in A Midsummer Night's Dream. Oberon sends Puck to gather "a little western flower" that maidens call "Love-in-idleness". Oberon's account is that he diverted an arrow from Cupid's bow aimed at "a fair vestal, throned by the west" (supposedly Queen Elizabeth I) to fall upon the plant "before milk-white, now purple with love's wound". The "imperial vot'ress" passes on "fancy-free", destined never to fall in love. The juice of the heartsease now, claims Oberon, "on sleeping eyelids laid, Will make man or woman madly dote upon the next live creature that it sees." Equipped with such powers, Oberon and Puck control the fates of various characters in the play to provide Shakespeare's essential dramatic and comic structure for the play.

Habitat: The Heartsease, or Wild Pansy, very different in habit from any other kind of Viola, is abundantly met with almost throughout Britain. Though found on hedgebanks and waste ground, it seems in an especial degree a weed of cultivation, found most freely in cornfields and garden ground. It blossoms almost throughout the entire floral season, expanding its attractive little flowers in the early days of summer and keeping up a succession of blossom until late in autumn.

Description: The Heartsease is as variable as any of the other members of the genus, but whatever modifications of form it may present, it may always be readily distinguished from the other Violets by the general form of its foliage, which is much more cut up than in any of the other species and by the very large leafy stipules at the base of the true leaves. The stem, too, branches more than is commonly found in the other members of the genus. Besides the free branching of the stem, which is mostly 4 to 8 inches in height, it is generally very angular. The leaves are deeply cut into rounded lobes, the terminal one being considerably the largest. In the other species of Viola the foliage is ordinarily very simple in outline, heartshaped, or kidney-shaped, having its edge finely toothed.

The flowers (1/4 to 1 1/4 inch across) vary a great deal in colour and size, but are either purple, yellow or white, and most commonly there is a combination of all these colours in each blossom. The upper petals are generally most showy in colour and purple in tint, while the lowest and broadest petal is usually a more or less deep tint of yellow. The base of the lowest petal is elongated into a spur, as in the Violet.

The flowers are in due course succeeded by the little capsules of seeds, which when ripe, open by three valves. Though a near relative of the Violet, it does not produce any of the curious bud-like flowers - cleistogamous flowers - characteristic of the Violet, as its ordinary showy flowers manage to come to fruition so that there is no necessity for any others. Darwin found that the humble bee was the commonest insect visitor of the Heartsease, though the moth Pluvia visited it largely - another observer mentions Thrips small wingless insects - as frequent visitors to the flowers. Darwin considered that the cultivated Pansy rarely set seed if there were no insect visitors, but that the little Field Pansy can certainly fertilize itself if necessary.

The flower protects itself from rain and dew by drooping its head both at night and in wet weather, and thus the back of the flower and not its face receives the moisture.

It is a very widely distributed plant, found not only throughout Britain, but in such diverse places as Arctic Europe, North Africa, Siberia and N.W. India. Several of the varieties have been distinguished as subspecies: the most marked of these are *V. arvensis*, most common in cornfields, with white or yellowish flowers, with spreading petals; and lutea, which has a branched rootstock, short stems, with underground runners, and blue, purple or yellow flowers with spreading petals much longer than the sepals.

'Love in Idleness' is still in use in Warwickshire. In ancient days the plant was much used for its potency in love charms, hence perhaps its name of Heartsease. It is this flower that plays such an important part as a love-charm in the Midsummer Night's Dream.

The celebrated Quesnay, founder of the 'Economists,' physician to Louis XV, was called by the king his 'thinker,' and given, as an armorial bearing, three pansy flowers.

In many old Herbals the plant is called Herba Trinitatis, being dedicated by old writers to the Trinity, because it has in each flower three colours.

Stepmother is a familiar name for it in both France and Germany, from a fanciful reference to the different-shaped petals, supposed to represent a stepmother, her own daughters and her stepchildren.

Historical Medicinal Uses - For Entertainment ONLY

Part Used Medicinally and Preparation for Market: The whole herb, collected in the wild state and dried.

The Wild Pansy may be collected any time from June to August, when the foliage is in the best condition.

Constituents: The herb contains an active chemical principle, Violine (a substance similar to Emetin, having an emeto-cathartic action), mucilage, resin, sugar, salicylic acid and a bitter principle. When bruised, the plant, and especially the root, smells like peach kernels or prussic acid. The seeds are considered to have the same therapeutic activity as the leaves and flowers.

Medicinal Action and Uses: The Pansy has very similar properties to the Violet.

It was formerly in much repute as a remedy for epilepsy, asthma and numerous other complaints, and the flowers were considered cordial and good in diseases of the heart, from which may have arisen its popular name of Heartsease as much as from belief in it as a love potion.

Gerard states:

'It is good as the later physicians write for such as are sick of ague, especially children and infants, whose convulsions and fits of the falling sickness it is thought to cure. It is commended against inflammation of the lungs and chest, and against scabs and itchings of the whole body and healeth ulcers.'

A strong decoction of syrup of the herb and flowers was recommended by the older herbalists for skin diseases and a homoeopathic medicinal tincture is still made from it with spirits of wine, using the entire plant, and given in small diluted doses for the cure of cutaneous eruptions.

It was formerly official in the United States Pharmacopoeia, and is still employed in America in the form of an ointment and poultice in eczema and other skin troubles, and internally for bronchitis.

Some years ago attention was called to this herb by a writer in the Medical Journal as a valuable remedy for the cutaneous disorder called crusta lactes, or Scald head, in children. For this purpose, 1/2 drachm of dried leaves, or a handful of the fresh herb boiled in milk, was recommended to be given every morning and evening: poultices formed of the leaves were likewise applied with success. By several medical writers its use is said to have proved very efficacious in this complaint.

On the Continent, the herbaceous parts of the plant have been employed for their mucilaginous, demulcent and expectorant properties. The root and seeds are also emetic and purgative, which properties as well as the expectorant action of the plant are doubtless due to the presence of the violine.

Pansy leaves are used on the Continent in place of litmus in acid and alkali tests.

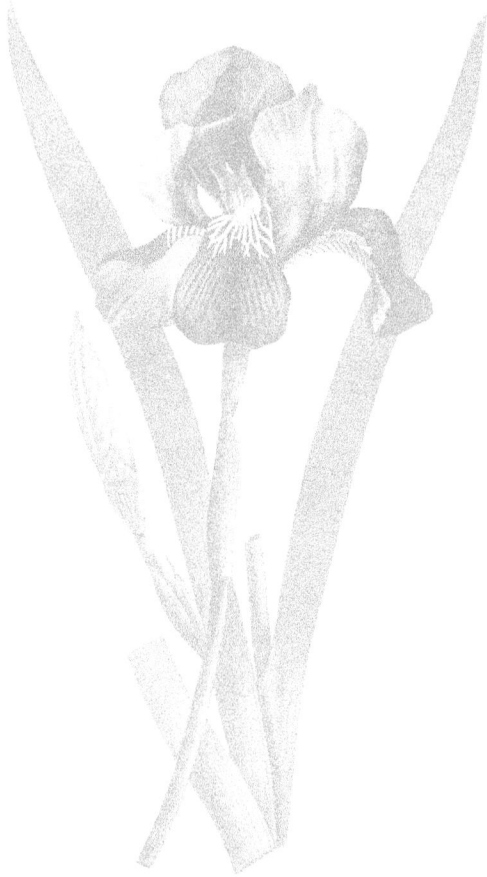

Henbane

Quick Facts

Latin/Linnaen:	*Hyoscamus Niger*
Family:	*Solanaceae*
Old English :	Belene
Synonyms:	Henbane, Hyoscyamus, Hog's-bean, Jupiter's-bean, Symphonica. Cassilata, Cassilago, Deus Caballinus, (Anglo-Saxon) Henbell, (French) Jusquiame.
Action:	Henbane preparations produce a parasympatholytic or anticholinergic effect by competitive inhibition of acetylcholine. This inhibition affects the muscarinic action of acetylcholine but not its nicotine like effects on ganglia and motor end-plates. Henbane preparations exert peripheral actions on the autonomic nervous system and on smooth muscle, as well as the central nervous system. Because of their parasympatholytic properties, they cause relaxation of organs containing smooth muscle, particularly in the region of the gastrointestinal tract. Furthermore, they relieve muscular tremors of central nervous origin. The spectrum of actions includes a sedative effect.
Parts Used:	Leaf
Indicated For:	Spasms of the gastrointestinal tract
Dosage:	Unless otherwise prescribed: Average single dosage: 0.5 of standardized henbane powder corresponding to 0.25-0.35mg total alkaloid. Maximum single dosage: 1g of standardized henbane powder corresponding to 0.5-0.7mg total alkaloid. Maximum daily dosage: 3g of standardized henbane powder corresponding to 1.5-2.1mg total alkaloid, calculated as hyoscyamine.
Preparation:	Standardized henbane powder and galenical preparations for internal application.
Cautions:	POISONOUS
	Contraindications: Tachycardiac arrhythmias, prostatic adenoma with urine retention, narrow-angle glaucoma, acute pulmonary edema, mechanical stenosis in any part of the gastrointestinal tract, megacolon. Side Effects: Dryness of the mouth, disturbances of optic conditions, tachycardia, difficulty in urination. Interactions: Enhancement of anticholinergic action by tricyclic antidepressants, amantadine, antihistimines, phenothiazines, procainamide

and quinidine.

Other Uses: None Known

Descripton

Henbane (*Hyoscyamus niger*, also known as stinking nightshade or black henbane, is a plant of the family *Solanaceae* that originated in Eurasia, though it is now globally distributed.

It was historically used in combination with other plants, such as mandrake, deadly nightshade, and datura as an anaesthetic potion, as well as for its psychoactive properties in "magic brews." These psychoactive properties include visual hallucinations and a sensation of flight. Its usage was originally in continental Europe, Asia and the Arab world, though it did spread to England in the Middle Ages. The use of henbane by the ancient Greeks was documented by Pliny. The plant, recorded as Herba Apollinaris, was used to yield oracles by the priestesses of Apollo.

The name henbane dates at least to A.D. 1265. The origins of the word are unclear but "hen" probably originally meant death rather than referring to chickens. Hyoscyamine, scopolamine, and other tropane alkaloids have been found in the foliage and seeds of the plant. Common effects of henbane ingestion in humans include hallucinations, dilated pupils, restlessness, and flushed skin. Less common symptoms such as tachycardia, convulsions, vomiting, hypertension, hyperpyrexia and ataxia have all been noted.

Henbane can be toxic, even fatal, to animals in low doses. Not all animals are susceptible, however; the larvae of some Lepidoptera species including Cabbage Moth eat henbane.

It was sometimes one of the ingredients in gruit, traditionally used in beers as a flavouring, until replaced by hops in the 11th to 16th centuries (for example, the Bavarian Purity Law of 1516 outlawed ingredients other than barley, hops, and water).

In 1910, an American homeopath living in London, Hawley Harvey Crippen, allegedly used scopolamine, an alkaloid extracted from henbane, to poison his wife.

Henbane is thought to have been the "hebenon" poured into the ear of Hamlet's father (although other candidates for hebenon exist.

Cultivation

Hardiness Zone:	5-10
Soil pH:	6.6-8.5
Soil type:	Light, moderately rich and well drained soil.
Cultivation:	Sow seed once the ground is warm in spring, or for fall planting in late summer, early fall.
Sunlight:	Full sun
Habitat:	Native to southern Europe and across western Asia. In the wild it can be found along waste ground and in places with stony soil.

Henbane occurs as an annual and as a biennial. Henbane leaves should be collected when the plant is in full flower. Some people report irritation from handling henbane, so care is advised.

Historical Notes

Henbane is found throughout Central and Southern Europe and in Western Asia, extending to India and Siberia. As a weed of cultivation it now grows also in North America and Brazil. It had become naturalized in North America prior to 1672, as we find it mentioned in a work published in that year among the plants 'sprung up since the English planted and kept cattle in New England.'

It is not considered truly indigenous to Great Britain, but occurs fairly frequently in parts of Scotland, England and Wales, and also in Ireland, and has been found wild in sixty British counties, chiefly in waste, sandy places, by road-sides, on rubbish heaps and near old buildings, having probably first escaped from the old herb gardens. It is frequently found on chalky ground and particularly near the sea. It appears to have been more common in Gerard's time (Queen Elizabeth's reign) than it is now.

Henbane (Hyoscyamus niger, Linn.) is a member of the important order Solanaceae, to which belong the Potato, Tobacco and Tomato, and also the valuable Belladonna.

There are about eleven species of the genus Hyoscyamus, distributed from the Canary Islands over Europe and Northern Africa to Asia. All those which have been investigated contain similar principles and possess similar properties.

The medicinal uses of Henbane date from remote ages; it was well known to the Ancients, being particularly commended by Dioscorides (first century A.D.), who used it to procure sleep and allay pains, and Celsus (same period) and others made use of it for the same purpose, internally and externally, though Pliny declared it to be 'of the nature of wine and therefore offensive to the understanding.' There is mention of it in a work by Benedictus Crispus (A.D. 681) under the names of Hyoscyamus and Symphonica. In the tenth century, we again find its virtues recorded under the name of Jusquiasmus (the modern French name is Jusquiame). There is frequent mention made of it in AngloSaxon works on medicine of the eleventh century, in which it is named 'Henbell,' and in the old glossaries of those days it also appears as Caniculata, Cassilago and Deus Caballinus.

Later it fell into disuse. It was omitted from the London Pharmacopoeia of 1746 and 1788, and only restored in 1809, its re-introduction being chiefly due to experiments and recommendations by Baron Storch, who gave it in the form of an extract, in cases of epilepsy and other nervous and convulsive diseases.

It is supposed that this is the noxious herb referred to by Shakespeare in Hamlet:

'Sleeping within mine orchard,

My custom always of the afternoon

Upon my secure hour thy uncle stole,

With juice of cursed hebenon in a vial,

And in the porches of mine ear did pour

The leprous distillment.'

Other authorities argue that the name used here is a varied form of that by which the Yew is known in at least five of the Gothic languages, and which appears in Marlowe and other Elizabethan writers as 'hebon.' There can be little doubt that Shakespeare took both the name and the use of this plant from Marlowe, who mentions 'juice of hebon' as a deadly poison. Hebenus, according to Gower, is a 'sleepy tree.' Spenser, too, makes 'heben' a tree, and speaks of 'the deadly heben bow,' a weapon that could hardly be made of Henbane. 'This tree,' wrote Lyte in his Herball, 1578, 'is altogether venomous and against man's nature; such as do only sleepe under the shadow thereof become sicke and sometimes they die,' whereas he recommends the juice of Henbane as an application for earache.

Speaking of Henbane, Gerard says:

'The leaves, the seeds and the juice, when taken internally cause an unquiet sleep, like unto the sleep of drunkenness, which continueth long and is deadly to the patient. To wash the feet in a decoction of Henbane, as also the often smelling of the flowers causeth sleep.'

Culpepper says:

'I wonder how astrologers could take on them to make this an herb of Jupiter: and yet Mizaldus, a man of penetrating brain, was of that opinion as well as the rest: the herb is indeed under the dominion of Saturn and I prove it by this argument: All the herbs which delight most to grow in saturnine places are saturnine herbs. Both Henbane delights most to grow in saturnine places, and whole cart loads of it may be found near the places where they empty the common Jakes, and scarce a ditch to be found without it growing by it. Ergo, it is a herb of Saturn. The leaves of Henbane do cool all hot inflammations in the eyes.... It also assuages the pain of the gout, the sciatica, and other pains in the joints which arise from a hot cause. And applied with vinegar to the forehead and temples, helps the headache and want of sleep in hot fevers.... The oil of the seed is helpful for deafness, noise and worms in the ears, being dropped therein; the juice of the herb or root doth the same. The decoction of the herb or seed, or both, kills lice in man or beast. The fume of the dried herb stalks and seeds, burned, quickly heals swellings, chilblains or kibes in the hands or feet, by holding them in the fume thereof. The remedy to help those that have taken Henbane is to drink goat's milk, honeyed water, or pine kernels, with sweet wine; or, in the absence of these, Fennel seed, Nettle seed, the seed of Cresses, Mustard or Radish; as also Onions or Garlic taken in wine, do all help to free

them from danger and restore them to their due temper again. Take notice, that this herb must never be taken inwardly; outwardly, an oil, ointment, or plaister of it is most admirable for the gout . . . to stop the toothache, applied to the aching side....'

The leaves or roots eaten produce maniacal delirium, if nothing worse. Another old writer says:

'If it be used either in sallet or in pottage, then doth it bring frenzie, and whoso useth more than four leaves shall be in danger to sleepe without waking.'

It is poisonous in all its parts, and neither drying nor boiling destroys the toxic principle. The leaves are the most powerful portion, even the odour of them when fresh will produce giddiness and stupor. Accidental cases of poisoning by Henbane are, however, not very common, as the plant has too unpleasant a taste and smell to be readily mistaken for any esculent vegetable, but its roots, which are thick and somewhat like those of salsafy, have sometimes been gathered and eaten. In one case recorded, a woman pulled up a quantity of Henbane roots which she found in a field, supposing them to be parsnips. She boiled them in soup, which was eaten by the family. The whole of the nine persons who had partaken of them suffered severely, being soon seized with indistinctness of vision, giddiness and sleepiness, followed by delirium and convulsions.

It is also recorded that the whole of the inmates of a monastery were once poisoned by using the roots instead of chicory. The monks partaking of the roots for supper were all more or less affected during the night and following day, being attacked with a sort of delirious frenzy, accompanied in many cases by such hallucinations that the establishment resembled a lunatic asylum.

The herb was used in magic and diabolism, for its power of throwing its victims into convulsions. It was employed by witches in their midnight brews, and from the leaves was prepared a famous sorcerer's ointment.

Anodyne necklaces were made from the root and were hung about the necks of children as charms to prevent fits and to cause easy teething.

In mythology, we read that the dead in Hades were crowned with it as they wandered hopelessly beside the Styx.

The herb is also called Hog's-bean, and both its botanical name Hyoscyamus and the tenth-century Jusquiasmus are derived from the Greek words hyos and cyamos, signifying 'the bean of the hog,' which animal is supposed to eat it with impunity. An old AngloSaxon name for it was 'Belene,' probably from the bell-shaped flowers; then it became known as 'Hen-bell,' and from the time that its poisonous properties were recognized this name was changed to 'Henbane,' because the seeds were thought to be fatal to poultry. Dr. Prior is inclined to think that the name Henbane is derived from the Spanish hinna (a mule), e.g. 'henna bell,' referring to the similarity of its seed-vessel to the bell hung upon the neck of the mules.

Although swine are said to feed upon the leaves and suffer no ill effects, this plant should not be allowed to grow in places to which cattle have access, though they seldom touch it, and its effects seem less violent on most of the larger domestic animals than on man, sheep will sometimes eat it when young, and it has occasionally been noticed that no bad effects have followed. Cows, however, have been poisoned by having Henbane mixed with their forage, it is said for the purpose of fattening them. A small quantity of the seeds of the Stramonium or Thornapple, as well as those of Henbane, are also sometimes added, the idea appears to be that the tendency to stupor and repose caused by these plants is conducive to fattening. In some districts, horse-dealers mix the seeds of Henbane with their oats, in order to fatten their animals.

Description: H. niger is susceptible of considerable diversity of character, causing varieties which have by some been considered as distinct species. Thus the plant is sometimes annual, the stem almost unbranched, smaller and less downy than in the biennial form, the leaves shorter and less hairy and the flowers often yellow, without any purple markings. The annual plant also flowers in July or August, the biennial in May and June.

The annual and biennial form spring indifferently from the same crop of seed, the former growing during summer to a height of from 1 to 2 feet, and flowering and perfecting seed, the latter producing the first season only a tuft of radical leaves, which disappear in winter, leaving underground a thick, fleshy root, from the crown of which arises in spring a branched, flowering stem, usually much taller and more vigorous than the flowering stems of the annual plants. The annual form is apparently produced by the weaker and later developed seeds formed in the fruit at the ends of the shoots; it is considered to be less active than the typical species and differs in being of dwarfed growth and having rather paler flowers. The British drug of commerce consists of dense flowering shoots only, and of larger size.

Both varieties are used in medicine, but the biennial form is the one considered official. The leaves of this biennial plant spread out flat on all sides from the crown of the root like a rosette; they are oblong and egg-shaped, with acute points, stalked and more or less sharply toothed, often more than a foot in length, of a greyish-green colour and covered with sticky hairs. These leaves perish at the appearance of winter. The flowering stem pushes up from the root-crown in the following spring, ultimately reaching from 3 to 4 feet in height, and as it grows, becoming branched and furnished with alternate, oblong, unequally lobed, stalkless leaves, which are stem-clasping and vary considerably in size, but seldom exceed 9 or 10 inches in length. These leaves are pale green in colour, with a broad conspicuous mid-rib, and are furnished on both sides (but particularly on the veins on the under surface) with soft, glandular hairs, which secrete a resinous substance that causes the fresh leaves to feel unpleasantly clammy and sticky. Similar hairs occur on the sub-cylindrical branches. The flowers are shortly stalked, the lower ones growing in the fork of the branches, the upper ones stalkless, crowded together in one sided, leafy spikes, which are rolled back at the top before flowering, the hairy, leafy, coarsely-toothed bracts becoming smaller upwards. The flowers have a hairy, pitcher shaped calyx, which remains round the fruit and is strongly veined, with five stiff, broad, almost prickly lobes. The corollas are obliquely funnel-shaped, upwards of an inch across, of a dingy yellow or buff, marked with a close network of lurid purple veins. A variety sometimes occurs in which the corolla is not marked with these purple veins. The seed-capsule opens transversely by a convex lid and contains numerous small seeds. Perhaps the most striking feature of the plant are these curious seed-vessels, a very detailed description of which is given in the works of Flavius Josephus, as it was upon this capsule that one of the ornaments of the Jewish High Priests' head-dress was modelled. The whole plant has a powerful, oppressive, nauseous odour.

Cultivation: Henbane is in such demand for medicinal purposes that it is necessary to cultivate it, the wild plants not yielding a sufficient supply. Both varieties were formerly cultivated in England, but at present the biennial is almost solely grown. English grown Henbane has always been nearly sufficient to provide enough fresh leaves for the preparation of the juice, or green extract, but large quantities, chiefly of the annual kind, were imported before the War (WWI) from Germany, Austria and Russia, in the form of dry leaves.

Henbane will grow on most soils, in sandy spots near the sea, on chalky slopes, and in cultivation flourishing in a good loam.

It is, however, very capricious in its growth, the seeds being prone to lie dormant for a season or more, refusing to germinate at all in some places, and the crop varying without any apparent reason, sometimes dying in patches. In some maritime localities it can be grown without any trouble. It requires a light, moderately rich and well-drained soil for successful growth and an open, sunny situation, but does not want much attention beyond keeping the ground free from weeds.

The seed should be sown in the open early in May or as soon as the ground is warm, as thinly as possible, in rows 2 to 2 1/2 feet apart, the seedlings thinned out to 2 feet apart in the rows, as they do not stand transplanting well. Only the larger seedlings should be reserved, especially those of a bluish tint. The soil where the crop is to be, must have been well manured, and must be kept moist until the seeds have germinated, and also during May and June of the first year. It is also recommended to sow seeds of biennial Henbane at their natural ripening time, August, in porous soil.

The ground must never be water-logged, especially in the first winter; it runs to stalk in a wet season. Drought and late frosts stunt the growth and cause it to blossom too early, and if the climatic conditions are unsuitable, especially in a dry spring and summer, the biennial Henbane will flower in its first year, while the growth is quite low, but well manured soil may prevent this.

Care must be taken in selecting the seed: commercial Henbane seed is often kiln-dried and useless for sowing. In order to more readily ensure germination, it is advisable to soak the seeds in water for twenty-four hours before planting: the unfertile seeds will then float on the top of the water and may thus be distinguished. Ripe seed should be grey, and yellowish or brown seeds should be rejected, as they are immature. Let the seeds dry and then sift out the smallest, keeping only the larger seeds.

Henbane seed being very small and light should be well mixed with fine dry soil as it is sown.

As seedlings often die off, a reserve should be kept in a box or bed to fill gaps, even though they do not always transplant success fully.

If it is desired to raise a crop of the annual variety the plants, being smaller and not branching so freely, may be grown at a distance of 18 inches apart each way, but the annual is very little cultivated in this country (UK).

If any annuals come up among the biennials sown, the flowers should be cut off until the leaves get larger and the stem branches.

There is usually some difficulty in growing Henbane owing to its destruction by insects: sometimes the whole of the foliage is destroyed by the larvae of a leaf-mining fly, Pegomyia Hyoscyami, and the crop is rendered worthless in a week. And when the large autumnal leaves of the first-year plants of the biennial variety decay, the large terminal bud is often destroyed by one of the various species of macro-lepidopterous caterpillars which hide themselves in the ground. The crown or bud should be covered as soon as the leaves have rotted away with soil mixed with soot or naphthaline, to prevent the depredations of these and other insects.

Floods may also rot the plants in winter, if grown on level ground. Potato pests are fond of the prickly leaves and will leave a potato patch to feed on the Henbane plant.

If mildew develops on the foliage in summer, dust the plants with powdered sulphur or spray with 1/2 oz. of liver of sulphur in 2 gallons of water.

When it is desired to preserve seed for propagation, it is well to cut off the top flowering shoots at an early stage of flowering (these may be dried and sold as flowering tops), and allow only about six seed-capsules to ripen. This will ensure strong seed to the capsules left, and this seed will probably produce biennial Henbane, weaker seeds being apt to produce the less robust and less valuable annual Henbane.

Seeds sown as soon as ripe in August may germinate in autumn, and thus constitute a biennial by growing on all through the winter and flowering the next summer.

Although the cultivation of Henbane in sandy ground near the sea, especially on the rich soil of estuaries, would probably pay well, it is hardly a profitable plant to grow in small gardens, more especially as the yield of dried leaf is very small. It is estimated that about 15 cwt. of dry herb are obtained from an acre of ground.

Parts Used, Preparation for Market: Henbane leaves are official in all pharmacopoeias. Some require that it be collected from uncultivated plants, others that it be not used after keeping for more than a year.

The official drug, according to the British Pharmacopoeia, consists of the fresh leaves, flowering tops and branches of the biennial variety of *H. niger*, and the same parts of the plant carefully dried.

The drug is preferably given in the form of the fluid extract or tincture. The smaller branches and leaves of the plant, with the leaves and flowers, is the drug from which the green extract and juice of Henbane are prepared, whilst the leaves and flowering tops are separated from the branches and dried and used for making tincture. The inspissated juice of the fresh leaves is considered exceedingly variable in its operation, and is not so much recommended.

The commercial drug presents three varieties, distinguished by the trade names 'Annual,' 'First Biennial' (the leaves from the biennial plant in its first year), and 'Biennial,' or 'Second Biennial,' the official drug, which is scarce and high-priced, the first two kinds commanding lower prices.

When grown in this country (UK), the official Henbane plant, as already mentioned, is usually biennial. The leaves of the first year's growth are collected and sold under the name of 'First Biennial Henbane.' This variety consists of large, stalked leaves, attaining 10 inches or more in length, and is of course free from flower.

Under certain conditions the biennial plant will flower in the first year: this is also collected and sold as 'Annual (English) Henbane.' It closely resembles the biennial, but the flowering tops are usually less dense, and the drug often contains portions of the stem. Such plants are much stronger than the foreign imported annual, and being more carefully dried are richer in alkaloids.

Formerly the second year's growth of the biennial plant was thought to contain a considerably larger percentage of alkaloid than either the first year's growth of the same plant, or the annual plant, and only the actual flowering tops of such plants were official, but it is now held that leaves from the English-grown species of all the above are practically of equal alkaloidal value, though the imported drug is of much less value.

Much Henbane is imported from Germany and Russia; this is probably collected mostly from annual plants, and often arrives in very poor condition, sometimes mixed with other species of Henbane. In consequence, English Henbane has always commanded a much higher price. Foreign annual Henbane is usually a much more slender plant than the English, and as imported its alkaloidal value is lower than that of the English-grown varieties. This may be due to the large proportion of stem, sand, etc., that the drug contains, the whole plant being cut and dried. It is probable that the well-dried leaves alone of all the varieties are of approximately equal alkaloidal strength.

Harvesting: Much of the efficacy of Henbane depends upon the time at which it is gathered. The leaves should be collected when the plant is in full flower. In the biennial plant, those of the second year are preferred to those of the first; the latter are less clammy and foetid, yield less extractive, and are medicinally considered less efficient. Sometimes, however, the plant is destroyed by a severe winter in England, and then no leaves of the second year's growth are obtainable, and it has been suggested that this is, perhaps, one of the causes of the great uncertainty of the medicine as found in commerce.

The leaves of the biennial variety are collected in June or the first week of July and those of the annual in August.

The leaves and flowering tops which constitute the 'Second Biennial Henbane' are collected either with or without the smaller branches to which they are attached and carefully dried, unless they are required for the preparation of the juice or green extract, when they should be sent to the distillery at once on cutting.

The herb when required in the fresh state should be cut the first week in June, because in the second week the leaf-mining insect attacks the leaves, leaving only patches of white epidermis.

The herb requires very careful drying, as its properties are liable to be in great measure destroyed if kept too long in a damp state.

The fresh herb loses 80 to 86 per cent of its weight on drying, 100 lb. yielding 14 to 20 lb. of dry herb.

The fresh leaves have, when bruised, a strong, disagreeable narcotic odour, somewhat like that of tobacco: their taste is mucilaginous and very slightly acrid. The characteristic odour disappears to a large extent on drying, but the bitter taste then becomes more pronounced.

When the dried leaves are thrown upon the fire they burn with a crackling noise from the nitrate they contain, and at the same time they emit a strong odour.

The dried drug consists principally of the flowering tops. In commerce, it is commonly found in irregular rounded or flattened masses, in which the coarsely-toothed hairy bracts, the yellowish corolla with deep purple lines and two-celled ovary, with numerous ovules, can easily be identified.

The root is not employed in medicine, but experiments have shown that the seeds not only possess all the properties of the plant, but have ten times the strength of the leaves. They are also employed in pharmacy, having been much used in the Middle Ages. At the present time, they are much prescribed by the Mohammedan doctors of India.

The seed should be gathered in August; it may be kiln-dried for medicinal purposes, but the treatment renders it useless for culture, and if required for propagation seeds should be sun-dried. The capsules should be harvested before the lids split off, the seeds then being shaken out and dried in the sun.

Constituents: The chief constituent of Henbane leaves is the alkaloid Hyoscyamine, together with smaller quantities of Atropine and Hyoscine, also known as Scopolamine.

The proportion of alkaloid in the British Pharmacopoeia dried drug varies from 0.045 to 0.14 per cent. Higher yields are exceptional. The amount of Hyoscyamine is many times greater than that of Hyoscine.

Other constituents of Henbane are a glucosidal bitter principle called hyoscytricin, choline, mucilage, albumin, calcium oxalate and potassium nitrate. On incineration, the leaves yield about 12 per cent of ash. By destructive distillation, the leaves yield a very poisonous empyreumatic oil.

The chief constituent of the seeds is about 0.5 to 0.6 per cent of alkaloid, consisting of Hyoscyamine, with a small proportion of Hyoscine. The seeds also contain about 20 per cent of fixed oil.

Historical Medicinal Uses - For Entertainment ONLY

Medicinal Action and Uses: Antispasmodic, hypnotic, mild diuretic. The leaves have long been employed as a narcotic medicine. It is similar in action to belladonna and stramonium, though milder in its effects.

The drug combines the therapeutic actions of its two alkaloids, Hyoscyamine and Hyoscine. Because of the presence of the former, it tends to check secretion and to relax spasms of the involuntary muscles, while through the narcotic effects of its hyoscine it lessens pain and exercises a slight somnifacient action.

Its most important use is in relief of painful spasmodic affections of the unstriped muscles, as in lead colic and irritable bladder. It will also relieve pain in cystitis.

It is much employed to allay nervous irritation, in various forms of hysteria or irritable cough, the tincture or juice prepared from the bruised, fresh leaves and tops being given in mixtures as an antispasmodic in asthma.

Combined with silver nitrate, it is especially useful in the treatment of gastric ulcer and chronic gastric catarrh.

It is used to relieve the griping caused by drastic purgatives, and is a common ingredient of aperient pills, especially those containing aloes and colocynth.

In small repeated doses Henbane has been found to have a tranquillizing effect upon persons affected by severe nervous irritability, producing a tendency to sleep, not followed by the disorder of the digestive organs and headache, which too frequently result from the administration of repeated doses of opium, to which Henbane is often preferred when an anodyne or sedative is required. The comparatively small amount of atropine present does not give rise to the excitation and delirium occasioned by belladonna. It is, therefore, used in insomnia, especially when opium cannot be given. Except for this, it acts like atropine.

A watery solution of the extract applied to the eye has a similar effect to that of atropine, in dilating the pupil and thus preparing the eye for an operation, or assisting the cure of its internal inflammation. This dilution leaves no injurious effect afterwards.

In the form of extract or tincture, it is a valuable remedy, either as an anodyne, a hypnotic or a sedative, and will take effect when other drugs fail. When used for such a purpose, it is the active principle, Hyoscine, that is employed. This is very powerful - only a very small amount is used, from $1/200$ to $1/70$ of a grain of the Hydrobromate of Hyoscine. This drug comes under Table I of the Poisons Schedule. In poisonous doses Henbane in any form causes dimness of sight, faintness, delirium, and sometimes death.

Hyoscine, in combination with other drugs, has of late come into use in the treatment known as Twilight Sleep. This is on account of its sedative action on brain and spine, causing loss of recollection and insensibility. Hyoscine is also used to a considerable extent in asylum practice, for the treatment of acute mania and delirium tremens.

A sedative application for external use is prepared by macerating Henbane leaves in alcohol, mixing the strong tincture with olive oil and heating in a water-bath, until the alcohol is dissipated. A compound liniment of Henbane, when applied to the skin, is of great service for relieving obstinate rheumatic pains.

The fresh leaves, crushed and applied as a poultice, or fomentation, will similarly relieve local pains of gout or neuralgia. They have been employed also to allay pain in cancerous ulcers, irritable sores and swellings, but their use for this purpose is of doubtful real advantage, and seems only a palliative. The extract, in form of suppositories, is also frequently used to alleviate the pain of haemorrhoids.

Preparations and Dosages: Powdered leaves, 2 to 10 grains. Fluid extract, 2 to 10 drops. Tincture, B.P. and U.S.P., 1/2 to 1 drachm. Juice, B.P., 1/2 to 1 drachm. Solid extract, 2 to 8 grains. Hyoscyamine, 1/8 to 1 grain.

The seeds possess all the properties of the plant. Their expressed oil was formerly used externally.

Henbane seeds are used in some parts of the country as a domestic remedy for toothache; the smoke obtained by heating the seeds on a hot plate is applied to the mouth by means of a funnel, or a poultice is sometimes made from the crushed drug. The seeds were a favourite remedy for toothache in the Middle Ages, but their use is dangerous, having caused convulsions and even insanity in some instances. Both leaves and seeds have also been smoked in a pipe as a remedy for neuralgia and rheumatism, but with equal risk, being too uncertain and violent in their effect to be safe.

Children have been known to eat the seeds with serious results.

Sir Hans Sloane records the case of four children who, having eaten some of the capsules in mistake for filberts, exhibited all the symptoms of narcotic poisoning, continuing for two days and nights in a profound sleep.

In the case of adults, twenty seeds have been proved insufficient to prove fatal, though they induced grave results, the effects being the same as in poisoning by atropine or belladonna, the remedies to be employed being an emetic of mustard, followed by large draughts of warm water, strong tea or coffee, with powdered charcoal; stimulants (whisky, etc.), if necessary; the patient to be roused if drowsy;

heat and friction to be applied to the extremities and finally, in acute cases, artificial respiration.

Gerard writes with regard to the use of the seed of Henbane by mountebanks for obstinate toothache:

'Drawers of teeth who run about the country and pretend they cause worms to come forth from the teeth by burning the seed in a chafing dish of coals, the party holding his mouth over the fume thereof, do have some crafty companions who convey small lute strings into the water, persuading the patient that these little creepers came out of his mouth, or other parts which it was intended to ease.'

Another old writer says: 'These pretended worms are no more than an appearance of worms which is always seen in the smoak of Henbane seed.' As a matter of fact, the small white, cylindrical embryos of the seed are forced out of some of them by the heat (especially if the seed be put into a basin with boiling water), and these were mistaken by ignorant sufferers for 'worms' coming out of their teeth.

Other Species of Hyoscyamus

Henbane, except for the use of the unofficial forms, is scarcely subject to adulteration in the entire condition. It, however, frequently contains an excessive amount of stem, which reduces its alkaloidal percentage and value.

In the south of Europe, RUSSIAN HENBANE (*H. albus*) - a native of the region of the Mediterranean, and so called from the pale colour of its flowers - is used as the official Henbane, and is regarded as equal in medicinal value. In France it is used indiscriminately with *H. niger*, though here it is not recognized as having identical properties. It is easily distinguished by the bracts, as well as the leaves being all stalked, and by the pale-yellow colour of the flower. According to Pharmacographia, the Hyoscyamus of the Ancients was probably H. albus, and the white variety was preferred for internal use in the practice of more modern times. Both the black and the white occur in our first Pharmacopoeia, but the use of the former was confined to external applications, such as unguentum populeum, while the latter was an ingredient of the famous electuary, Philonium Romanum, the original of the Confection of Opium. In France, too, White Henbane had the preference, though it was held to be milder in operation: only the seeds were official, whereas in the black variety only the leaves were official.

The alkaloidal contents of *H. muticus*, EGYPTIAN HENBANE, from Egypt and the East Indies, often exceeds 1.25 per cent. This is mostly pure Hyoscyamine: its medicinal action is thus different, and its use as a substitute is dangerous.

The drug is readily distinguished, consisting chiefly of very light and light-coloured stems, often as thick as the finger, and capsules which are equally light-coloured and far more elongated than those of *H. niger*. The calyx limb is also further prolonged beyond the capsule. The leaves are much narrower; they are coarsely toothed or lobed at the summit, but lack the very large and sharp lateral lobe of the European Henbane.

The presence of *H. muticus*, as an admixture of the official imported drug, may be detected by the presence of characteristic branching non-glandular hairs, which are found on both the stems and leaves.

H. muticus is one of the most important medicinal herbs produced in Egypt, and is a valuable source of the alkaloids, Hyoscyamine, Hyoscine and Atropine, Hyoscyamine, practically pure, occurring in the drug in considerably greater proportion than in the European herb, the Egyptian-grown plant being much richer than the Indian, and being chiefly imported into this country for the manufacture of Hyoscyamine.

The drug occurs in three forms, as a mixture of broken stem, leaf and fruit, in which stem predominates - as leaves with little stem, and as seeds; the first named is the variety usually met with.

Although *H. muticus* is grown in Egypt, a British Protectorate before the War (WWI), the Germans had a monopoly of the supply. The Imperial Institute, during the War (WWI), investigated *H. muticus* as a source of atropine, and reported that if a sufficient supply of the drug could be imported, it would be an additional inducement to British manufacturers to take up the preparation of atropine. As a result, pressed bales have reached this country in fair supply, and the manufacture of atropine is now carried on here in increased quantities.

It has been grown in this country, but not to any great extent. In 1916 it was reported that it was proposed to experiment with the seed of this plant in certain districts in the West Indian islands.

In Egypt the drug is called Sakran, meaning 'the drunken.' In India it is considerably used as a narcotic.

Scopola carniolica, a common plant in Austria and Hungary, Bavaria and southwest Russia, which appears in our trade lists of plants recommended for our pleasure gardens, also yields the alkaloid Hyoscine (Scopolamine) and is worth attention. By selective cultivation, its yield of alkaloid might be raised.

In 1916 (reported in the Chemist and Druggist, Feb. 17, 1924) Wild Hyoscyamus was discovered growing in Montana, U.S.A., the plant growing to the height of about 6 feet near Bearmouth, also Big Timber and other nearby places. It is assumed that it was introduced by some foreigners who were working on a building at Big Timber, Montana. From here it spread and became such a pest that every property-owner was ordered to rid his place of it. The climate and soil seem to suit it and the plants yield the normal quantity of alkaloid.

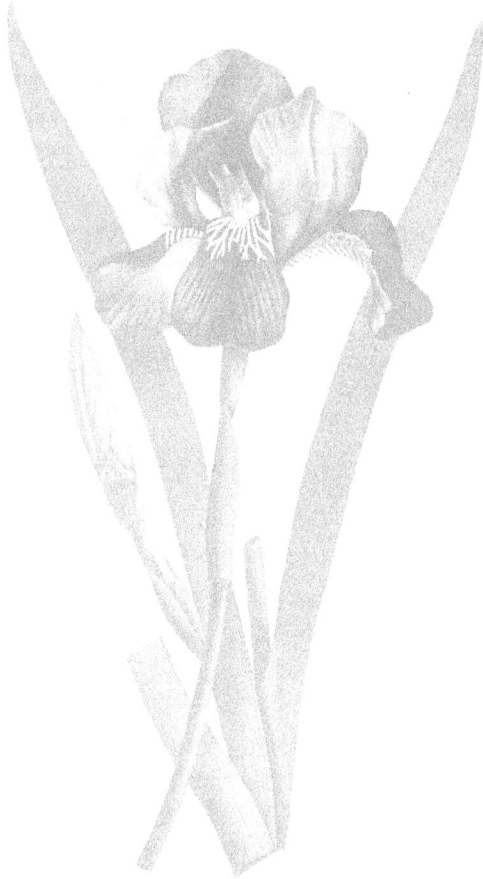

Hops

Humulus Lupulus L.

Quick Facts

Latin/Linnaen:	*Humulus Lupulus*
Family:	*Cannabaceae*
Old English :	Hymele
Synonyms:	Flower
Action:	Calming, sleep promoting
Parts Used:	Flower Head
Indicated For:	Mood disturbances such as restlessness and anxiety, sleep disturbances.
Dosage:	Unless otherwise prescribed: Single dose of drug 0.5g.
Preparation:	Cut drug, powdered drug or dry extract powder for infusions or decoctions or other preparations. Liquid and solid preparations for internal use.
Cautions:	
Other Uses:	Dye: The leaves and flower-heads have been used also to produce a fine brown dye.

Descripton

Humulus lupulus (Common hop) is a species of *Humulus* in the *Cannabaceae* family.

Common hop is a dioecious, perennial herbaceous climbing plant which sends up new shoots in early spring and dies back to the cold-hardy rhizome in autumn. It is native to the temperate Northern Hemisphere.

The flower cones of the plant, known as hops, are used in the production of beer to impart bitterness and flavor, and for their preservative qualities. The extract is antimicrobial, which makes it useful for making natural deodorant. Hops also contain the potent phytoestrogen, 8-prenylnaringenin that may have a relative binding affinity to estrogen receptors. Hop also contains myrcene, humulene, xanthohumol, myrcenol, linalool, tannins, resin.

Cultivation

Hardiness Zone:	4-9
Soil pH:	5.5-8.0
Soil type:	Deep well drained sandy loamy soil is ideal.
Cultivation:	Started by planting rhizomes in the spring.
Sunlight:	Full sun
Habitat:	Native to England, now grown in much of the world.

Hop is a climbing vine which grows well on a trellis. The hop cones are ready to harvest when they change from a leathery feel to a papery feel.

Historical Notes

The Hop (*Humulus Lupulus*, Linn.) is a native British plant, having affinities, botanically speaking, with the group of plants to which the Stinging Nettles belong. The sole representative of its genus in these islands, it is found wild in hedges and copses from York southwards, being only considered an introduced species in Scotland, and rare and not indigenous in Ireland. It is found in most countries of the North temperate zone.

The root is stout and perennial. The stem that arises from it every year is of a twining nature, reaching a great length, flexible and very tough, angled and prickly, with a tenacious fibre, which has enabled it to be employed to some extent in Sweden in the manufacture of a coarse kind of cloth, white and durable, though the fibres are so difficult of separation, that the stems require to be steeped in water a whole winter. Paper has also been made from the stem, or bine, as it is termed.

The leaves are heart-shaped and lobed, on foot-stalks, and as a rule placed opposite one another on the stem, though sometimes the upper leaves are arranged singly on the stem, springing from alternate sides. They are of a dark-green colour with their edges finely toothed.

The flowers spring from the axils of the leaves. The Hop is dioecious, i.e. male and female flowers are on separate plants. The male flowers are in loose bunches or panicles, 3 to 5 inches long. The female flowers are in leafy cone-like catkins, called strobiles. When fully developed, the strobiles are about 1 1/4 inch long, oblong in shape and rounded, consisting of a number of overlapping, yellowish-green bracts, attached to a separate axis. If these leafy organs are removed, the axis will be seen to be hairy and to have a little zigzag course. Each of the bracts enfolds at the base a small fruit (achene), both fruit and bract being sprinkled with yellow translucent glands, which appear as a granular substance. Much of the value of Hops depends on the abundance of this powdery substance, which contains 10 per cent of Lupulin, the bitter principle to which Hops owe much of their tonic properties.

As it is, these ripened cones of the female Hop plant that are used in brewing, female plants only are cultivated, since from these alone can the fruits be obtained. Those with undeveloped seeds are preferred to ensure which the staminate plants are excluded, only a few male plants being found scattered over a plantation of hops.

We find the Hop first mentioned by Pliny, who speaks of it as a garden plant among the Romans, who ate the young shoots in spring, in the same way as we do asparagus, and as country people frequently do in England at the present day. The young tops of Hop used formerly to be brought to market tied up in small bundles for table use. The tender first foliage, blanched, is a good potherb.

The origin of the name of the Hop genus, Humulus, is considered doubtful, though it has been assumed by some writers that it is derived from humus, the rich moist ground in which the plant grows. The specific name Lupulus, is derived from the Latin, lupus (a wolf), because, as Pliny explains, when produced among osiers, it strangles them by its light, climbing embraces, as the wolf does a sheep. The English name Hop comes from the Anglo-Saxon hoppan (to climb).

Hops appear to have been used in the breweries of the Netherlands in the beginning of the fourteenth century. In England they were not used in the composition of beer till nearly two centuries afterwards. The liquor prepared from fermented malt formed the favourite drink of our Saxon and Danish forefathers. The beverage went by the name of Ale (the word derived from the Scandinavian öl - the Viking's drink) and was brewed either from malt alone, or from a mixture of the latter with Honey and flavoured with Heath tops, Ground Ivy, and various other bitter and aromatic herbs, such as Marjoram, Buckbean, Wormwood, Yarrow, Woodsage or Germander and Broom. They knew not, however, the ale to which Hops give both flavour and preservation. For long after the introduction of Hops, the liquor flavoured in the old manner retained the name of Ale, while the word of German and Dutch origin, Bier or Beer, was given only to that made with the newly-introduced bitter catkins.

It has been stated that the planting of Hops in this country was forbidden in the reign of Henry VI, but half a century later the cultivation was introduced from Flanders, though only to a limited extent, and it did not become sufficient for the needs of the kingdom till the end of the seventeenth century. The prejudice against the use of Hops was at first great. Henry VIII forbade brewers to put hops and sulphur into ale, Parliament having been petitioned against the Hop as 'a wicked weed that would spoil the taste of the drink and endanger the people.' In the fifth year of Edward VI, however, privileges were granted to Hop growers, though in the reign of James I the plant was still not sufficiently cultivated to supply the consumption, as we find a statute of 1608 against the importation of spoiled Hops.

Hops were at first thought to engender melancholy.

'Hops,' says John Evelyn, in his Pomona (1670), 'transmuted our wholesome ale into beer, which doubtless much alters its constitution. This one ingredient, by some suspected not unworthily, preserves the drink indeed, but repays the pleasure in tormenting diseases and a shorter life.'

Cultivation: It has been estimated that in pre-war (pre-WWI) times 70 per cent of the Hops used in brewing was home produce and 30 per cent imported, chiefly from the United States and Germany.

Hops are also grown in France, South Russia, Australia and New Zealand.

The cultivation of Hops in the British Islands is restricted to England, where it is practically confined to half a dozen counties: four in the south-east (Kent, Surrey, Hants and Sussex) and two in the western Midland counties (Worcester and Hereford). As a rule, over 60 per cent of home-grown Hops are grown in Kent.

In the years 1898-1907, the average annual acreage of Hops under cultivation in this country was 48,841 acres (being 51,127 acres in 1901 and 33,763 acres in 1907). The average annual yield per acre for these ten years was 8.84 cwt., and the average annual home produce 434,567 cwt. In 1907 Kent had under cultivation 28,169 acres; Hereford, 6,143; Sussex, 4,243; Worcester, 3,622; Hants; 1,842, and Surrey, 744.

Hops require deep, rich soil, on dry bottom, with south or south-west aspect - free circulation of air is necessary. The ground is generally well pulverized and manured to considerable depth by plough or spade before planting. Hops in Kent are usually planted in October or November, the plants being placed 6 feet apart each way, thus giving 1,210 plant centres to the acre. The plants are usually set in 'stools' of from three to five, a few inches apart. They are obtained from cuttings or suckers taken from the healthiest old shoots, which are usually planted out closely in nursery lines a year before being planted permanently.

Very little growth takes place the first year. Some planters still grow potatoes or mangels between the rows of the first year, as the plants do not bear much till the second year, but this is considered a mistake, as it exhausts the ground.

As a rule, the plants are not full bearing till the third year, when four to six poles from 14 to 18 feet long are required for each stool. The most used timber for

Hop poles is Spanish Chestnut, which is largely grown for this special purpose in coppices in hopgrowing districts. Ash is also used. The poles are set to the plants in spring, before growth commences, and removed when the latter are cut away in autumn. The plants are then dressed with manure, and the soil between the stools stirred lightly. Much of the Hop-land is ploughed between the rows, but it is better to dig Hop-land if possible, the tool used being the Kent spud.

Experiments in Hop manuring have been conducted in connexion with the South-East Agricultural College, Wye. The main results have been to demonstrate the necessity of a liberal supply of phosphates, if the full benefit is to be reaped from application of nitrogenous manures. Manuring is applied in the winter and dug or ploughed in. London manure from stables is used to an enormous extent. Rags, fur waste, sprats, wood waste and shoddy, are also put on in the winter. In the summer, rape dust, guano, nitrate of soda and various patent Hopmanures are chopped in with the Canterbury hoe. Fish guano, or desiccated fish, is largely used; it is very stimulating and more lasting than some of the forcing manures.

Hop-land is ploughed or dug between November and March. After this, the plants are trimmed or 'dressed,' i.e. all the old bine ends are cut off with a sharp curved Hop-knife and the plant centres kept level with the ground. Much attention is required to keep the bines in their places on the poles, strings or wire during the summer.

The Hop cones - or strobiles - are fit to gather when a brown-amber colour and of a firm consistence. The stalks are then cut at the base and removed with the poles and laid horizontally on frames of wood, to each of which is attached a large sack into which the Hops fall as they are picked. When picked, the Hops are at once taken to the kiln or roast-house, and dried, as they are liable to become spoiled in a few hours, especially when picked moist. During the process of drying which is carried out in a similar manner to the drying of malt, great care is required to prevent overheating, by which the essential oil would become volatilized. The Hops are spread 8 to 12 inches deep, on hair-cloth, also being sometimes exposed to fumes of burning sulphur. When the ends of the stalks shrivel, they are removed from the kiln and laid on a woodenfloor till quite cool, when they are packed in bales, known as 'pockets.'

The difficulties attendant upon the cultivation of Hops have been aggravated and the expenses increased in recent years by the regularly recurring attacks of aphis blight, due to the insect Aphis humuli, which make it necessary to spray or syringe every Hop plant, every branch and leaf with insecticidal solutions three or four times and sometimes more often in each season. Quassia and soft soap solutions are usually employed: the soft soap serves as a vehicle to retain the bitterness of the quassia upon the bines and leaves, making them repulsive to the Aphides, which are thus starved out. The solution is made from 4 to 8 lb. of quassia chips to 100 gallons of water.

Another pest, the Red Spider (Tetranychus telarius) is most destructive in very hot summers. Congregating on the under surfaces of the leaves, the red spiders exhaust the sap and cause the leaves to fall. The Quassia and Soft Soap Hopwash is of little avail in the case of Red Spider. Some success has attended the use of a solution consisting of 8 to 10 lb. of soft soap to 100 gallons of water, with 3 pints of paraffin added. It must be applied with great force, to break through the webs with which the spiders protect themselves.

Hop washing is done by means of large garden engines worked by hand or by horse engines: even steam-engines have sometimes been employed.

Among fungoid parasites, Mould or Mildew is frequently the cause of loss to Hop planters. It is due to the action of the fungus Podosphaera castagnei, and the mischief is more especially that done to the cones. The remedy is sulphur, employed usually in the form of flowers of sulphur, from 40 to 60 lb. per acre being applied at each sulphuring, distributed by means of a blast pipe. The first sulphuring takes place when the plants are fairly up the poles and is repeated three or four weeks later, and even again if indications of mildew are present. Sulphur is also successfully employed in the form of an alkaline sulphur, such as a solution of liver of sulphur, a variety of potassium sulphide.

Historical Medicinal Uses - For Entertainment ONLY

Parts Used Medicinally: (a) The strobiles, collected and dried as described. (b) The Lupulin, separated from the strobiles by sifting.

Chemical Constituents: The aromatic odour of the Hop strobiles is due to a volatile oil, of which they yield about 0.3 to 1.0 per cent. It appears to consist chiefly of the sesquiterpene Humulene. Petroleum spirit extracts 7 to 14 per cent of a powerfully antiseptic soft resin, and ether extracts a hard resin. The petroleum spirit extract contains the two crystalline bitter principles (a) Lupamaric acid (Humulone), (b) Lupamaric acid (Lupulinic acid). These bodies are chiefly contained in the glands at the base of the bracts. The leafy organs contain about 5 per cent of tannin which is not a constituent of the glands. Hops yield about 7 per cent Ash.

The oil and the bitter principle combine to make Hops more useful than Chamomile, Gentian or any other bitter in the manufacture of beer: hence the medicinal value of extra-hopped or bitter beer. The tannic acid contained in the strobiles adds to the value of Hops by causing precipitation of vegetable mucilage and consequently the cleansing of beer.

Fresh Hops possess a bitter aromatic taste and a strong characteristic odour. The latter, however, changes and becomes distinctly unpleasant as the Hops are kept. This change is ascribed to oxidation of the soft resin with production of Valerianic acid. On account of the rapid change in the odour of Hops, the recently dried fruits should alone be used: these may be recognized by the characteristic odour and distinctly green colour. Those which have been subjected to the treatment of sulphuring are not to be used in pharmacy. This process is conducted with a view of improving the colour and odour of the Hops, since sulphuric acid is found to retard the production of the Valerianic odour and to both preserve and improve the colour of the Hops.

Lupulin, which consists of the glandular powder present on the seeds and surface of the scales, may be separated by shaking the strobiles. The drug occurs in a granular, brownish-yellow powder, with the strong odour and bitter aromatic taste characteristic of Hops. The glands readily burst on the application of slight pressure and discharge their granular oleo-resinous contents. Commercial Lupulin is often of a very inferior quality, and consists of the sifted sweepings from the floors of hop-kilns. It should contain not more than 40 per cent of matter insoluble in ether and not yield more than 12 per cent of ash on incineration. A dark colour and disagreeable odour indicates an old drug.

The chief constituent of Lupulin is about 3 per cent of volatile oil, which consists chiefly of Humulene, together with various oxygenated bodies to which the oil owes its peculiar odour. Other constituents are the two Lupamaric acids, cholene and resin.

Lupulin is official both in the British Pharmacopoeia and the United States Pharmacopoeia.

Medicinal Action and Uses: Hops have tonic, nervine, diuretic and anodyne properties. Their volatile oil produces sedative and soporific effects, and the Lupamaric acid or bitter principle is stomachic and tonic. For this reason Hops improve the appetite and promote sleep.

The official preparations are an infusion and a tincture. The infusion is employed as a vehicle, especially for bitters and tonics: the tincture is stomachic and is used to improve the appetite and digestion. Both preparations have been considered to be sedative, were formerly much given in nervousness and hysteria and at bedtime to induce sleep; in cases of nervousness, delirium and inflammation being considered to produce a most soothing effect, frequently procuring for the patient sleep after long periods of sleeplessness in overwrought conditions of the brain.

The bitter principle in the Hop proves one of the most efficacious vegetable bitters obtainable. An infusion of 1/2 oz. Hops to 1 pint of water will be found the proper quantity for ordinary use. It has proved of great service also in heart disease, fits, neuralgia and nervous disorders, besides being a useful tonic in indigestion, jaundice, and stomach and liver affections generally. It gives prompt ease to an irritable bladder, and is said to be an excellent drink in cases of delirium tremens. Sherry in which some Hops have been steeped makes a capital stomachic cordial.

A pillow of warm Hops will often relieve toothache and earache and allay nervous irritation.

An infusion of the leaves, strobiles and stalks, as Hop Tea, taken by the wineglassful two or three times daily in the early spring, is good for sluggish livers. Hop Tea in the leaf, as frequently sold by grocers, consists of Kentish Hop leaves, dried, crushed under rollers and then mixed with ordinary Ceylon or Indian Tea. The infusion combines the refreshment of the one herb with the sleep inducing virtues of the other.

Hop juice cleanses the blood, and for calculus trouble nothing better can be found than the bitter principle of the Hop. A decoction of the root has been esteemed as of equal benefit with Sarsaparilla.

As an external remedy, an infusion of Hops is much in demand in combination with chamomile flowers or poppy heads as a fomentation for swelling of a painful nature, inflammation, neuralgic and rheumatic pains, bruises, boils and gatherings. It removes pain and allays inflammation in a very short time. The Hops may also be applied as a poultice.

The drug Lupulin is an aromatic bitter and is reputed to be mildly sedative, inducing sleep without causing headache.

It is occasionally administered as a hypnotic, either in pills with alcohol, or enclosed in a cachet.

Preparations of Lupulin are not much used in this country (UK), although official, but in the United States they are considered preferable for internal use.

RECIPES FOR HERB BEERS

Formerly every farmhouse inn had a brewing plant and brewhouse attached to the buildings, and all brewed their own beer till the large breweries were established and supplanted home-brewed beers. Many of these farmhouses then began to brew their own 'stingo' from wayside herbs, employing old rustic recipes that had been carried down from generation to generation. The true value of vegetable bitters and of herb beers have yet to be recognized by all sections of the community. Workmen in puddling furnaces and potteries in the Midland and Northern counties find, however, that a tea made of tonic herbs is cheaper and less intoxicating than ordinary beer and patronize the herb beers freely, Dandelion Stout ranking as one of the favourites. It is also made in Canada.

Dandelion is a good ingredient in many digestive or diet drinks. A dinner drink may be made as follows: Take 2 OZ. each of dried Dandelion and Nettle herbs and 1 OZ. of Yellow Dock. Boil in 1 gallon of water for 15 minutes and then strain the liquor while hot on to 2 Lb. of sugar, on the top of which is sprinkled 2 tablespoonsful of powdered Ginger. Leave till milk-warm, then add boiled water gone cold to bring the quantity up to 2 gallons. The temperature must then not be above 75 degrees F. Now dissolve 1/2 oz. solid yeast in a little of the liquid and stir into the bulk. Allow to ferment 24 hours, skim and bottle, and it will be ready for use in a day or two.

A good, pleasant-tasting botanic beer is also made of the Nettle alone. Quantities of the young fresh tops are boiled in a gallon of water, with the juice of two lemons, a teaspoonful of crushed ginger and 1 Lb. of brown sugar. Fresh yeast is floated on toast in the liquor, when cold, to ferment it, and when it is bottled the result is a specially wholesome sort of ginger beer.

Meadow Sweet was also formerly much in favour. The mash when worked with barm made a pleasant drink, either in the harvest field or at the table. It required little sugar, some even made it without any sugar at all.

Another favourite brew was that of armsful of Meadowsweet, Yarrow, Dandelion and Nettles, and the mash when 'sweetened with old honey' and well worked with barm, and then bottled in big stoneware bottles, made a drink strong enough to turn even an old toper's head.

Old honeycomb from the thatch of an ancient cottage, filled with rich and nearly black honey, when boiled into syrup and then strained, was used in the making of herb beer, while the wax was put at the mouths of the hives for the bees.

Dandelion, Meadowsweet and Agrimony, equal quantities of each, would also be boiled together for 20 minutes (about 2 oz. each of the dried herbs to 2 gallons of water), then strained and 2 lb. of sugar and 1/2 pint of barm or yeast added. This was bottled after standing in a warm place for 12 hours. This recipe is still in use.

A Herb Beer that needs no yeast is made from equal quantities of Meadowsweet, Betony, Agrimony and Raspberry leaves (2 oz. of each) boiled in 2 gallons of water for 15 minutes, strained, then 2 lb. of white sugar added and bottled when nearly cool.

In some outlying islands of the Hebrides there is still brewed a drinkable beer by making two-thirds Heath tops with one-third of malt.

HOP BITTERS, as an appetizer, to be taken in tablespoonful doses three times in the day before eating, may be made as follows: Take 2 oz. of Buchu leaves and 1/2 lb. of Hops. Boil these in 5 quarts of water in an iron vessel for an hour. When lukewarm add essence of Wintergreen (Pyrola) 2 oz. and 1 pint alcohol.

Another way of making Hop Bitters is to take 1/2 oz. Hops, 1 oz. Angelica Herb and 1 oz. Holy Thistle. Pour 3 pints of boiling water on them and strain when cold. A wineglassful may be taken four times a day.

To make a good **HOP BEER**, put 2 oz. Hops in 2 quarts of water for 15 minutes. Then strain and dissolve 1 lb. of sugar in the liquor. To this add 4 quarts of cold water and 2 tablespoonful of fresh barm. Allow to stand for 12 hours in a warm place and it will then be ready for bottling.

Horehound

Quick Facts

Latin/Linnaen:	*Marrubium vulgare*
Family:	*Lamiaceae*
Old English :	Hune
Synonyms:	White Horehound or Common Horehound
Action:	Marrubinic acid works as a choleretic
Parts Used:	Fresh or dried aerial parts.
Indicated For:	Loss of appetite and dyspepsia, such as bloating and flatulence.
Dosage:	Unless otherwise prescribed: Daily dosage: 4.5g of drug; 2-6tbs of pressed juice; equivalent preparations.
Preparation:	Comminuted herb, freshly expressed plant juice and other galenical preparations for internal use.
Cautions:	
Other Uses:	**Candy**: Horehound is used to make hard lozenge candies that are considered by folk medicine to aid digestion, soothe sore throats, and relieve inflammation

Description

Marrubium vulgare (White Horehound or Common Horehound) is a flowering plant in the family *Lamiaceae*, native to Europe, northern Africa and Asia.

It is a gray-leaved herbaceous perennial plant, somewhat resembling mint in appearance, which grows to 25–45 cm tall. The leaves are 2–5 cm long with a densely crinkled surface, and are covered in downy hairs. The flowers are white, borne in clusters on the upper part of the main stem.

Horehound was introduced to southern Australia in the 19th century as a medicinal herb. It became a weed of native grasslands and pastures where it was introduced with settlers' livestock, and was first declared under noxious weeds legislation. It now appears to have reached its full potential distribution.

It occupies disturbed or overgrazed ground, and is favoured by grazing because it is highly unpalatable to livestock. It may persist in native vegetation that has been grazed.

Cultivation

Hardiness Zone:	4-10
Soil pH:	4.5-8.3
Soil type:	Well drained
Cultivation:	Sow seeds in spring, or divide plants.
Sunlight:	Full sun
Habitat:	Native to Europe, but now found throughout the world.

Horehound is a good companion plant to tomatoes and peppers. Horehound can be invasive like mint plants.

Historical Notes

White Horehound is a perennial herbaceous plant, found all over Europe and indigenous to Britain. Like many other plants of the Labiate tribe, it flourishes in waste places and by roadsides, particularly in the counties of Norfolk and Suffolk, where it is also cultivated in the corners of cottage gardens for making tea and candy for use in coughs and colds. It is also brewed and made into Horehound Ale, an appetizing and healthful beverage, much drunk in Norfolk and other country districts.

The plant is bushy, producing numerous annual, quadrangular and branching stems, a foot or more in height, on which the whitish flowers are borne in crowded, axillary, woolly whorls. The leaves are much wrinkled, opposite, petiolate, about 1 inch long, covered with white, felted hairs, which give them a woolly appearance. They have a curious, musky smell, which is diminished by drying and lost on keeping. Horehound flowers from June to September.

The Romans esteemed Horehound for its medicinal properties, and its Latin name of *Marrubium* is said to be derived from Maria urbs, an ancient town of Italy. Other authors derive its name from the Hebrew marrob (a bitter juice), and state that it was one of the bitter herbs which the Jews were ordered to take for the Feast of Passover.

The Egyptian Priests called this plant the 'Seed of Horus,' or the 'Bull's Blood,' and the 'Eye of the Star.' It was a principal ingredient in the negro Caesar's[3] antidote for vegetable poisons.

Gerard recommends it, in addition to its uses in coughs and colds, to 'those that have drunk poyson or have been bitten of serpents,' and it was also administered for 'mad dogge's biting.'

It was once regarded as an anti-magical herb.

According to Columella, Horehound is a serviceable remedy against Cankerworm in trees, and it is stated that if it be put into new milk and set in a place pestered with flies, it will speedily kill them all.

Cultivation: White Horehound is a hardy plant, easily grown, and flourishes best in a dry, poor soil. It can be propagated from seeds sown in spring, cuttings, or by dividing the roots (the most usual method). If raised from seed, the seedlings should be planted out in the spring, in rows, with a space of about 9 inches or more between each plant. No further culture will be needed than weeding. It does not blossom until it is two years old.

Until recently, it was chiefly collected in Southern France, where it is much cultivated. It is in steady demand, and it would probably pay to cultivate it more in this country.

White Horehound is distinguished from other species by its woolly stem, the densely felted hairs on the leaves, and the tentoothed teeth of the calyx.

---

[3] There was a negro slave named Caesar in 1749 who concocted an antidote to posion. He was referred to fondly as Dr. Caesar, but there was still much pushback from white doctor's of the time, who disputed the efficacy of the cure, or stated that it must have been invented by white doctors.

Constituents: The chief constituent is a bitter principle known as Marrubium, with a little volatile oil, resin, tannin, wax, fat, sugar, etc.

Historical Medicinal Uses - For Entertainment ONLY

Medicinal Action and Uses: White Horehound has long been noted for its efficacy in lung troubles and coughs. Gerard says of this plant:

'Syrup made of the greene fresh leaves and sugar is a most singular remedie against the cough and wheezing of the lungs . . . and doth wonderfully and above credit ease such as have been long sicke of any consumption of the lungs, as hath beene often proved by the learned physitions of our London College.'

And Culpepper says:

'It helpeth to expectorate tough phlegm from the chest, being taken with the roots of Irris or Orris.... There is a syrup made of this plant which I would recommend as an excellent help to evacuate tough phlegm and cold rheum from the lungs of aged persons, especially those who are asthmatic and short winded.'

Preparations of Horehound are still largely used as expectorants and tonics. It may, indeed, be considered one of the most popular pectoral remedies, being given with benefit for chronic cough, asthma, and some cases of consumption.

Horehound is sometimes combined with Hyssop, Rue, Liquorice root and Marshmallow root, 1/2 oz. of each boiled in 2 pints of water, to 1 1/2 pint, strained and given in 1/2 teacupful doses, every two to three hours.

For children's coughs and croup, it is given to advantage in the form of syrup, and is a most useful medicine for children, not only for the complaints mentioned, but as a tonic and a corrective of the stomach. It has quite a pleasant taste.

Taken in large doses, it acts as a gentle purgative.

The powdered leaves have also been employed as a vermifuge and the green leaves, bruised and boiled in lard, are made into an ointment which is good for wounds.

For ordinary cold, a simple infusion of Horehound (Horehound Tea) is generally sufficient in itself. The tea may be made by pouring boiling water on the fresh or dried leaves, 1 oz. of the herb to the pint. A wineglassful may be taken three or four times a day.

Candied Horehound is best made from the fresh plant by boiling it down until the juice is extracted, then adding sugar before boiling this again, until it has become thick enough in consistence to pour into a paper case and be cut into squares when cool.

Two or three teaspoonsful of the expressed juice of the herb may also be given as a dose in severe colds.

Preparations and Dosages: Fluid extract, 1/2 to 1 drachm. Syrup, 2 to 4 drachms. Solid extract, 5 to 15 grains.

Horsetail

Equisetum arvense.

J. E. S. Fecit.

Quick Facts

Latin/Linnaen:	*Equisetum arvense*
Family:	*Equisetaceae*
Old English :	æquiseia
Synonyms:	Field Horsetail or Common Horsetail
Action:	Anti-oxidant, mild diuretic
Parts Used:	Herb
Indicated For:	Internal: Post traumatic and static edema. Irrigation therapy for bacterial and inflammatory diseases of the lower urinary tract and renal gravel. External: Supportive treatment for poorly healing wounds.
Dosage:	Unless otherwise prescribed: Internal: Average daily dosage: 6g of herbs; equivalent preparations. External use in compresses: 10g of herbs in 1litre of water
Preparation:	Internal: Comminuted herb for infusions and other galenical preparations for oral administration. For irrigation therapy, ensure an abundant fluid intake. External: Comminuted herb for decoctions and other galenical preparations.
Cautions:	No irrigation therapy in case of edema due to impaired heart and kidney function.
Other Uses:	None of note.

Description

Equisetum arvense, the Field Horsetail or Common Horsetail, is an herbaceous perennial plant, native throughout the arctic and temperate regions of the northern hemisphere. It has separate sterile non-reproductive and fertile spore-bearing stems, growing from a perennial underground rhizomatous stem system. The fertile stems are produced in early spring and are non-photosynthetic, while the green sterile stems start to grow after the fertile stems have wilted, and persist through the summer until the first autumn frosts.

The sterile stems are 10–90 cm tall and 3–5 mm diameter, with jointed segments around 2–5 cm long with whorls of side shoots at the segment joints; the side shoots have a diameter of about 1 mm. Some stems can have as many as 20 segments. The fertile stems are succulent-textured, off-white, 10–25 cm tall and 3–5 mm diameter, with 4–8 whorls of brown scale leaves, and an apical brown spore cone 10–40 mm long and 4–9 mm broad.

It has a very high diploid number of 216 (108 pairs of chromosomes).

The plant contains several substances which can be used medicinally. It is rich in the minerals silicon (10%), potassium, and calcium. The buds are eaten as a vegetable in Japan and Korea in spring time. All other Equisetum species are toxic. In polluted conditions, it may synthesize nicotine. Externally it was traditionally used for chilblains and wounds. It was also once used to polish pewter and wood (gaining the name pewterwort) and to strengthen fingernails. It is also an abrasive. It was used by Hurdy-Gurdy players to dress the wheels of their instruments by removing resin build up.

Cultivation

Hardiness Zone:	2-10
Soil pH:	4.5-6.5
Soil type:	All types, moist
Cultivation:	Horsetail is a spore bearing plant whose rhizomes grow to

	depth of up to 6 feet.
Sunlight:	Part sun-part shade
Habitat:	Native to Europe and north Africa

Horsetail can be hard to control so care should be taken before deciding on planting it. Could be planted in a sunken pot that will contain its rhizomes.

Historical Notes

None of note.

Ivy

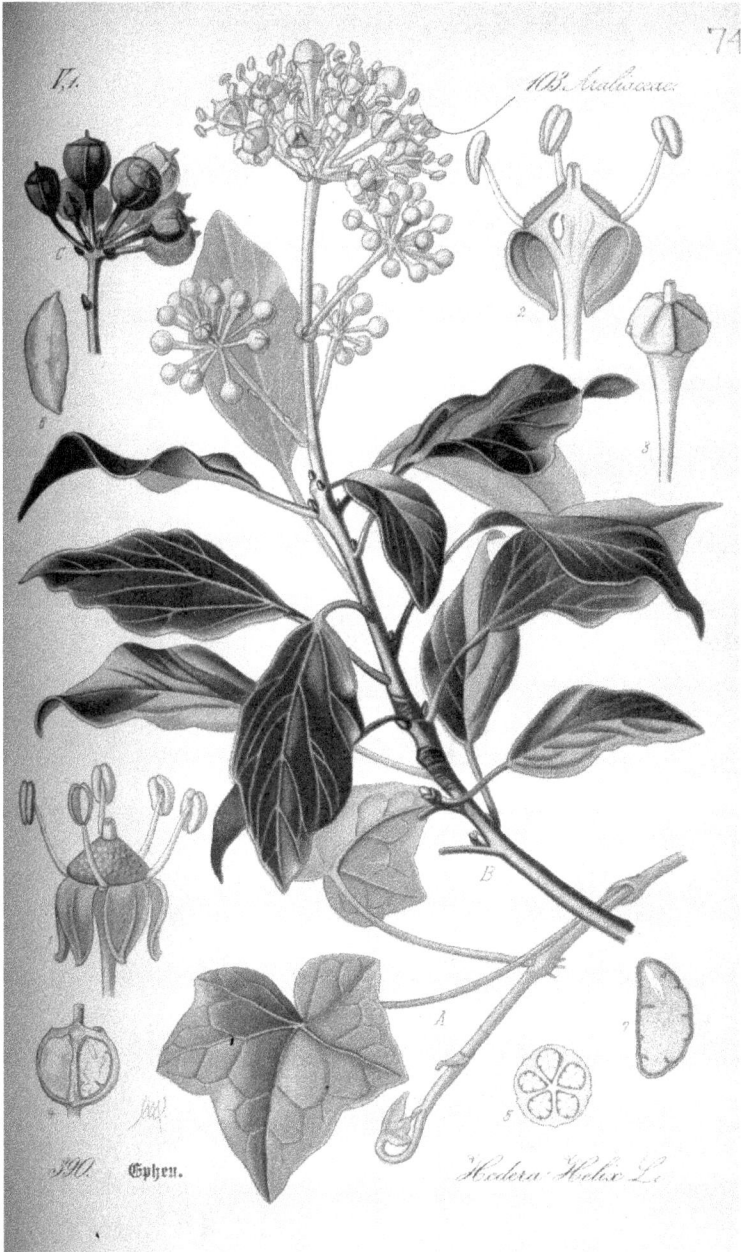

Quick Facts

Latin/Linnaen:	*Hedera Helix*
Family:	*Araliaceae*
Old English :	Iue, Ife, Efic, Ifig, Ifign
Synonyms:	Common ivy, English ivy, Hedera acuta, Hedera arborea ("tree ivy"), Hedera baccifera, Hedera grandifolia, English Ivy, Bindwood, and Lovestone.
Action:	Expectorant, Antispasmodic, Irritative to skin and mucosa
Parts Used:	Leaf
Indicated For:	Catarrhs of the respiratory passages, symptomatic treatment of chronic inflammatory bronchial conditions.
Dosage:	Unless otherwise prescribed: Average daily dosage: 0.3g of drug; equivalent preparations.
Preparation:	Comminuted drug and other galenical preparations for internal use.
Cautions:	
Other Uses:	

Description

Hedera helix (Common Ivy, English Ivy) is a species of ivy native to most of Europe and western Asia. It is labeled as an invasive species in a number of areas where it has been introduced.

It is an evergreen climbing plant, growing to 20–30 m high where suitable surfaces (trees, cliffs, walls) are available, and also growing as ground cover where there are no vertical surfaces. It climbs by means of aerial rootlets which cling to the substrate.

The leaves are alternate, 50–100 mm long, with a 15–20 mm petiole; they are of two types, with palmately five-lobed juvenile leaves on creeping and climbing stems, and unlobed cordate adult leaves on fertile flowering stems exposed to full sun, usually high in the crowns of trees or the top of rock faces.

The flowers are produced from late summer until late autumn, individually small, in 3–5 cm diameter umbels, greenish-yellow, and very rich in nectar, an important late autumn food source for bees and other insects.

The fruit are purple-black to orange-yellow berries 6–8 mm diameter, ripening in late winter, and are an important food for many birds, though somewhat poisonous to humans.

There are one to five seeds in each berry, which are dispersed by birds eating the berries.

There are three subspecies:

1. Hedera helix subsp. helix.
   a. Central, northern and western Europe. Plants without rhizomes. Purple-black ripe fruit.
2. Hedera helix subsp. poetarum Nyman (syn. Hedera chrysocarpa Walsh).
   a. Southeast Europe and southwest Asia (Italy, Balkans, Turkey). Plants without rhizomes. Orange-yellow ripe fruit.
3. Hedera helix subsp. Rhizomatifera
   a. McAllister. Southeast Spain. Plants rhizomatiferous. Purple-black ripe fruit.

The closely related species *Hedera canariensis* and *Hedera hibernica* are also often treated as subspecies of *H. helix*, though they differ in chromosome number so do not hybridise readily. *H. helix* can be best distinguished by the shape and colour of its leaf trichomes, usually smaller and slightly more deeply lobed leaves and somewhat less vigorous growth, though identification is often not easy.

It ranges from Ireland northeast to southern Scandinavia, south to Spain, and east to Ukraine and northern Turkey.

The northern and eastern limits are at about the -2°C winter isotherm, while to the west and southwest, it is replaced by other species of ivy.

It is widely cultivated as an ornamental plant. Within its native range, the species is greatly valued for attracting wildlife. The flowers are visited by over 70 species of nectar-feeding insects, and the berries eaten by at least 16 species of birds. The foliage provides dense evergreen shelter, and is also browsed by deer.

Over 30 cultivars have been selected for such traits as yellow, white, variegated (e.g. 'Glacier'), and/or deeply lobed leaves (e.g. 'Sagittifolia'), purple stems, and slow, dwarfed growth.

Cultivation

Hardiness Zone:	5-10
Soil pH:	5.2-7.8
Soil type:	Well drained fertile soil, but can tolerate clay.
Cultivation:	Best propagated from cuttings, divisions.
Sunlight:	Full sun to partial shade
Habitat:	Native to Europe and western Asia. Invasive in North America and Australia.

Invasive species

The plant is considered invasive and destructive in parts of Australia and the United States. Its sale, transport or propagation is banned in several places. Like other exotic species, the invasion is due to human actions. *H. helix* is labeled as an invasive species in many parts of the United States, and its sale or import is banned in the state of Oregon. Ivies are plants adapted to the laurel forest, a type of cloud forest habitat. European Ivy for example, is believed to have been spread by birds in Europe, that helped to colonize large areas again where it had disappeared during the glaciations.

Laurus nobilis and *Ilex aquifolium* are widespread relics of the laurisilva forests that originally covered much of the Mediterranean Basin when the climate of the region was more humid. Ivy also is a relict plant and one of the survivors of the laurel forest flora in Europe tertiary era. Disappeared during the glaciations, Ivy re-colonized large areas when the weather was favorable again. The ecological requirements of the species, are those of the laurel forest and like most of their counterparts laurifolia in the world, it is a vigorous species with a great ability to populate the habitat that is conducive. Ivy responded to favourable climatic periods and expanded across the available habitat. Ivy occur as opportunistic species across wide distribution with close vicariant relatives and few species, indicating the recent divergence of this species. The extant Ivy species of this group are relatively young. The expansion is favored by seeds spread by birds

Historical Notes

The plant is found over the greater part of Europe and Northern and Central Asia, and is said to have been particularly abundant at Nyssa, the fabled home of Bacchus in his youth. There are many varieties, but only two accepted species, i.e. Hedera Helix and the Australian species, which is confined to the southern Continent.

This well-known evergreen climber, with its dark-green, glossy, angular leaves is too familiar to need detailed description. It climbs by means of curious fibres resembling roots, which shoot out from every part of the stem, and are furnished with small disks at the end, which adapt themselves to the roughness of the bark or wall against which the plant grows and to which it clings firmly. These fibres on meeting with soil or deep crevices become true roots, obtaining nourishment for the plant, but when dilated at the extremity, they merely serve to attach the stems and do not absorb nourishment from the substance to which they adhere. The Ivy is therefore liable to injure the trees around which it twines by abstracting the juices of the stem.

When it attains the summit of a tree or wall, it grows out in a bushy form, and the leaves instead of being five-lobed and angular, as they are below, become ovate, with entire margins. Ivy only produces flowers when the branches get above their support, the flowering branches being bushy and projecting a foot or two from the climbing stems, with flowers at the end of every shoot.

Professor Henslow has an interesting note on the Ivy and its shoots, in his Floral Rambles in Highways and Byways:

'The shoots turn to the darker side, as may be seen when Ivy reaches the top of a wall, from both sides; wherever the sun may be the shoots lie flat upon the top. The roots themselves only come out from the darker side of the shoots, so that both of these acquired habits have their purposes. When the Ivy is going to flower, the shoots now turn to the

light and stand out freely into the air; moreover the form of the leaf changes from a finepointed one to a much smaller oval type. As the shoot now has to support itself, if a section be made and compared with one of the same diameter which is supported by the adhesive roots, it will be found that it has put on more wood with less pith, than in that of the supported stem. It at once, so to speak, feels the strain and makes wood sufficient to meet it.'

The form of Ivy which creeps over the ground on banks and in woods, etc., never blossoms. The branches root into the soil, but they are of the ordinary kind deriving nourishment from it. On endeavouring to train this kind on a wall, it was found to have practically lost the power of climbing; for it kept continually falling away from the wall instead of adhering to it; just as cucumbers refuse to climb by their tendrils, if the stem and branches are supported artificially.

The flowers of Common Ivy are small, in clusters of nearly globular umbels and of a yellowish-green, with five broad and short petals and five stamens. They seldom open before the latter end of October, and often continue to expand till late in December. Though they have little or no scent, they yield abundance of nectar and afford food to bees late in the autumn, when they can get no other.

The berries, which do not become ripe till the following spring, provide many birds, especially wood pigeons, thrushes and blackbirds with food during severe winters. When ripe, they are about the size of a pea, black or deep purple, smooth and succulent, and contain two to five seeds. They have a bitter and nauseous taste, and when rubbed, an aromatic and slightly resinous odour.

History: Ivy was in high esteem among the ancients. Its leaves formed the poet's crown, as well as the wreath of Bacchus, to whom the plant was dedicated, probably because of the practice of binding the brow with Ivy leaves to prevent intoxication, a quality formerly attributed to the plant. We are told by old writers that the effects of intoxication by wine are removed if a handful of Ivy leaves are bruised and gently boiled in wine and drunk.

It is the Common Ivy that is alluded to in the Idylls of Theocritus, but the Golden Ivy of Virgil is supposed to be the yellowberried variety (Hedera Chrysocarpa), now so rare.

The Greek priests presented a wreath of Ivy to newly-married persons, and the Ivy has throughout the ages been regarded as the emblem of fidelity. The custom of decorating houses and churches with Ivy at Christmas was forbidden by one of the early Councils of the Church, on account of its pagan associations, but the custom still remains.

The Roman agricultural writers much recommended Ivy leaves as cattle food, but they are not relished by cows, though sheep and deer will sometimes eat them in the winter. The broad leaves being evergreen afford shelter to birds in the winter, and many prefer Ivy to other shrubs, in which to build their nests.

The wood when it attains a sufficient size is employed by turners in Southern Europe, but being very soft is seldom used in England except for whetting the knives of leatherdressers. It is very porous, and the ancients thought it had the property of separating wine from water by filtration, an error arising from the fact that wood absorbs the colour of the liquid in its passage through the pores. On the Continent it has sometimes been used in thin slices as a filter.

In former days, English taverns bore over their doors the sign of an Ivy bush, to indicate the excellence of the liquor supplied within: hence the saying 'Good wine needs no bush.'

Ivy is very hardy; not only are the leaves seldom injured by frost, but they suffer little from smoke, or from the vitiated air of manufacturing towns. The plant lives to a great age, its stems become woody and often attain a considerable size - Ivy trunks of a foot in diameter are often to be seen where the plant has for many years climbed undisturbed over rocks and ruins.

The spring months are the best times for planting.

Historical Medicinal Uses - For Entertainment ONLY

The medicinal virtues of Ivy are little regarded nowadays. Its great value is as an ornamental covering for unsightly buildings and it is said to be the only plant which does not make walls damp. It acts as a curtain, the leaves from the way they fall, forming a sort of armour and holding and absorbing the rain and moisture.

Medicinal Action and Uses: Robinson tells us that a drachm of the flowers decocted in wine restrains dysentery, and that the yellow berries are good for those who spit blood and against the jaundice.

Culpepper says of the Ivy:

'It is an enemy to the nerves and sinews taken inwardly, but most excellent outwardly.'

To remove sunburn it is recommended to smear the face with tender Ivy twigs boiled in butter; according to the old English Leechbook of Bald.

Ethnomedical uses: In the past, the leaves and berries were taken orally as an expectorant to treat cough and bronchitis. In 1597, the British herbalist John Gerard recommended water infused with ivy leaves as a wash for sore or watering eyes. The leaves can cause severe contact dermatitis in some people. People who have this allergy (strictly a Type IV hypersensitivity) are also likely to react to carrots and other members of the Apiaceae as they contain the same allergen, falcarinol.

Lady's Mantle

Frauenmantel. 440. Alchemilla vulgaris L.

Quick Facts

Latin/Linnaen:	*Alchemilla Vulgaris*
Family:	*Rosaceae*
Old English :	Leonfoot
Synonyms:	Lion's Foot, Bear's Foot. Nine Hooks, Leontopodium, Stellaria, (French) Pied-de-lion, (German) Frauenmantle.
Action:	Astringent
Parts Used:	Above ground plant parts.
Indicated For:	Light and nonspecific diarrhea.
Dosage:	Unless otherwise prescribed: Average daily dosage: 5-10g of herb; equivalent preparations.
Preparation:	Cut herb for infusions and decoctions, as well as other galenical preparations for internal use.
Cautions:	
Other Uses:	

Description

Alchemilla is a genus of herbaceous perennial plants in the *Rosaceae*, and a popular garden herb with the common name Lady's Mantle. There are about 300 species, the majority native to cool temperate and subarctic regions of Europe and Asia, with a few species native to the mountains of Africa, North America and South America.

Most species of *Alchemilla* are clump-forming or mounded, perennials with basal leaves arising from woody rhizomes. Some species have leaves with lobes that radiate from a common point and others have divided leaves--both are typically fan-shaped with small teeth at the tips. The long-stalked, gray-green to green leaves are often covered with soft hairs, which hold water drops on the surface and along the edges. Green to bright chartreuse flowers are small, have no petals and appear in clusters above the foliage in late spring and summer.

Cultivation

Hardiness Zone:	3-9
Soil pH:	6-8
Soil type:	Well drained fertile soil.
Cultivation:	Plant division, or by seed.
Sunlight:	Full sun to part shade, prefers the shade
Habitat:	Native to North America, Europe and Asia

Historical Notes

The Lady's Mantle and the Parsley Piert, two small, inconspicuous plants, have considerable reputation as herbal remedies. They both belong to the genus *Alchemilla* of the great order *Rosaceae*, most of the members of which are natives of the American Andes, only a few being found in Europe, North America and Northern and Western Asia. In Britain, we have only three species, *Alchemilla vulgaris*, the Common Lady's Mantle, *A. arvensis*, the Field Lady's Mantle or Parsley Piert, and *A. alpina*, less frequent and only found in mountainous districts.

The Common Lady's Mantle is generally distributed over Britain, but more especially in the colder districts and on high-lying ground, being found up to an altitude of 3,600 feet in the Scottish Highlands. It is not uncommon in moist, hilly pastures and by streams, except in the south-east of England, and is abundant in Yorkshire, especially in the Dales. It is indeed essentially a plant of the north, freely found beyond the Arctic circle in Europe, Asia and also in Greenland and Labrador, and only on high mountain ranges, such as the Himalayas, if found in southern latitudes.

The plant is of graceful growth and though only a foot high and green throughout- flowers, stem and leaves alike, and therefore inconspicuous - the rich form of its foliage and the beautiful shape of its clustering blossoms make it worthy of notice.

The rootstock is perennial - black, stout and short - and from it rises the slender erect stem. The whole plant is clothed with soft hairs. The lower, radical leaves, large and handsome, 6 to 8 inches in diameter, are borne on slender stalks, 6 to 18 inches long and are somewhat kidneyshaped in general outline, with their margins cut into seven or mostly nine broad, but shallow lobes, finely toothed at the edges, from which it has obtained one of its local names: 'Nine Hooks.' The upper leaves are similar and either stalkless, or on quite short footstalks and are all actually notched and toothed. A noticeable feature is the leaflike stipules, also toothed, which embrace the stem.

The flowers, which are in bloom from June to August, are numerous and small, only about 1/8 inch in diameter, yellow-green in colour, in loose, divided clusters at the end of the freely-branching flower-stems, each on a short stalk, or pedicle. There are no petals, the calyx is four-cleft, with four conspicuous little bracteoles that have the appearance of outer and alternate segments of the calyx. There are four stamens, inserted on the mouth of the calyx, their filaments jointed.

The rootstock is astringent and edible and the leaves are eaten by sheep and cattle.

The common name, Lady's Mantle (in its German form, Frauenmantle), was first bestowed on it by the sixteenth-century botanist, Jerome Bock, always known by the Latinized version of his name: Tragus. It appears under this name in his famous History of Plants, published in 1532, and Linnaeus adopted it. In the Middle Ages, this plant had been associated, like so many flowers, with the Virgin Mary (hence it is Lady's Mantle, not Ladies' Mantle), the lobes of the leaves being supposed to resemble the scalloped edges of a mantle. In mediaeval Latin we also find it called *Leontopodium* (lion's foot), probably from its spreading root-leaves, and this has become in modern French, Pied-de-lion. We occasionally find the same idea expressed in two English local names, 'Lion's foot' and 'Bear's foot.' It has also been called 'Stellaria,' from the radiating character of its lower leaves, but this belongs more properly to quite another group of plants, with star-like blossoms of pure white.

A yellow fungus sometimes attacks the plant known as Uromyces alchemillae, and has the curious effect of causing abnormal length of the leaf-stalk and rendering the blade of the leaf smaller and of a paler green colour; this fungus produces the same effect in other plants.

The generic name *Alchemilla* is derived from the Arabic word, Alkemelych (alchemy), and was bestowed on it, according to some old writers, because of the wonder-working powers of the plant. Others held that the alchemical virtues lay in the subtle influence the foliage imparted to the dewdrops that lay in its furrowed leaves and in the little cup formed by its joined stipules, these dewdrops constituting part of many mystic potions.

Historical Medicinal Uses - For Entertainment ONLY

Part Used Medicinally: The whole herb, gathered in June and July when in flower and when the leaves are at their best, and dried.

The root is sometimes also employed, generally fresh.

Medicinal Action and Uses: The Lady's Mantle has astringent and styptic properties, on account of the tannin it contains. It is 'of a very drying and binding character' as the old herbalists expressed it, and was formerly considered one of the best vulneraries or wound herbs.

Culpepper says of it:

'Lady's Mantle is very proper for inflamed wounds and to stay bleeding, vomitings, fluxes of all sorts, bruises by falls and ruptures. It is one of the most singular wound herbs and therefore highly prized and praised, used in all wounds inward and outward, to drink a decoction thereof and wash the wounds therewith, or dip tents therein and put them into the wounds which wonderfully drieth up all humidity of the sores and abateth all inflammations thereof. It quickly healeth green wounds, not suffering any corruption to remain behind and cureth old sores, though fistulous and hollow.'

In modern herbal treatment, it is employed as a cure for excessive menstruation and is taken internally as an infusion 1 oz. of the dried herb to 1 pint of boiling water) in teacupful doses as required and the same infusion is also employed as an injections.

A strong decoction of the fresh root, by some considered the most valuable part of the plant, has also been recommended as excellent to stop all bleedings, and the root dried and reduced to powder is considered to answer the same purpose and to be good for violent purgings.

In Sweden, a tincture of the leaves has been given in cases of spasmodic or convulsive diseases, and an old authority states that if placed under the pillow at night, the herb will promote quiet sleep.

Fluid extract, dose, 1/2 to 1 drachm.

Horses and sheep like the plant, and it has therefore been suggested as a profitable fodder plant, but the idea has proved unpractical. Grazing animals will not eat the leaves till the moisture in them is dissipated.

Other Species: *Alchemilla alpine*, a mountain variety, found on the banks of Scotch rivulets. The leaves are deeply divided into five oblong leaflets and are thickly covered with lustrous silky hairs. A form of this plant in which the leaflets are connate for one-third of their length is known as *A. conjuncta*.

Lily of the Valley

Quick Facts

Latin/Linnaen:	*Convallaria majalis*
Family:	*Asparagaceae*
Old English :	Glovewort, Glofwyrt
Synonyms:	Dog's Tongue, May Lily, Convallaria, Our Lady's Tears, Convall-Lily, Lily Constancy, Ladder-to-Heaven, Jacob's Ladder, Male Lily.
Action:	Positive inotropic on the myocardium, economizes heart performance, lowers the elevated left-ventricular diastolic pressure, as well as pathologically elevated venous pressure, tonic for the veins, natriuretic, kaliuretic.
Parts Used:	Above ground parts of plant.
Indicated For:	Mild cardiac insufficiency, heart insufficiency due to old age, chronic cor pulmonale.
Dosage:	Unless otherwise prescribed: Average daily dosage; 0.6g standardized lily-of-the-valley powder; equivalent preparations.
Preparation:	Comminuted herb, as well as galenical preparations thereof for internal use.
Cautions:	Contraindications: Therapy with digitalis glycosides, potassium deficiency. Side Effects: Nausea, vomiting, cardiac arrhythmias. Interactions with other drugs: Increased effectiveness and also side effects of simultaneously administered quinidine, calcium, saleretics, laxatives, and extended therapy with glucocorticoids.
Other uses:	**Dye:** The leaves yield a green dye, with lime water.

Description

Convallaria majalis, commonly known as the lily-of-the-valley, is a poisonous woodland flowering plant native throughout the cool temperate Northern Hemisphere in Asia and Europe.

A limited native population occurs in Eastern USA (*Convallaria majalis var. montana*). There is, however, some debate as to the native status of the American variety.

C. majalis is an herbaceous perennial plant that forms extensive colonies by spreading underground stems called rhizomes. New upright shoots are formed at the ends of stolons in summer, these upright dormant stems are often called pips. These grow in the spring into new leafy shoots that still remain connected to the other shoots under ground, often forming extensive colonies. The stems grow to 15–30 cm tall, with one or two leaves 10–25 cm long, flowering stems have two leaves and a raceme of 5–15 flowers on the stem apex. The flowers are white tepals (rarely pink), bell-shaped, 5–10 mm diameter, and sweetly scented; flowering is in late spring, in mild winters in the Northern Hemisphere it is in early March. The fruit is a small orange-red berry 5–7 mm diameter that contains a few large whitish to brownish colored seeds that dry to a clear translucent round bead 1–3 mm wide. Plants are self-sterile, and colonies consisting of a single clone do not set seed.

Cultivation

Hardiness Zone:	2-9
Soil pH:	5.5-7
Soil type:	Rich moist soil
Cultivation:	Can be grown from pips or divisions.
Sunlight:	Prefers dappled shade, but can tolerate full shade and sun.
Habitat:	Native to Europe, now common in North America and Asia. Can be invasive in good conditions.

Lily of the Valley does well in a moist woodland setting. It can spread invasively if given good conditions. Very fragrant flower, but not very showy.

Plant towards the end of September. The ground for Lily-of-the-Valley should be thoroughly stirred to a depth of 15 inches, early in September, laying it up rough for a few weeks, then breaking it down and adding some rotten manure, or if that cannot be obtained, some kind of artificial manure must be used, but this is better applied later on, hoeing it in just as growth appears. Plant the crowns about 6 inches apart and work fine, rich soil, with some leaf mould if possible, in between. Leave at least 9 inches between the rows. Keep the crowns well below the surface and above all plant firmly.

In some soils the plants will last longer in the best form than in others, but should be transplanted about every fourth year and in light, porous soils it may be necessary to do so every third year. Periodic transplanting, deep culture and liberal feeding produce fine blooms. Autumn is the best time for remaking beds, which are best done in entirely fresh soil. Cut the roots from the old bed out into tufts 6 inches or 9 inches square, and divide into pieces 3 inches square. Replant the tufts the original 6 inches apart. It is best to prepare the entire beds before replanting. Replanted by October, the crowns will be well settled in by winter rains, and the quality of the spikes will show a marked difference in early spring.

Historical Notes

Lily of the Valley is a native of Europe, being distributed also over North America and Northern Asia, but in England it is very local as a wild flower. In certain districts it is to be found in abundance, but in many parts it is quite unknown. It is rare in Scotland and doubtfully native and only naturalized in Ireland. It grows mostly in the dryer parts of woods - especially ash woods - often forming extensive patches, and is by no means peculiar to valleys, though both the English and botanical names imply that it is so.

Culpepper reports that in his time these little Lilies grew plentifully on Hampstead Heath, but Green, writing about 100 years ago, tells us that 'since the trees on Hampstead Heath, near London, have been destroyed, it has been but sparingly found there.'

The Lily-of-the-Valley, with its broad leaves and fragrant little, nodding, white, bell-shaped flowers, is familiar to everyone.

In early spring days, the creeping rhizome, or underground stem, sends up quill-like shoots emerging from a scaly sheath. As they lengthen and uncoil, they are seen to consist of two leaves, their stalks sheathing one within the other, rising directly from the rhizome on long, narrowing foot-stalks, one leaf often larger than the other. The plain, oval blades, with somewhat concave surfaces, are deeply ribbed and slant a little backwards, thus catching the rain and conducting it by means of the curling-in base of the leaf, as though in a spout, straight down the foot-stalk to the root. At the back of the leaves, lightly enclosed at the base in the same scaly sheath, is the flower-stalk, quite bare of leaves itself and bearing at its summit a number of buds, greenish when young, each on a very short stalk, which become of the purest white, and as they open turn downwards, the flowers hanging, like a pearl of fairy bells, each bell with the edges turned back with six small scallops. The six little stamens are fastened inside the top of the bell, and in the centre hangs the ovary. There is no free honey in the little flowers, but a sweet, juicy sap is stored in a tissue round the base of the ovary and proves a great attraction to bees, who also visit the flower to collect its pollen and who play an important part in the fertilization of the flowers.

By September, the flowers have developed into scarlet berries, each berry containing vermilion flesh round a pale, hard seed. Though the plant produces fruit freely under cultivation, its propagation is mainly effected by its quickly-creeping underground stem, and in the wild state its fruit rarely comes to maturity. Its specific name, *Majalis*, or *Maialis*, signifies 'that which belongs to May,' and the old astrological books place the plant under the dominion of Mercury, since Maia, the daughter of Atlas, was the mother of Mercury or Hermes.

There is an old Sussex legend that St. Leonard fought against a great dragon in the woods near Horsham, only vanquishing it after a mortal combat lasting many hours, during which he received grievous wounds, but wherever his blood fell, Lilies-of-theValley sprang up to commemorate the desperate fight, and these woods, which bear the name of St. Leonard's Forest to this day, are still thickly carpeted with them.

Legend says that the fragrance of the Lily-of-the-Valley draws the nightingale from hedge and bush, and leads him to choose his mate in the recesses of the glade.

The Lily-of-the-Valley is one of the British-grown plants included in the Pharmacopoeia, and its medicinal virtues have been tested by very long experience. Although not in such general use as the Foxglove, it is still prescribed by physicians with success. Its use dates back to ancient times, for Apuleius in his Herbal written in the fourth century, declares it was found by Apollo and given by him to Æsculapius, the leech.

In recent years it has been largely employed in experiments relating to the forcing of plants by means of anaesthetics such as chloroform and ether. It has been found that the winter buds, placed in the vapour of chloroform for a few hours and then planted, break into leaf and flower considerably before others not tested in this manner, the resulting plants being, moreover, exceptionally fine.

Parts Used Medicinally: The whole plant, collected when in flower and dried, and also the root, herb and flowers separately. The inflorescence is said to be the most active part of the herb, and is preferred on that account, being the part usually employed.

The flowers are dried on the scape or flower-stalk, the whole stalk being cut before the lowermost flowers are faded. A good price is obtainable for the flowers, and in Lincolnshire, Derbyshire, Westmorland and other counties, where the plant grows freely wild, they would pay for collecting. During the process of drying, the white flowers assume a brownish-yellow tinge, and the fragrant odour almost entirely disappears, being replaced by a somewhat narcotic scent, the taste of the flowers is bitter.

If Lily-of-the-Valley flowers are thrown into oil of sweet almonds or olive oil, they impart to it their sweet smell, but to become really fragrant the infusion has to be repeated a dozen times with the same oil, using fresh flowers for each infusion.

Historical Medicinal Uses - For Entertainment ONLY

Constituents: The chief constituents of Lily-of-the-Valley are two glucosides, Convallamarin, the active principle, a white crystalline powder, readily soluble in water and in alcohol, but only slightly in ether, which acts upon the heart like

Digitalin, and has also diuretic action, and Convallarin, which is crystalline in prisms, soluble in alcohol, slightly soluble in water and has a purgative action. There are also present a trace of volatile oil, tannin, salts, etc.

Medicinal Action and Uses: Lily-of-the-Valley is valued as a cardiac tonic and diuretic. The action of the drug closely resembles that of Digitalis, though it is less powerful; it is used as a substitute and strongly recommended in valvular heart disease, also in cases of cardiac debility and dropsy. It slows the disturbed action of a weak, irritable heart, whilst at the same time increasing its power. It is a perfectly safe remedy. No harm has been known to occur from taking it in full and frequent doses, it being preferable in this respect to Digitalis, which is apt to accumulate in the blood with poisonous results.

It proved most useful in cases of poisonous gassing of our men at the Front.

It is generally administered in the form of a tincture. The infusion of 1/2 oz. of herb to 1 pint of boiling water is also taken in tablespoonful doses. Fluid extracts are likewise prepared from the rhizome, whole plant and flowers and the flowers have been used in powdered form.

A decoction of the flowers is said to be useful in removing obstructions in the urinary canal, and it has been also recommended as a substitute for aloes, on account of its purgative quality.

Preparations and Dosages: Fluid extract, herb, 10 to 30 drops. Fluid extract, whole plant, 10 to 30 drops. Fluid extract, flowers, 1/2 to 1 drachm.

Russian peasants have long employed the Lily-of-the-Valley for certain forms of dropsy proceeding from a faulty heart.

Special virtues were once thought to be possessed by water distilled from the flowers, which was known as Aqua aurea (Golden Water), and was deemed worthy to be preserved in vessels of gold and silver. Coles (1657) gives directions for its preparation:

'Take the flowers and steep them in New Wine for the space of a month; which being finished, take them out again and distil the wine three times over in a Limbeck. The wine is more precious than gold, for if any one that is troubled with apoplexy drink thereof with six grains of Pepper and a little Lavender water they shall not need to fear it that moneth.'

Dodoens (1560) pointed out how this water 'doth strengthen the Memorie and comforteth the Harte,' and about the same time, Joachim Camerarius, a renowned physician of Nuremberg, gave a similar prescription, which Gerard quotes, saying that:

'a Glasse being filled with the flowers of May Lilies and set in an Ant Hill with the mouth close stopped for a month's space and then taken out, ye shall find a liquor in the glasse which being outwardly applied helps the gout very much.'

This spirit was also considered excellent as an embrocation for sprains, as well as for rheumatism.

We are told by old writers that a decoction of the bruised root, boiled in wine, is good for pestilential fevers, and that bread made of barley meal mixed with the juice is an excellent cure for dropsy, also that an ointment of the root and lard is good for ulcers and heals burns and scalds without leaving a scar.

Culpepper said of the Lily-of-the-Valley:

'It without doubt strengthens the brain and renovates a weak memory. The distilled water dropped into the eyes helps inflammations thereof. The spirit of the flowers, distilled in wine, restoreth lost speech, helps the palsy, and is exceedingly good in the apoplexy, comforteth the heart and vital spirits.'

The powdered flowers have been said to excite sneezing, proving serviceable in the relief of headache and earache; but to some sick people the scent of the flowers has proved harmful.

In some parts of Germany, a wine is still prepared from the flowers, mixed with raisins.

Loveage

Quick Facts

Latin/Linnaen:	*Levisticum officinale*
Family:	*Apiaceae*
Old English :	Lufestice
Synonyms:	Lovage
Action:	The ligustilide containing essential oil is antispasmodic.
Parts Used:	Root
Indicated For:	Irrigation therapy for inflammation of the lower urinary tract for prevention of kidney gravel.
Dosage:	Unless otherwise prescribed: Daily dosage: 4-8g of drug; equivalent preparations
Preparation:	Comminuted herb and other galenical preparations for internal use.
Cautions:	**Contraindications**: Preparation of lovage should not be used if acute inflammation of the kidney parenchyma with impaired kidney function exists. **Note**: Intense exposure to the sun and ultraviolet light should be avoided during extended use of lovage root.
Other Uses:	**Culinary:** The leaves can be used in salads, or to make soup, and the roots can be eaten as a vegetable or grated for use in salads. Its flavor and smell is very similar to celery.

Beverage: Lovage tea can be applied to wounds as an antiseptic, or drunk to stimulate digestion. The seeds can be used as a spice, similar to fennel seeds In the UK, an alcoholic lovage cordial is traditionally mixed with brandy in the ratio of 2:1 as a winter drink. Lovage is second only to capers in its quercetin content.

The roots, which contain a heavy, volatile oil, are used as a mild aquaretic (Aquaresis is the excretion of water without electrolyte loss.)

Description

Lovage (*Levisticum officinale*) is a tall perennial plant, the sole species in the genus *Levisticum*, in the family *Apiaceae*, subfamily *Apioideae*, tribe *Apieae*.

The exact native range is disputed; some sources cite it as native to much of Europe and southwestern Asia, others from only the eastern Mediterranean region in southeastern Europe and southwestern Asia, and yet others only to southwestern Asia in Iran and Afghanistan, citing European populations as naturalised. It has been long cultivated in Europe, the leaves being used as an herb, the roots as a vegetable, and the seeds as a spice, especially in southern European cuisine.

Lovage is an erect herbaceous perennial plant growing to 1.8–2.5 m tall, with a basal rosette of leaves and stems with further leaves, the flowers being produced in umbels at the top of the stems. The stems and leaves are shiny glabrous green to yellow-green. The larger basal leaves are up to 70 cm long, tripinnate, with broad triangular to rhomboidal, acutely pointed leaflets with a few marginal teeth; the stem leaves are smaller, and less divided with few leaflets. The flowers are yellow to greenish-yellow, 2–3 mm diameter, produced in globose umbels up to 10–15 cm diameter; flowering is in late spring. The fruit is a dry two-parted schizocarp 4–7 mm long, mature in autumn.

Etymology

The name 'lovage' is from "love-ache", ache being a medieval name for parsley; this is a folk-etymological corruption of the older French name levesche, from late Latin levisticum, in turn thought to be a corruption of the earlier Latin ligusticum, "of Liguria" (northwest Italy), where the herb was grown extensively. In modern botanical usage, both Latin forms are now used, for different, but closely related genera, with *Levisticum* for (culinary) Lovage, and *Ligusticum* for Scots Lovage, a similar species from northern Europe, and related species. In Germany and Holland, one of the common names of Lovage is Maggikraut (German) or Maggiplant (Dutch) because the plant's taste is reminiscent of Maggi soup seasoning.

Cultivation

Hardiness Zone:	3-5
Soil pH:	5.0-7.6
Soil type:	Tolerant of most soil.
Cultivation:	By seed or rood division.
Sunlight:	Full sun-partial shade
Habitat:	Native to the Mediterranean

Lovage looks like a giant celery plant. One plant will be sufficient for most uses.

Historical Notes

It is not considered to be indigenous to Great Britain, and when occasionally found growing apparently wild, it is probably a garden escape. It is a native of the Mediterranean region, growing wild in the mountainous districts of the south of France, in northern Greece and in the Balkans.

The Garden Lovage is one of the old English herbs that was formerly very generally cultivated, and is still occasionally cultivated as a sweet herb, and for the use in herbal medicine of its root, and to a less degree, the leaves and seeds.

It is a true perennial and hence is very easy to keep in garden cultivation; it can be propagated by offsets like Rhubarb, and it is very hardy. Its old-time repute has suffered by the substitution of the medicinally more powerful Milfoil and Tansy, just as was the case when 'Elecampane' superseded Angelica in medical use. The public-house cordial named 'Lovage,' formerly much in vogue, however, owed such virtue as it may have possessed to Tansy. Freshly-gathered leafstalks of Lovage (for flavouring purposes) should be employed in long split lengths.

Description: This stout, umbelliferous plant has been thought to resemble to some degree our Garden Angelica, and it does very closely resemble the Spanish Angelica heterocarpa in foliage and perennial habit of growth. It has a thick and fleshy root, 5 or 6 inches long, shaped like a carrot, of a greyish-brown colour on the outside and whitish within. It has a strong aromatic smell and taste. The thick, erect hollow and channelled stems grow 3 or 4 feet or even more in height. The large, dark green radical leaves, on erect stalks, are divided into narrow wedge-like segments, and are not unlike those of a coarse-growing celery; their surface is shining, and when bruised they give out an aromatic odour, somewhat reminiscent both of Angelica and Celery. The stems divide towards the top to form opposite whorled branches, which in June and July bear umbels of yellow flowers, similar to those of Fennel or Parsnip, followed by small, extremely aromatic fruits, yellowish-brown in colour, elliptical in shape and curved, with three prominent winged ribs. The odour of the whole plant is very strong. Its taste is warm and aromatic, and it abounds with a yellowish, gummy, resinous juice.

It is sometimes grown in gardens for its ornamental foliage, as well as for its pleasant odour, but it is not a striking enough plant to have claimed the attention of poets and painters, and no myths or legends are connected with it. The name of the genus, *Ligusticum*, is said to be derived from Liguria, where this species abounds.

Cultivation: Lovage is of easy culture. Propagation is by division of roots or by seeds. Rich moist, but well-drained soil is required and a sunny situation. In late summer, when the seed ripens, it should be sown and the seedlings transplanted, either in the autumn or as early in spring as possible, to their permanent quarters, setting 12 inches apart each way. The seeds may also be sown in spring, but it is preferable to sow when just ripe. Root division is performed in early spring.

The plants should last for several years, if the ground be kept well cultivated, and where the seeds are permitted to scatter the plants will come up without care.

Parts Used: The root, leaves and seeds for medicinal purposes.

The young stems, treated like Angelica, for flavouring and confectionery.

Constituents: Lovage contains a volatile oil, angelic acid, a bitter extractive, resins, etc. The colouring principle has been isolated by M. Niklis, who gives it the name of Ligulin, and suggests an important application of it that may be made in testing drinking water. If a drop of its alcoholic or aqueous solution is allowed to fall into distilled water, it imparts to the liquid its own fine crimson-red colour, which undergoes no change; but if limestone water be substituted, the red colour disappears in a few seconds and is followed by a beautiful blue, due to the alkalinity of the latter.

Historical Medicinal Uses - For Entertainment ONLY

Medicinal Action and Uses: Formerly Lovage was used for a variety of culinary purposes, but now its use is restricted almost wholly to confectionery, the young stems being treated like those of Angelica, to which, however, it is inferior, as its stems are not so stout nor so succulent.

The leafstalks and stem bases were formerly blanched like celery, but as a vegetable it has fallen into disuse.

An herbal tea is made of the leaves, when previously dried, the decoction having a very agreeable odour.

Lovage was much used as a drug plant in the fourteenth century, its medicinal reputation probably being greatly founded on its pleasing aromatic odour. It was never an official remedy, nor were any extravagant claims made, as with Angelica, for its efficacy in numberless complaints.

The roots and fruit are aromatic and stimulant, and have diuretic and carminative action. In herbal medicine they are used in disorders of the stomach and feverish attacks, especially for cases of colic and flatulence in children, its qualities being similar to those of Angelica in expelling flatulence, exciting perspiration and opening obstructions. The leaves eaten as salad, or infused dry as a tea, used to be accounted a good emmenagogue.

An infusion of the root was recommended by old writers for gravel, jaundice and urinary troubles, and the cordial, sudorific nature of the roots and seeds caused their use to be extolled in 'pestilential disorders.' In the opinion of Culpepper, the working of the seeds was more powerful than that of the root; he tells us that an infusion 'being dropped into the eyes taketh away their redness or dimness.... It is highly recommended to drink the decoction of the herb for agues.... The distilled water is good for quinsy if the mouth and throat be gargled and washed therewith.... The decoction drunk three or four times a day is effectual in pleurisy.... The leaves bruised and fried with a little hog's lard and laid hot to any blotch or boil will quickly break it.'

Several species of this umbelliferous genus are employed as domestic medicines. The root of *ligusticum sinense*, under the name of kao-pâu, is largely used by the Chinese, and in the north-western United States the large, aromatic roots of *ligusticum filicinum* (osha colorado cough-root) are used to a considerable extent as stimulating expectorants.

The old-fashioned cordial, 'Lovage,' now not much in vogue, though still occasionally to be found in public-houses, is brewed not only from the Garden Lovage, Ligusticum levisticum, but mainly from a species of Milfoil or Yarrow, Achillea ligustica, and from Tansy, Tanacetum vulgare, and probably owes its merit more to these herbs than to Lovage itself. From its use in this cordial, Milfoil has often been mistakenly called Lovage, though it is in no way related to the *Umbellifer* family.

Several other plants have been termed Lovage besides the true Lovage, and this has frequently caused confusion. Thus we have the scotch lovage, known also as Sea Lovage, or Scotch Parsley, and botanically as *Ligusticum scoticum*; the black lovage, or Alexanders, *Smyrnium Olusatrum*; bastard lovage, a species of the allied genus, *Laserpitum*, and water lovage, a species of the genus *Cenanthe*.

Laserpitum may be distinguished from its allies by the fruit having eight prominent, wing-like appendages. The species are perennial herbs, chiefly found in south-eastern Europe. Some of them are employed as domestic remedies, on account of their aroma.

The scent of the root of *meum athamanticum* (Jacq.), spignel (also called Spikenel or Spiknel), meu or bald-money, has much in common with that of both Lovage and Angelica, and the root has been eaten by the Scotch Highlanders as a vegetable. It is a perennial, smooth and very aromatic herb. The elongated root is crowned with fibres, the leaves, mostly springing from the root, are divided into leaflets which are further cut into numerous thread-like segments, which gives them a feathery appearance. The stem is about 6 or 8 inches high, and bears umbels of white or purplish flowers. The aromatic flavour of the leaves is somewhat like Melilot, and is communicated to milk and butter when cows feed on the herbage in the spring. The peculiar name of this plant, 'Baldmoney,' is said to be a corruption of Balder, the Apollo of the northern nations, to whom the plant was dedicated.

Mallow

Malvaceae.

Malva silvestris L.

Quick Facts

Latin/Linnaen:	*Malva Sylvestris*
Family:	*Malvaceae*
Old English :	Hocleaf, Geormenleaf
Synonyms:	Cheeses, High mallow and Tall mallow, (Mauve des bois by the French)
Action:	Demulcent
Parts Used:	Flower
Indicated For:	Irritations of the mucosa of the mouth and throat and associated dry, irritative cough.
Dosage:	Unless otherwise prescribed: Daily dosage: 5g of drug; equivalent preparations.
Preparation:	Comminuted herb for infusions and other preparations for internal use.
Cautions:	
Other Uses:	

Description

Malva sylvestris is a species of the Mallow genus Malva in the family of *Malvaceae* and is considered to be the type species for the genus. Known as common mallow to English speaking Europeans, it acquired the common names of cheeses, high mallow and tall mallow (mauve des bois by the French) as it migrated from its native home in Western Europe, North Africa and Asia through the English speaking world. *M. sylvestris* is a vigorously healthy plant with showy flowers of bright mauve-purple, with dark veins; a handsome plant, often standing 3 or 4 feet (1 m) high and growing freely in fields, hedgerows and in fallow fields.

Cultivation

Hardiness Zone:	3-9
Soil pH:	6.0-7.5
Soil type:	Moist average soil
Cultivation:	By seed, cuttings and root offsets.
Sunlight:	Full sun-partial shade
Habitat:	Native to Europe, occurs in damp areas like marshes.

Mallow is an easy plant to cultivate. Can become invasive.

Historical Notes

None of note.

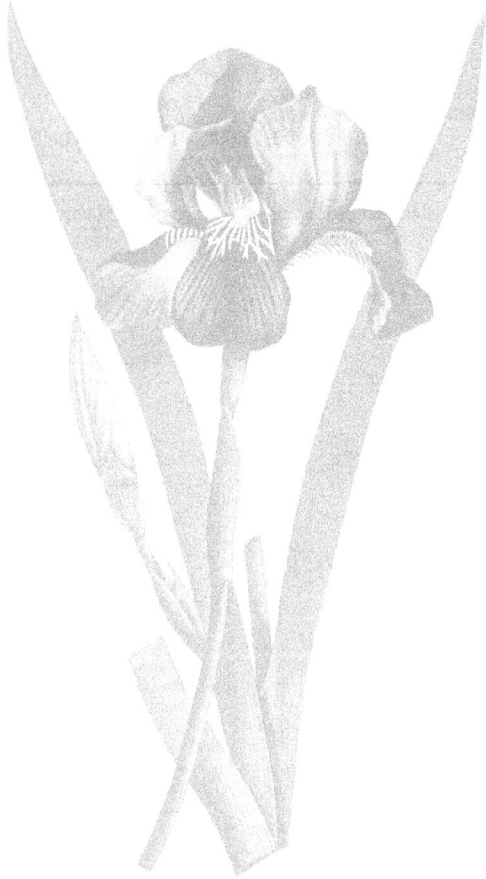

Marsh Mallow Leaf

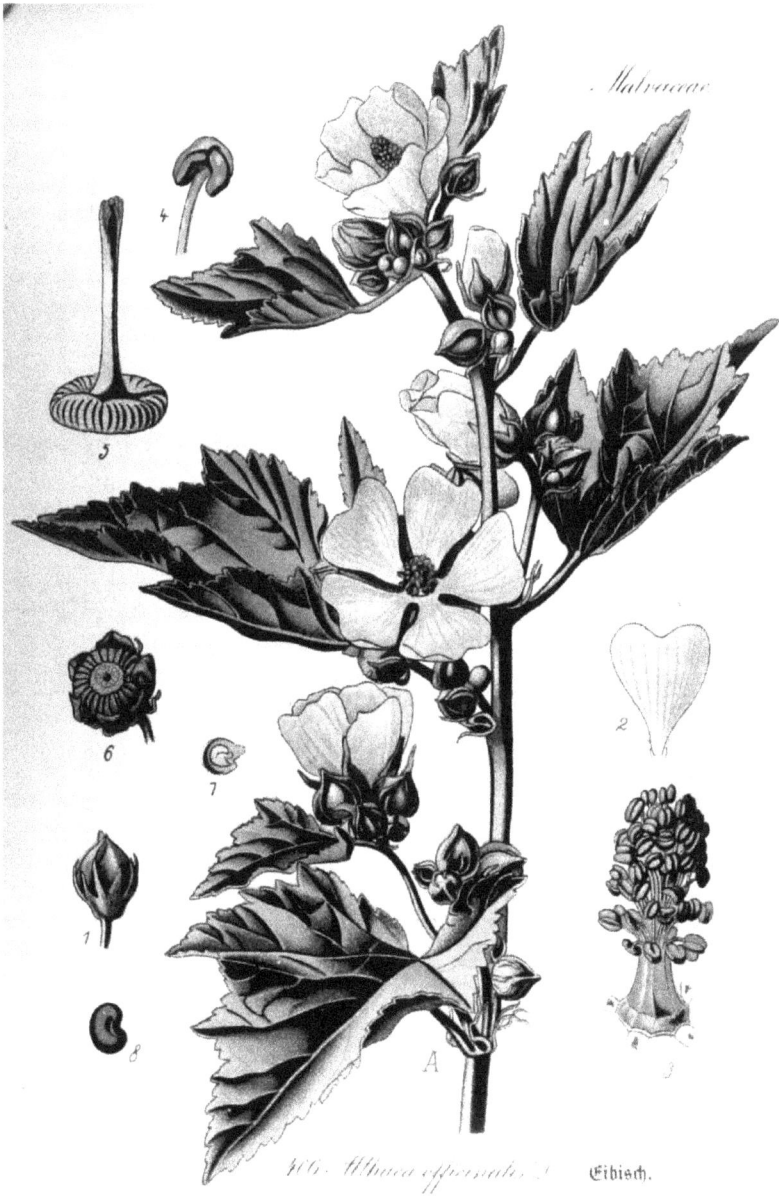

Quick Facts (Leaf)

Latin/Linnaen:	*Althaea Officinalis*
Family:	*Malvaceae*
Old English :	Merscmergylle
Synonyms:	Marshmallow, Marshmellow, Common Marshmallow, Mallards, Mauls, Schloss Tea, Cheeses, Mortification Koot, (French) Guimauve.
Action:	Alleviates local irritation
Parts Used:	**Leaf**
Indicated For:	Irritation of the oral and pharyngeal mucosa and associated dry cough.
Dosage:	Unless otherwise prescribed: Daily dosage: 5g of drug; equivalent preparations.
Preparation:	Cut leaves for aqueous extracts as well as other galenical preparations for internal use.
Cautions:	Absorption of other drugs taken simultaneously may be delayed.
Other Uses:	**Culinary:** The root extract (halawa extract) is sometimes used as flavouring in the making of a Middle Eastern snack called halva.
	The flowers and young leaves can be eaten, and are often added to salads or are boiled and fried.

Quick Facts (Root)

Latin/Linnaen:	*Althaea Officinalis*
Family:	*Malvaceae*
Old English :	Merscmergylle

Synonyms:	Marshmallow, Marshmellow, Common Marshmallow
Action	Alleviates local irritation, Inhibits mucociliary activity, Stimulates phagocytosis
Parts Used:	**root**
Indicated For:	(a) Irritation of the oral and pharyngeal mucosa and associated dry cough. (b)Mild inflammation of the gastric mucosa.
Dosage:	Unless otherwise prescribed: Daily dosage: 6g of roots, equivalent preparations. Marshmallow syrup: single dose: 10g.
Preparation:	Cut or ground root for aqueous extracts as well as other galenical preparations for internal use. Marshmallow syrup to be used only for use (a).
Cautions:	Marshmallow syrup: diabetics need to allow for sugar concentration.
Other Uses:	

Description

Althaea officinalis (Marshmallow, Marsh Mallow, or Common Marshmallow) is a species indigenous to Africa, which is used as a medicinal plant and ornamental plant. A confection made from the root since ancient Egyptian time evolved into today's marshmallow treat.

The stems, which die down in the autumn, are erect, 3 to 4 feet (1.2 m) high, simple, or putting out only a few lateral branches. The leaves, shortly petioled, are roundish, ovate-cordate, 2 to 3 inches (76 mm) long, and about 1 1/4 inch broad, entire or three to five lobed, irregularly toothed at the margin, and thick. They are soft and velvety on both sides, due to a dense covering of stellate hairs. The flowers are shaped like those of the common Mallow, but are smaller and of a pale colour, and are either axillary, or in panicles, more often the latter.

The stamens are united into a tube, the anthers, kidney-shaped and one-celled. The flowers are in bloom during August and September, and are followed, as in other species of this order, by the flat, round fruit which are popularly called 'cheeses.'

The common Mallow is frequently called by country people 'Marsh Mallow,' but the true Marsh Mallow is distinguished from all the other Mallows growing in Great Britain, by the numerous divisions of the outer calyx (six to nine cleft), by the hoary down which thickly clothes the stems and foliage, and by the numerous panicles of blush-coloured flowers, paler than the Common Mallow. The roots are perennial, thick, long and tapering, very tough and pliant, whitish yellow outside, white and fibrous within. The whole plant, particularly the root, abounds with a mild mucilage, which is emollient to a much greater degree than the common Mallow. The generic name, Althaea, is derived from the Greek altho (to cure), from its healing properties. The name of the family, *Malvaceae*, is derived from the Greek malake (soft), from the special qualities of the Mallows in softening and healing.

Marshmallow is traditionally used as a treatment for the irritation of mucous membranes, including use as a gargle for mouth and throat ulcers, and gastric ulcers.

Cultivation

Hardiness Zone:	3-10
Soil pH:	5.5-8.5
Soil type:	Tolerant of most soils, prefers rich moist soil.
Cultivation:	By seed or root division.
Sunlight:	Full sun
Habitat:	Native to Europe, western Asia and northern Africa.

Marsh Mallow is tolerant of most growing conditions and can be grown in coastal regions.

It can be raised from seed, sown in spring, but cuttings will do well, and offsets of the root, carefully divided in autumn, when the stalks decay, are satisfactory, and will grow of their own accord.

Plant about 2 feet apart. It will thrive in any soil or situation, but grows larger in moist than in dry land, and could well be cultivated on unused ground in damp localities near ditches or streams.

Historical Notes

The root has been used since the Middle Ages in the treatment of sore throat. The later French version of the recipe, called pâte de guimauve (or "guimauve" for short), included an eggwhite meringue and was often flavored with rose water. Pâte de guimauve more closely resembles contemporary commercially available marshmallows, which no longer contain any actual marshmallow.

Most of the Mallows have been used as food, and are mentioned by early classic writers with this connection. Mallow was an esculent vegetable among the Romans; a dish of Marsh Mallow was one of their delicacies. Prosper Alpinus stated in 1592 that a plant of the Mallow kind was eaten by the Egyptians. Many of the poorer inhabitants of Syria subsist for weeks on herbs, of which Marsh Mallow is one of the most common. When boiled first and fried with onions and butter, the roots are said to form a palatable dish, and in times of scarcity consequent upon the failure of the crops, this plant, which fortunately grows there in great abundance, is collected heavily as a foodstuff.

Marsh Mallow is a native of most countries of Europe, from Denmark southward. It grows in salt marshes, in damp meadows, by the sides of ditches, by the sea and on the banks of tidal rivers.

In this country it is local, but occurs in most of the maritime counties in the south of England, ranging as far north as Lincolnshire. In Scotland it has been introduced.

The stems, which die down in the autumn, are erect, 3 to 4 feet high, simple, or putting out only a few lateral branches. The leaves, shortly petioled, are roundish, ovate-cordate, 2 to 3 inches long, and about 1 1/4 inch broad, entire or three to five lobed, irregularly toothed at the margin, and thick. They are soft and velvety on both sides, due to a dense covering of stellate hairs. The flowers are shaped like those of the common Mallow, but are smaller and of a pale colour, and are either axillary, or in panicles, more often the latter.

The stamens are united into a tube, the anthers, kidney-shaped and one-celled. The flowers are in bloom during August and September, and are followed, as in other species of this order, by the flat, round fruit called popularly 'cheeses.'

In Job XXX. 4 we read of Mallow being eaten in time of famine, but it is doubtful whether this was really a true mallow. Canon Tristram thinks it was some saline plant; perhaps the Orache, or Sea-Purslane.

Horace and Martial mention the laxative properties of the Marsh Mallow leaves and root, and Virgil tells us of the fondness of goats for the foliage of the Mallow.

Historical Medicinal Uses - For Entertainment ONLY
Pliny said:

'Whosoever shall take a spoonful of the Mallows shall that day be free from all diseases that may come to him.'

All Mallows contain abundant mucilage, and the Arab physicians in early times used the leaves as a poultice to suppress inflammation.

Dioscorides extols it as a remedy, and in ancient days it was not only valued as a medicine, but was used, especially the Musk Mallow, to decorate the graves of friends.

Preparations of Marsh Mallow, on account of their soothing qualities, are still much used by country people for inflammation, outwardly and inwardly, and are used for lozenge-making. French druggists and English sweetmeat-makers prepare a confectionary paste (Pâét, de Guimauve) from the roots of Marsh Mallow, which is emollient and soothing to a sore chest, and valuable in coughs and hoarseness. The 'Marsh Mallows' usually sold by confectioners here are a mixture of flour, gum, egg-albumin, etc., and contain no mallow.

In France, the young tops and tender leaves of Marsh Mallow are eaten uncooked, in spring salads, for their property in stimulating the kidneys, a syrup being made from the roots for the same purpose.

Parts Used: Leaves, roots and flowers. The leaves are picked in August, when the flowers are just coming into bloom. They should be stripped off singly and gathered only on a fine day, in the morning, after the dew has been dried off by the sun.

Constituents: Marsh Mallow contains starch, mucilage, pectin, oil, sugar, asparagin, phosphate of lime, glutinous matter and cellulose.

RECIPES

Marsh Mallow Water

'Soak one ounce of marsh mallow roots in a little cold water for half an hour; peel off the bark, or skin; cut up the roots into small shavings, and put them into a jug to stand for a couple of hours; the decoction must be drunk tepid, and may be sweetened with honey or sugar-candy, and flavoured with orange-flower water, or with orange juice. Marshmallow water may be used with good effect in all cases of inveterate coughs, catarrhs, etc.' (Francatelli's Cook's Guide.)

For Gravel, etc.

'Put the flower and plant (all but the root) of Marsh Mallows in a jug, pour boiling water, cover with a cloth, let it stand three hours - make it strong. If used for gravel or irritation of the kidney, take 1/2 pint as a tea daily for four days, then stop a few days, then go on again. A teaspoonful of gin may be added when there is no tendency to inflammation.' (From a family recipe-book.)

The powdered or crushed fresh roots make a good poultice that will remove the most obstinate inflammation and prevent mortification. Its efficacy in this direction has earned for it the name of Mortification Root. Slippery Elm may be added with advantage, and the poultice should be applied to the part as hot as can be borne and renewed when dry. An infusion of 1 oz. of leaves to a pint of boiling water is also taken frequently in wineglassful doses. This infusion is good for bathing inflamed eyes.

An ointment made from Marsh Mallow has also a popular reputation, but it is stated that a poultice made of the fresh root, with the addition of a little white bread, proves more serviceable when applied externally than the ointment. The fresh leaves, steeped in hot water and applied to the affected parts as poultices, also reduce inflammation, and bruised and rubbed upon any place stung by wasps or bees take away the pain, inflammation and swelling. Pliny stated that the green leaves, beaten with nitre and applied, drew out thorns and prickles in the flesh.

The flowers, boiled in oil and water, with a little honey and alum, have proved good as a gargle for sore throats. In France, they form one of the ingredients of the Tisane de quatre fleurs, a pleasant remedy for colds.

Medicinal Action and Uses: The great demulcent and emollient properties of Marsh Mallow make it useful in inflammation and irritation of the alimentary canal, and of the urinary and respiratory organs. The dry roots boiled in water give out half their weight of a gummy matter like starch. Decoctions of the plant, especially of the root, are very useful where the natural mucus has been abraded from the coats of the intestines, The decoction can be made by adding 5 pints of water to 1/4 lb. of dried root, boiling down to 3 pints and straining: it should not be made too thick and viscid. It is excellent in painful complaints of the urinary organs, exerting a relaxing effect upon the passages, as well as acting curatively. This decoction is also effective in curing bruises, sprains or any ache in the muscles or sinews. In haemorrhage from the urinary organs and in dysentery, it has been recommended to use the powdered root boiled in milk. The action of Marsh Mallow root upon the bowels is unaccompanied by any astringency.

Preparations and Dosage: Fluid extract leaves. 1/2 to 2 drachms.

Boiled in wine or milk, Marsh Mallow will relieve diseases of the chest, constituting a popular remedy for coughs, bronchitis, whooping-cough, etc., generally in combination with other remedies. It is frequently given in the form of a syrup, which is best adapted to infants and children.

Mint

MXXXVIII.

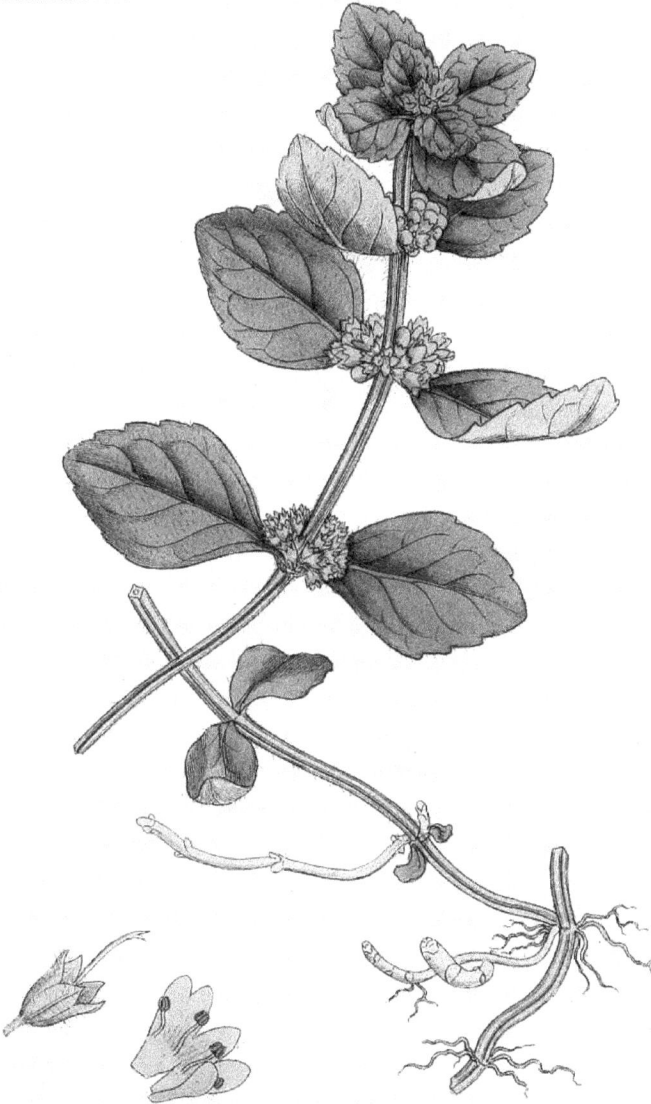

E. B. 2119.   Mentha arvensis, var. genuina.   Corn Mint, var. *a.*

Quick Facts

Latin/Linnaen:	*Mentha Arvensis*
Family:	*Lamiaceae*
Old English :	Minte
Synonyms:	Field Mint, Pudina in Hindi, Wild Mint, Corn Mint
Action:	Carminative, cholagogue, antibacterial, secretolytic, cooling
Parts Used:	Oil
Indicated For:	Internal: flatulence, functional gastrointestinal and gallbladder disorders, catarrhs of the upper respiratory tract. External: myalgia and neuralgic ailments.
Dosage:	Unless otherwise prescribed: Internal: Average daily dosage: 3-6 drops; Inhalation: 3-4 drops in hot water; External: Several drops rubbed into the skin; equivalent preparations. 5-20 percent in oil and semi-solid preparations; 5-10 percent in aqueous-alcoholic preparations; In nasal ointments, 1-5 percent essential oil.
Preparation:	Essential oil and other galenical preparations for internal and external applications.
Cautions:	Contraindications: Internal: obstruction of the bile ducts, inflammation of the gallbladder, severe liver damage. External: For infants and young children, mint oil-containing preparations should not be used on areas of the face and especially the nose.
Other Uses:	**Beverage:** A herb tea can be made from the fresh or dried leaves.

Description

Mentha arvensis (Field Mint, Pudina in Hindi), Wild Mint or Corn Mint, is a species of mint with a circumboreal distribution. It is native to the temperate regions of Europe and western and central Asia, east to the Himalaya and eastern Siberia, and North America.

It is an herbaceous perennial plant growing to 10–60 cm (rarely to 100 cm) tall. The leaves are in opposite pairs, simple, 2–6.5 cm long and 1–2 cm broad, hairy, and with a coarsely serrated margin. The flowers are pale purple (occasionally white or pink), in clusters on the stem, each flower 3–4 mm long.

Cultivation

Hardiness Zone:	4-10
Soil pH:	Prefers slightly acidic soil.
Soil type:	Tolerant of most soil, even heavy clay.
Cultivation:	By seed or root division.
Sunlight:	Full sun-partial shade
Habitat:	Native to Europe, Asia and North America

Mint can be highly invasive and you could consider growing it annually in containers if you don't have land to devote to letting mint spread.

Historical Notes

It is a perennial, the root-stock, as in all the Mints, creeping freely, so that when the plant has once taken hold of the ground it becomes very difficult to eradicate it, as its long creeping roots bind the soil together and ultimately overrun a considerable area. It is generally an indication that the drainage of the land has been neglected. It is abundantly distributed throughout Britain, though less common in the northern counties and flourishes in fields and moist ground, and Peppermint growers must be ever watchful for its appearance.

The Corn Mint (*Mentha arvensis*) is the type species of the Japanese Menthol plant, but is not endowed with useful medicinal properties, great care indeed, as has been mentioned, having to be taken to eradicate it from Peppermint plantations, for if mingled with that valuable herb in distilling its strong odour affects the quality of the oil.

It is a branched, downy plant. From the low, spreading, quadrangular stems that lie near the ground, the flowering stems are each year thrown up, 6 to 12 inches high. The leaves, springing from the stems, in pairs, are stalked, their outlines freely toothed. The upper leaves are smaller than the lower, and the flowers are arranged in rings (whorls) in their axils. The flowers themselves are small individually, but the delicacy of their colour and the dense clusters in which they grow, give an importance collectively, as ring after ring of the blossoms form as a whole a conspicuous head. The flowering season lasts throughout August and September.

This mint varies considerably in appearance in different plants, like all the other native species of mint, some being much larger than others, with a more developed foliage and a much greater hairiness of all the parts. It has a strong odour that becomes more decided still when the leaves are bruised in any way.

It is said that the effect of this plant, when animals eat it, is to prevent coagulation of their milk, so that it can hardly be made to yield cheese.

Mistletoe

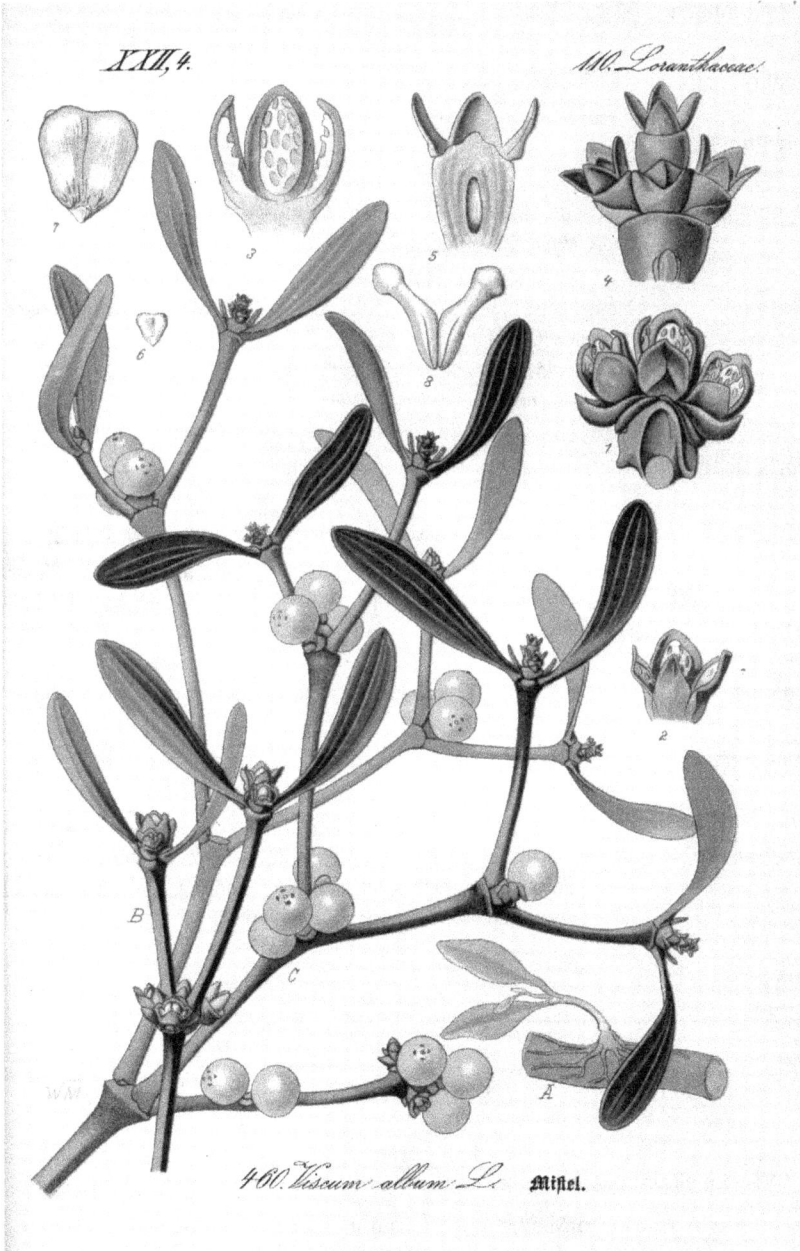

460. *Viscum album* L. Miftel.

Quick Facts

Latin/Linnaen:	*Viscum Album*
Family:	*Santalaceae*
Old English :	Mistel
Synonyms:	European Mistletoe or Common Mistletoe, Birdlime Mistletoe. Herbe de la Croix, Mystyldene, Lignum Crucis.
Action:	Intracutaneous injections cause local inflammation which can lead to necrosis. Cytostatic, non specific immune stimulation. Note: The blood pressure lowering effects and the therapeutic effectiveness for mild forms of hypertonia need further investigation.
Parts Used:	Younger branches with flowers and fruits.
Indicated For:	For treating degenerative inflammation of the joints by stimulating cuti-visceral reflexes following local inflammation brought about by intradermal injections. As palliative therapy for malignant tumors through non specific stimulation.
Dosage:	Unless otherwise prescribed: According to directions of the manufacturer.
Preparation:	Fresh plant, cut and powdered herb for the preparation of solutions for injections.
Cautions:	Contraindications: Protein hypersensitivity, chronic progressive infections. Side Effects: Chills, high fever, headaches, angina, orthostatic circulatory disturbances and allergic reactions.
Other Uses:	

Description

Viscum album is a species of mistletoe, the species originally so-named, and also known as European Mistletoe or Common Mistletoe to distinguish it from other related species. It is native to Europe and western and southern Asia. Witches' Broom looks similar but is an abnormal growth of the tree.

It is a hemi-parasitic shrub, which grows on the stems of other trees. It has stems 30–100 centimetres (12–39 in) long with dichotomous branching. The leaves are in opposite pairs, strap-shaped, entire, leathery textured, 2–8 centimetres (0.79–3.1 in) long, 0.8–2.5 centimetres (0.31–0.98 in) broad and are a yellowish-green in colour. This species is dioecious and the flowers are inconspicuous, yellowish-green, 2–3 millimetres (0.079–0.12 in) diameter. The fruit is a white or yellow berry containing one (very rarely several) seed embedded in the very sticky, glutinous fruit pulp.

It is commonly found in the crowns of broad-leaved trees, particularly apple, lime, hawthorn and poplar.

Cultivation

Hardiness Zone:	6-8
Soil pH:	none
Soil type:	none
Cultivation:	You can try to plant the seed of mistletoe in a healthy mature tree by placing as deeply as possible into the bark.
Sunlight:	Full sun-partial shade
Habitat:	Native to Asia and Europe, not to be confused with Phoradendron Leucarpun (American Mistletoe), which has different properties.

Mistletoe is a parasitic plant which grows in the branches of apple, oak, pine and fir trees. If grown in a healthy mature tree, mistletoe should not have a significant impact on the tree. Mistletoe is not self fertile and needs a male and female plant to produce berries.

Historical Notes

The well-known Mistletoe is an evergreen parasitic plant, growing on the branches of trees, where it forms pendent bushes, 2 to 5 feet in diameter. It will grow and has been found on almost any deciduous tree, preferring those with soft bark, and being, perhaps, commonest on old Apple trees, though it is frequently found on the Ash, Hawthorn, Lime and other trees. On the Oak, it grows very seldom. It has been found on the Cedar of Lebanon and on the Larch, but very rarely on the Pear tree.

When one of the familiar sticky berries of the Mistletoe comes into contact with the bark of a tree - generally through the agency of birds - after a few days it sends forth a thread-like root, flattened at the extremity like the proboscis of a fly. This finally pierces the bark and roots itself firmly in the growing wood, from which it has the power of selecting and appropriating to its own use, such juices as are fitted for its sustenance: the wood of Mistletoe has been found to contain twice as much potash, and five times as much phosphoric acid as the wood of the foster tree. Mistletoe is a true parasite, for at no period does it derive nourishment from the soil, or from decayed bark, like some of the fungi do - all its nourishment is obtained from its host. The root becomes woody and thick.

Description: The stem is yellowish and smooth, freely forked, separating when dead into bone-like joints. The leaves are tongue-shaped, broader towards the end, 1 to 3 inches long, very thick and leathery, of a dull yellow-green colour, arranged in pairs, with very short footstalks. The flowers, small and inconspicuous, are arranged in threes, in close short spikes or clusters in the forks of the branches, and are of two varieties, the male and female occurring on different plants. Neither male nor female flowers have a corolla, the parts of the fructification springing from the yellowish calyx. They open in May. The fruit is a globular, smooth, white berry, ripening in December.

Mistletoe is found throughout Europe, and in England is particularly common in Herefordshire and Worcestershire. In Scotland it is almost unknown.

The genus Viscum has thirty or more species. In South Africa there are several, one with very minute leaves, a feature common to many herbs growing in that excessively dry climate; one in Australia is densely woolly, from a similar cause. Several members of the family are not parasitic at all,being shrubs and trees, showing that the parasitic habit is an acquired one, and now, of course, hereditary.

Mistletoe is always produced by seed and cannot be cultivated in the earth like other plants, hence the ancients considered it to be an excrescence of the tree. By rubbing the berries on the smooth bark of the underside of the branches of trees till they adhere, or inserting them in clefts made for the purpose, it is possible to grow Mistletoe quite successfully, if desired.

The thrush is the great disseminator of the Mistletoe, devouring the berries eagerly, from which the Missel Thrush is said by some to derive its name. The stems and foliage have been given to sheep in winter, when fodder was scarce, and they are said to eat it with relish.

In Brittany, where the Mistletoe grows so abundantly, the plant is called Herbe de la Croix, because, according to an old legend, the Cross was made from its wood, on account of which it was degraded to be a parasite.

The English name is said to be derived from the Anglo-Saxon Misteltan, tan signifying twig, and mistel from mist, which in old Dutch meant birdlime; thus, according to Professor Skeat, Mistletoe means 'birdlime twig,' a reference to the fact that the berries have been used for making birdlime. Dr. Prior, however derives the word from tan, a twig, and mistl, meaning different, from its being unlike the tree it grows on. In the fourteenth century it was termed 'Mystyldene' and also Lignum crucis, an allusion to the legend just mentioned. The Latin name of the genus, Viscum, signifying sticky, was assigned to it from the glutinous juice of its berries.

History: Mistletoe was held in great reverence by the Druids. They went forth clad in white robes to search for the sacred plant, and when it was discovered, one of the Druids ascended the tree and gathered it with great ceremony, separating it from the Oak with a golden knife. The Mistletoe was always cut at a particular age of the moon, at the beginning of the year, and it was only sought for when the Druids declared they had visions directing them to seek it. When a great length of time elapsed without this happening, or if the Mistletoe chanced to fall to the ground, it was considered as an omen that some misfortune would befall the nation. The Druids held that the Mistletoe protected its possessor from all evil, and that the oaks on which it was seen growing were to be respected because of the wonderful cures which the priests were able to effect with it. They sent round their attendant youth with branches of the Mistletoe to announce the entrance of the new year. It is probable that the custom of including it in the decoration of our homes at Christmas, giving it a special place of honour, is a survival of this old custom.

The curious basket of garland with which 'Jack-in-the-Green' is even now occasionally invested on May-day is said to be a relic of a similar garb assumed by the Druids for the ceremony of the Mistletoe. When they had found it they danced round the oak to the tune of 'Hey derry down, down, down derry!' which literally signified, 'In a circle move we round the oak. ' Some oakwoods in Herefordshire are still called 'the derry'; and the following line from Ovid refers to the Druids' songs beneath the oak:

'---Ad viscum Druidce cantare solebant---.'

Shakespeare calls it 'the baleful Mistletoe,' an allusion to the Scandinavian legend that Balder, the god of Peace, was slain with an arrow made of Mistletoe. He was restored to life at the request of the other gods and goddesses, and Mistletoe was afterwards given into the keeping of the goddess of Love, and it was ordained that everyone who passed under it should receive a kiss, to show that the branch had become an emblem of love, and not of hate.

Historical Medicinal Uses - For Entertainment ONLY

Parts Used Medicinally: The leaves and young twigs, collected just before the berries form, and dried in the same manner as described for Holly.

Constituents: Mistletoe contains mucilage, sugar, a fixed oil, resin, an odorous principle, some tannin and various salts. The active part of the plant is the resin, Viscin, which by fermentation becomes a yellowish, sticky, resinous mass, which can be used with success as a birdlime.

The preparations ordinarily used are a fluid extract and the powdered leaves. A homoeopathic tincture is prepared with spirit from equal quantities of the leaves and ripe berries, but is difficult of manufacture, owing to the viscidity of the sap.

Medicinal Action and Uses: Nervine, antispasmodic, tonic and narcotic. Has a great reputation for curing the 'falling sickness' epilepsy - and other convulsive nervous disorders. It has also been employed in checking internal haemorrhage.

The physiological effect of the plant is to lessen and temporarily benumb such nervous action as is reflected to distant organs of the body from some central organ which is the actual seat of trouble. In this way the spasms of epilepsy and of other convulsive distempers are allayed. Large doses of the plant, or of its berries, would, on the contrary, aggravate these convulsive disorders. Young children have been attacked with convulsions after eating freely of the berries.

In a French work on domestic remedies, 1682, Mistletoe (gui de chêne) was considered of great curative power in epilepsy. Sir John Colbatch published in 1720 a pamphlet on The Treatment of Epilepsy by Mistletoe, regarding it as a specific for this disease. He procured the parasite from the Lime trees at Hampton Court, and recommended the powdered leaves, as much as would lie on a sixpence, to be given in Black Cherry water every morning. He was followed in this treatment by others who have testified to its efficacy as a tonic in nervous disorders, considering it the specific herb for St. Vitus's Dance. It has been employed in convulsions delirium, hysteria, neuralgia, nervous debility, urinary disorders, heart disease, and many other complaints arising from a weakened and disordered state of the nervous system.

Ray also greatly extolled Mistletoe as a specific in epilepsy, and useful in apoplexy and giddiness. The older writers recommended it for sterility.

The tincture has been recommended as a heart tonic in typhoid fever in place of Foxglove. It lessens reflex irritability and strengthens the heart's beat, whilst raising the frequency of a slow pulse.

Besides the dried leaves being given powdered, or as an infusion, or made into a tincture with spirits of wine, a decoction may be made by boiling 2 oz. of the bruised green plant with 1/2 pint of water, giving 1 tablespoonful for a dose several times a day. Ten to 60 grains of the powder may be taken as a dose, and homoeopathists give 5 to 10 drops of the tincture, with 1 or 2 tablespoonsful of cold water. Mistletoe is also given, combined with Valerian Root and Vervain, for all kinds of nervous complaints, cayenne pods being added in cases of debility of the digestive organs.

Fluid extract: dose, 1/4 to 1 drachm.

Country people use the berries to cure severe stitches in the side. The birdlime of the berries is also employed by them as an application to ulcers and sores.

It is stated that in Sweden, persons afflicted with epilepsy carry about with them a knife having a handle of Oak Mistletoe to ward off attacks.

Motherwort

324 Leonurus Cardiaca L.
Gemeines Herzgespann.

Quick Facts

Latin/Linnaen:	*Leonurus Cardiaca*
Family:	*Lamiaceae*
Old English :	Modorwyrt
Synonyms:	Throw-wort, Lion's Ear, Lion's Tail
Action:	
Parts Used:	Above ground plant parts
Indicated For:	Nervous cardiac disorders and as adjuvant for thyroid hyperfunction.
Dosage:	Unless otherwise prescribed: Average daily dosage: 4.5g herb; equivalent preparations
Preparation:	Comminuted herb for infusions and other galenical preparations for internal use.
Cautions:	
Other Uses:	

Description

Motherwort (*Leonurus cardiaca*) is an herbaceous perennial plant in the mint family, *Lamiaceae*. Other common names include Throw-wort, Lion's Ear, and Lion's Tail. The latter two are also common names for *Leonotis leonurus*. Originally from Central Asia it is now found worldwide, spread largely due to its use as a herbal remedy.

L. cardiaca has a square stem and opposite leaves. The leaves have serrated margins and are palmately lobed with long petioles; basal leaves are wedge shaped with three points and while the upper leaves are more latticed. Flowers appear in leaf axils on the upper part of the plant and it blooms between June - August. The flowers are small, pink to lilac in colour often with furry lower lips. The plant grows to about 60–100 cm in height. It can be found along roadsides and in vacant fields and other disturbed areas.

Cultivation

Hardiness Zone:	4-10
Soil pH:	7.7
Soil type:	Fertile moist soil
Cultivation:	Easily sown by seed
Sunlight:	Full sun-partial shade
Habitat:	Native to Europe and Asia, now common in the temperate parts of the world.

Motherwort grows in wasteland but can be cultivated in gardens. Its seeds are easily spread, so if you wish to contain it, remove stalks before seeds come.

When once planted in a garden, Motherwort will soon increase if the seeds are permitted to scatter. It is perfectly hardy and needs no special soil, and the roots will continue for many years.

Seedlings should be planted about a foot apart.

Historical Notes

Motherwort, the only British representative of the genus *Leonurus*, is a native of many parts of Europe, on banks and under hedges, in a gravelly or calcareous soil. It is often found in country gardens, where it was formerly grown for medicinal purposes, but it is rare to find it truly wild in England, and by some authorities it is not considered indigenous, but merely a garden escape.

It is distinguished from all other British labiates by the leaves, which are deeply and palmately cut into five lobes, or three-pointed segments, and by the prickly calyx-teeth of its flowers. When not in flower, it resembles Mugwort in habit.

From the perennial root-stock rise the square, stout stems, 2 to 3 feet high, erect and branched, principally below, the angles prominent. The leaves are very closely set, the radical ones on slender, long petioles, ovate, lobed and toothed, those on the stem, 2 to 3 inches long, petioled, wedge-shaped; the lower roundish, palmately five-lobed, the lobes trifid at the apex, the upper three-fid, coarsely serrate, reticulately veined, the veinlets prominent beneath, with slender, curved hairs. The uppermost leaves and bracts are very narrow and entire, or only with a tooth on each side, and bear in their axils numerous whorls of pinkish, or nearly white, sessile flowers, six to fifteen in a whorl. The corollas, though whitish on the outside, are stained with paler or darker purple within. They have rather short tubes and nearly flat upper lips, very hairy above, with long, woolly hairs. The two front stamens are the longest and the anthers are sprinkled with hard, shining dots.

The plant blossoms in August. It has rather a pungent odour and a very bitter taste. It is a dull green, the leaves paler below, pubescent, especially on the angles of the stem and the underside of the leaves, the hairs varying much in length and abundance.

The name of the genus, Leonurus, in Greek signifies a Lion's tail, from some fancied resemblance in the plant.

Part Used: The whole herb, dried, cut in August.

Medicinal Action and Uses: Diaphoretic, antispasmodic, tonic, nervine, emmenagogue. Motherwort is especially valuable in female weakness and disorders (hence the name), allaying nervous irritability and inducing quiet and passivity of the whole nervous system.

As a tonic, it acts without producing febrile excitement, and in fevers, attended with nervousness and delirium, it is extremely useful.

Old writers tell us that there is no better herb for strengthening and gladdening the heart, and that it is good against hysterical complaints, and especially for palpitations of the heart when they arise from hysteric causes, and that when made into a syrup, it will allay inward tremors, faintings, etc. There is no doubt it has proved the truth of their claims in its use as a simple tonic, not only in heart disease, neuralgia and other affections of the heart, but also in spinal disease and in recovery from fevers where other tonics are inadmissable.

In Macer's Herbal we find 'Motherwort' mentioned as one of the herbs which were considered all-powerful against 'wykked sperytis.'

The best way of giving it is in the form of a conserve, made from the young tops, says one writer. It may be given in decoctions, or a strong infusion, but is very unpleasant to take that way. The infusion is made from 1 oz. of herb to a pint of boiling water, taken in wineglassful doses.

Preparations and Dosages: Powdered herb, 1/2 to 1 drachm. Fluid extract, 1/2 to 1 drachm. Solid extract, 5 to 15 grains.

Culpepper wrote of Motherwort:

'Venus owns this herb and it is under Leo. There is no better herb to drive melancholy vapours from the heart, to strengthen it and make the mind cheerful, blithe and merry. May be kept in a syrup, or conserve, therefore the Latins call it cardiaca.... It cleansethe the chest of cold phlegm, oppressing it and killeth worms in the belly. It is of good use to warm and dry up the cold humours, to digest and disperse them that are settled in the veins, joints and sinews of the body and to help cramps and convulsions.'

And Gerard says:

'Divers commend it against infirmities of the heart. Moreover the same is commended for green wounds; it is also a remedy against certain diseases in cattell, as the cough and murreine, and for that cause divers husbandmen oftentimes much desire it.'

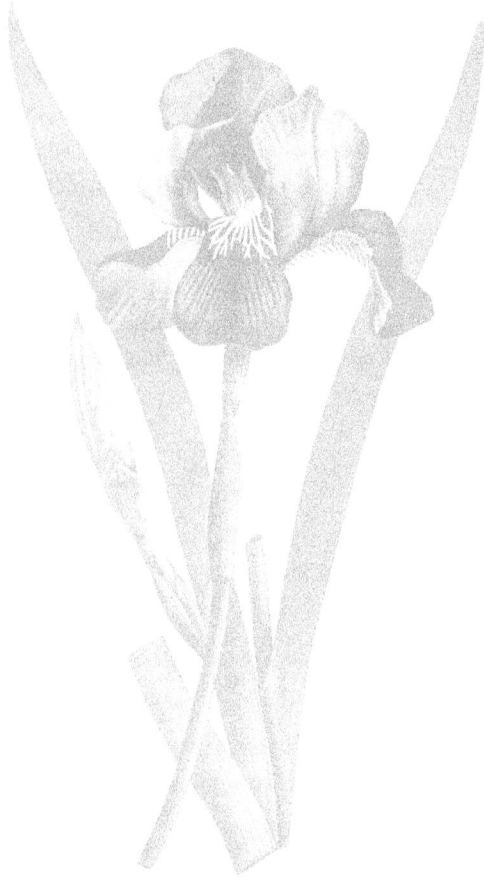

Mullein

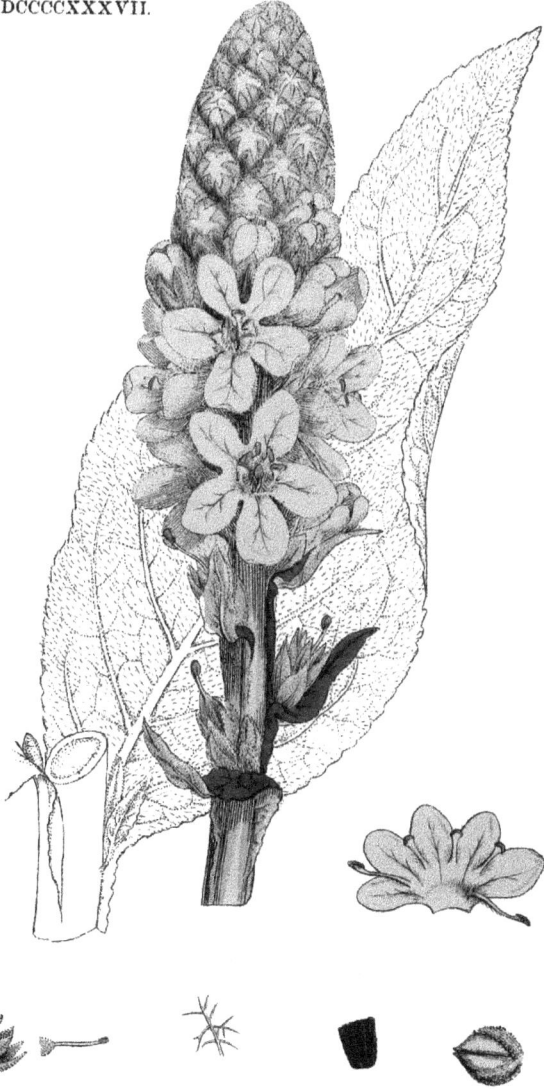

DCCCCXXXVII.

E.B. 549.   Verbascum Thapsus.   Great Mullein.

Quick Facts

Latin/Linnaen:	*Verbascum Thapsus* or *Densiflorum*
Family:	*Scrophulariaceae*
Old English :	
Synonyms:	Great or Common Mullein, Torches, Mullein Dock, Our Lady's Flannel, Velvet Dock, Blanket Herb, Velvet Plant, Woollen, Rag Paper, Candlewick Plant, Wild Ice Leaf, Clown's Lungwort, Bullock's Lungwort, Aaron's Rod, Jupiter's Staff, Jacob's Staff, Peter's Staff, Shepherd's Staff, Shepherd's Clubs, Beggar's Stalk, Golden Rod, Adam's Flannel, Beggar's Blanket, Clot, Cuddy's Lungs, Duffle, Feltwort, Fluffweed, Hare's Beard, Old Man's Flannel, Hag's Taper.
Action:	Alleviating irritation, Expectorant
Parts Used:	Flower
Indicated For:	Catarrhs of the respiratory tract.
Dosage:	Unless otherwise prescribed: Daily dosage: 3-4g of herb; equivalent preparations.
Preparation:	Comminuted herb for teas and other galenical preparations for internal use.
Cautions:	
Other Uses:	**Hair Dye:** An infusion of the flowers was used by the Roman ladies to dye their hair a golden colour.

Description

Verbascum thapsus (Great or Common Mullein) is a species of mullein native to Europe, northern Africa and Asia, and introduced in the Americas and Australia.

It is a hairy biennial plant that can grow to 2 m or more tall. Its small yellow flowers are densely grouped on a tall stem, which bolts from a large rosette of leaves. It grows in a wide variety of habitats, but prefers well-lit disturbed soils, where it can appear soon after the ground receives light, from long-lived seeds that persist in the soil seed bank. It is a common weedy plant that spreads by prolifically producing seeds, but rarely becomes aggressively invasive, since its seed require open ground to germinate. It is a very minor problem for most agricultural crops, since it is not a very competitive species, being intolerant of shade from other plants and unable to survive tilling. It also hosts many insects, some of which can be harmful to other plants. Although individuals are easy to remove by hand, populations are difficult to eliminate permanently.

It is widely used for herbal remedies with emollient and astringent properties. It is especially recommended for coughs and related problems, but also used in topical applications against a variety of skin problems. The plant was also used to make dyes and torches.

Cultivation

Hardiness Zone:	4-10
Soil pH:	5-7.5
Soil type:	Tolerant of poor soil and drought
Cultivation:	Sow seeds in fall
Sunlight:	Full sun
Habitat:	Native to Europe and Asia, now common in temperate parts of the world.

Mullein often grows along roadsides and in pastures and hillsides. Mullein can become invasive, so if it is grown, it is best to deadhead the plant. It is an incredibly tall plant, especially under garden conditions, some reaching 12 feet.

Historical Notes

Mullein, is a widely distributed plant, being found all over Europe and in temperate Asia as far as the Himalayas, and in North America is exceedingly abundant as a naturalized weed in the eastern States. It is met with throughout

Britain (except in the extreme north of Scotland) and also in Ireland and the Channel Islands, on hedge-banks, by roadsides and on waste ground, more especially on gravel, sand or chalk. It flowers during July and August.

The natural order Scrophulariaceae is an important family of plants comprising 200 genera and about 2,500 species, occurring mostly in temperate and sub-tropical regions, many of them producing flowers of great beauty, on which account they are frequently cultivated among favourite garden and greenhouse flowers. Of this group are the Calceolaria, Mimulus, Penstemon, Antirrhinum and Collinsia. Among its British representatives it embraces members so diverse as the Foxglove and Speedwell, the Mullein and Figworts, the Toadflax and the semi-parasites, Eyebright, Bartsia, Cowwheat, and the Red and Yellow Rattles.

Most of the flowers are capable of self-fertilization in default of insect visits.

Unlike the Labiatae, to which they are rather closely related, plants belonging to this order seldom contain much volatile oil, though resinous substances are common. The most important constituents are glucosides, and many of them are poisonous or powerfully active.

A number of the *Scrophulariaceae* are or have been valued for their curative properties and are widely employed both in domestic and in regular medicine.

The genus *Verbascum*, to which the Mullein belongs, contains 210 species, distributed in Europe, West and Central Asia and North Africa, six of which are natives of Great Britain. The Mulleins, like the Veronicas, are exceptions to the general character of the *Scrophulariaceae*, having nearly regular, open corollas, the segments being connected only towards the base, instead of having the more fantastic flowers of the Snapdragon and others. They are all tall, stout biennials, with large leaves and flowers in long, terminal spikes.

In the first season of the plant's growth, there appears only a rosette of large leaves, 6 to 15 inches long, in form somewhat like those of the Foxglove, but thicker - whitish with a soft, dense mass of hairs on both sides, which make them very thick to the touch. In the following spring, a solitary, stout, pale stem, with tough, strong fibres enclosing a thin rod of white pith, arises from the midst of the felted leaves. Its rigid uprightness accounts for some of the plant's local names: 'Aaron's Rod,' 'Jupiter's' or 'Jacob's Staff,' etc.

The leaves near the base of the stem are large and numerous, 6 to 8 inches long and 2 to 2 1/2 inches broad, but become smaller as they ascend the stem, on which they are arranged not opposite to one another, but on alternate sides. They are broad and simple in form, the outline rather waved, stalkless, their bases being continued some distance down the stem, as in the Comfrey and a few other plants, the midrib from a quarter to half-way up the blade being actually joined to the stem. By these 'decurrent' leaves (as this hugging of the stem by the leaves is botanically termed) the Great Mullein is easily distinguished from other British species of Mullein - some with white and some with yellow flowers. The leaf system is so arranged that the smaller leaves above drop the rain upon the larger ones below, which direct the water to the roots. This is a necessary arrangement, since the Mullein grows mostly on dry soils. The stellately-branched hairs which cover the leaves so thickly act as a protective coat, checking too great a giving off of the plant's moisture, and also are a defensive weapon of the plant, for not only do they prevent the attacks of creeping insects, but they set up an intense irritation in the mucous membrane of any grazing animals that may attempt to browse upon them, so that the plants are usually left severely alone by them. The leaves are, however, subject to the attacks of a mould, *Peronospora sordida*. The hairs are not confined to the leaves alone, but are also on every part of the stem, on the calyces and on the outside of the corollas, so that the whole plant appears whitish or grey. The homely but valuable Mullein Tea, a remedy of the greatest antiquity for coughs and colds, must indeed always be strained through fine muslin to remove any hairs that may be floating in the hot water that has been poured over the flowers, or leaves, for otherwise they cause intolerable itching in the mouth.

Towards the top of the stalk, which grows frequently 4 or even 5 feet high, and in gardens has been known to attain a height of 7 or 8 feet, the much-diminished woolly leaves merge into the thick, densely crowded flower-spike, usually a foot long, the flowers opening here and there on the spike, not in regular progression from the base, as in the Foxglove. The flowers are stalkless, the sulphur-yellow corolla, a somewhat irregular cup, nearly an inch across, formed of five rounded petals, united at the base to form a very short tube, being enclosed in a woolly calyx, deeply cut into five lobes. The five stamens stand on the corolla; three of them are shorter than the other two and have a large number of tiny white hairs on their filaments. These hairs are full of sap, and it has been suggested that they form additional bait to the insect visitors, supplementing the allurement of the nectar that lies round the base of the ovary. All kinds of insects are attracted by this plant, the Honey Bee, Humble Bee, some of the smaller wild bees and different species of flies, since the nectar and the staminal hairs are both so readily accessible, though the supply of nectar is not very great. The three short hairy stamens have only short, one-celled anthers - the two longer, smooth ones have larger anthers. The pollen sacs have an orangered inner surface, disclosed as the anthers open.

In some species, *Verbascum nigrum*, the Dark Mullein, and *V. blattaria*, the Moth Mullein, the filament hairs are purple. The rounded ovary is hairy and also the lower part of the style. The stigma is mature before the anthers and the style projects at the moment the flower opens, so that any insect approaching it from another blossom where it has got brushed by pollen, must needs strike it on alighting and thus insure crossfertilization, though, failing this, the flower is also able to fertilize itself. The ripened seed capsule is very hard and contains many seeds, which eventually escape through two valves and are scattered round the parent plant.

History: The down on the leaves and stem makes excellent tinder when quite dry, readily igniting on the slightest spark, and was, before the introduction of cotton, used for lamp wicks, hence another of the old names: 'Candlewick Plant.' An old superstition existed that witches in their incantations used lamps and candles provided with wicks of this sort, and another of the plant's many names, 'Hag's Taper', refers to this, though the word 'hag' is said to be derived from the Anglo-Saxon word Haege or Hage (a hedge) - the name 'Hedge Taper' also exists - and may imply that the sturdy spikes of this tall hedge plant, studded with pale yellow blossoms, suggested a tall candle growing in the hedge, another of its countryside names being, indeed, 'Our Lady's Candle.' Lyte (The Niewe Herball, 1578) tells us 'that the whole toppe, with its pleasant yellow floures sheweth like to a wax candle or taper cunningly wrought.'

'Torches' is another name for the plant, and Parkinson tells us:

'Verbascum is called of the Latines Candela regia, and Candelaria, because the elder age used the stalks dipped in suet to burne, whether at funeralls or otherwise.'

And Gerard (1597) also remarks that it is 'a plant whereof is made a manner of lynke (link) if it be talowed.' Dr. Prior, in The Popular Names of British Plants, states that the word Mullein was Moleyn in AngloSaxon, and Malen in Old French, derived from the Latin malandrium, i.e. the malanders or leprosy, and says:

'The term "malandre" became also applied to diseases of cattle, to lung diseases among the rest, and the plant being used as a remedy, acquired its name of "Mullein" and "Bullock's Lungwort." '

Coles, in 1657, in Adam in Eden, says that:

'Husbandmen of Kent do give it their cattle against the cough of the lungs, and I, therefore, mention it because cattle are also in some sort to be provided for in their diseases.'

The name 'Clown's Lung Wort refers to its use as a homely remedy. 'Ag-Leaf' and 'Ag-Paper' are other names for it. 'Wild Ice Leaf' perhaps refers to the white look of the leaves. Few English plants have so many local names.

The Latin name Verbascum is considered to be a corruption of barbascum, from the Latin barba (a beard), in allusion to the shaggy foliage, and was bestowed on the genus by Linnaeus.

Both in Europe and Asia the power of driving away evil spirits was ascribed to the Mullein. In India it has the reputation among the natives that the St. John's Wort once had here, being considered a sure safeguard against evil spirits and magic, and from the ancient classics we learn that it was this plant which Ulysses took to protect himself against the wiles of Circe.

The Cowslip and the Primrose are classed together by our old herbalists as Petty Mulleins, and are usually credited with much the same properties. Gerard recommends both the flowers and leaves of the primrose, boiled in wine, as a remedy for all diseases of the lungs and the juice of the root itself, snuffed up the nose, for megrim.

All the various species of Mullein found in Britain possess similar medicinal properties, but *V. thapsus*, the species of most common occurrence, is the one most employed.

For medicinal purposes it is generally collected from wild specimens, but is worthy of cultivation, not merely from its beauty as an ornamental plant, but also for its medicinal value, which is undoubted. In most parts of Ireland, besides growing wild, it is carefully cultivated in gardens, because of a steady demand for the plant by sufferers from pulmonary consumption.

Its cultivation is easy: being a hardy biennial, it only requires sowing in very ordinary soil and to be kept free from weeds. When growing in gardens, Mulleins will often be found to be infested with slugs, which can be caught wholesale by placing in borders slates and boards smeared with margarine on the underside. Examine in the morning and deposit the catch in a pail of lime and water.

Historical Medicinal Uses - For Entertainment ONLY

Parts Use: The leaves and flowers are the parts used medicinally.

Fresh Mullein leaves are also used for the purpose of making a homoeopathic tincture.

Constituents: The leaves are nearly odourless and of a mucilaginous and bitterish taste. They contain gum as their principal constituent, together with 1 to 2 per cent of resin, divisible into two parts, one soluble in ether, the other not; a readily soluble amaroid; a little tannin and a trace of volatile oil.

The flowers contain gum, resin, a yellow colouring principle, a green fatty matter (a sort of chlorophyll), a glucoside, an acrid, fatty matter; free acid and phosphoric acid; uncrystallizable sugar; some mineral salts, the bases of which are potassia and lime, and a small amount of yellowish volatile oil. They should yield not more than 6 per cent of ash. Their odour is peculiar and agreeable: their taste mucilaginous.

Medicinal Action and Uses: The Mullein has very markedly demulcent, emollient and astringent properties, which render it useful in pectoral complaints and bleeding of the lungs and bowels. The whole plant seems to possess slightly sedative and narcotic properties.

It is considered of much value in phthisis and other wasting diseases, palliating the cough and staying expectoration, consumptives appearing to benefit greatly by its use, being given in the form of an infusion, 1 oz. of dried, or the corresponding quantity of fresh leaves being boiled for 10 minutes in a pint of milk, and when strained, given warm, thrice daily, with or without sugar. The taste of the decoction is bland, mucilaginous and cordial, and forms a pleasant emollient and nutritious medicine for allaying a cough, or removing the pain and irritation of haemorrhoids.

A plain infusion of 1 oz. to a pint of boiling water can also be employed, taken in wineglassful doses frequently.

The dried leaves are sometimes smoked in an ordinary tobacco pipe to relieve the irritation of the respiratory mucus membranes, and will completely control, it is said, the hacking cough of consumption. They can be employed with equal benefit when made into cigarettes, for asthma and spasmodic coughs in general.

Fomentations and poultices of the leaves have been found serviceable in haemorrhoidal complaints.

Mullein is said to be of much value in diarrhoea, from its combination of demulcent with astringent properties, by this combination strengthening the bowels at the same time. In diarrhea the ordinary infusion is generally given, but when any bleeding of the bowels is present, the decoction prepared with milk is recommended.

On the Continent, a sweetened infusion of the flowers strained in order to separate the rough hairs, is considerably used as a domestic remedy in mild catarrhs, colic, etc.

A conserve of the flowers has also been employed on the Continent against ringworm, and a distilled water of the flowers was long reputed a cure for burns and erysipelas.

An oil produced by macerating Mullein flowers in olive oil in a corked bottle, during prolonged exposure to the sun, or by keeping near the fire for several days, is used as a local application in country districts in Germany for piles and other mucus membrane inflammation, and also for frost bites and bruises. Mullein oil is recommended for earache and discharge from the ear, and for any eczema of the external ear and its canal. Dr. Fernie (Herbal Simples) states that some of the most brilliant results have been obtained in suppurative inflammation of the inner ear by a single application of Mullein oil, and that in acute or chronic cases, two or three drops of this oil should be made to fall in the ear twice or thrice in the day.

Mullein oil is a valuable destroyer of disease germs. The fresh flowers, steeped for 21 days in olive oil, are said to make an admirable bactericide. Gerarde tells us that 'Figs do not putrifie at all that are wrapped in the leaves of Mullein.'

An alcoholic tincture is prepared by homoeopathic chemists, from the fresh herb with spirits of wine, which has proved beneficial for migraine or sick headache of long standing, with oppression of the ear. From 8 to 10 drops of the tincture are given as a dose, with cold water, repeated frequently.

Preparation and Dosage: Fluid extract, 1/2 to 1 drachm.

Formerly the flowers of several species of Mullein were officinal, but Mullein no longer has a place in the British Pharmacopoeia, though Verbascum Flowers were introduced into the 4th Edition of the United States National Formulary, as one of the ingredients in pectoral remedies, and the leaves, in fluid extract of Mullein leaves, made with diluted alcohol were directed to be used as a demulcent, the dose being 1 fluid drachm.

In more ancient times, much higher virtues were attributed to this plant. Culpepper gives us a list of most extraordinary cures performed by its agency, and Gerard remarks that:

'there be some who think that this herbe being but carryed about one, doth help the falling sickness, especially the leaves of the plant which have not yet borne flowers, and gathered when the sun is in Virgo and the moon in Aries, which thing notwithstanding is vaine and superstitious.'

A decoction of its roots was held to be an alleviation for toothache, and also good for cramps and convulsions, and an early morning draught of the distilled water of the flowers to be good for gout.

Mullein juice and powder made from the dried roots rubbed on rough warts was said to quickly remove them, though it was not recommended as equally efficacious for smooth warts. A poultice made of the seeds and leaves, boiled in hot wine, was also considered an excellent means to 'draw forth speedily thorns or splinters gotten into the flesh.' We also hear of the woolly leaves being worn in the stockings to promote circulation and keep the feet warm.

The flowers impart a yellow colour to boiling water and a rather permanent green colour with dilute sulphuric acid, the latter colour becoming brown upon the addition of alkalis. An infusion of the flowers was used by the Roman ladies to dye their hair a golden colour. Lyte tells us, 'the golden floures of Mulleyn stiped in lye, causeth the heare to war yellow, being washed therewithall,' and according to another old authority, Alexander Trallianus, the ashes of the plant made into a soap will restore hair which has become grey to its original colour.

The seeds are said to intoxicate fish when thrown into the water, and are used by poachers for that purpose, being slightly narcotic. According to Rosenthal

(Pharmaceutical Journal July, 1902), the seeds of *V. sinuatum* (Linn.), which are used in Greece as a fish poison, contain 6 to 13 per cent of Saponin. Traces of the same substance were found in the seeds of *V. phlomoides* (Linn.) and *V. thapsiforme* (Schrad.), common in the south of Europe, which have been used for the same purpose. *V. pulverulentum* of Madeira (also used as a fish poisoner) and *V. phlomoides* are employed as taenicides (expellers of tapeworm).

Myrrh

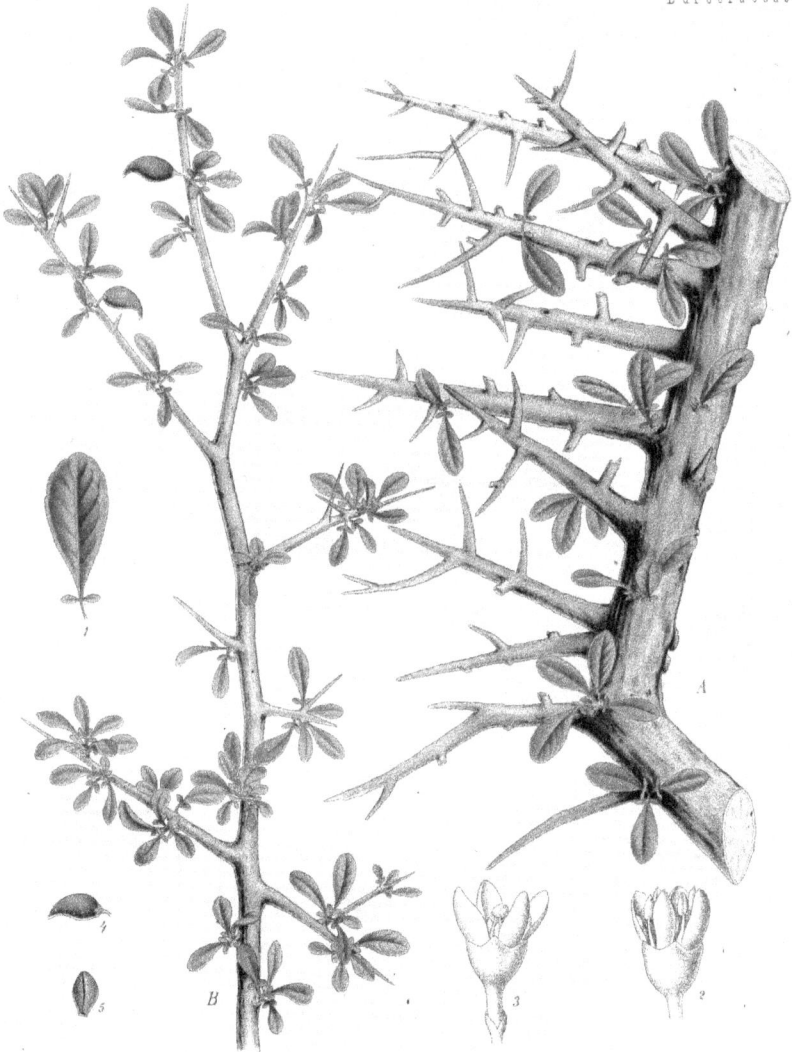

Burseraceae

Balsamodendron Myrrha Nees v. Es.

Quick Facts

Latin/Linnaen:	*Commiphora myrrha, Commiphora molmol* or *Balsamodendron Myrrha*
Family:	*Burseraceae*
Old English :	Murre
Synonyms:	Common Myrrh, Gum Myrrh, Somalian Myrrh, Balsamodendron Myrrha, Mirra, Morr, Didin, Didthin, Bowl.
Action:	Astringent
Parts Used:	Resin/gum
Indicated For:	Topical treatment of mild inflammations of the oral and pharyngeal mucosa.
Dosage:	Unless otherwise prescribed: Myrrh tincture: Dab 2-3 times daily with undiluted tincture; As a rinse or gargle: 5-10 drops in a glass of water. In dental powders: 10 percent of powdered resin.
Preparation:	Powdered resin, myrrh tincture and other galenical preparations for topical use.
Cautions:	
Other Uses:	Incense

Description

Common myrrh (*Commiphora myrrha*) or gum myrrh is a tree in the *Burseraceae* family. It is one of the primary trees used in the production of myrrh, a resin made from dried tree sap. The tree is native to the Arabian peninsula (Oman, Yemen) and to Africa (Djibouti, Ethiopia, Somalia, Northeast Kenya).

Commiphora myrrha is very spiny and it grows to a height of about 4 m. It grows at an altitude of between about 250–1300 m, with a yearly mean rainfall of about 230–300 mm. It does best in thin soil, primarily in areas with limestone.

Cultivation

Hardiness Zone:	10-11
Soil pH:	Mildly acidic-neutral
Soil type:	Well drained soil
Cultivation:	By seed or cuttings
Sunlight:	Full sun
Habitat:	Native to Northeastern Africa, Arabia, Somaliland.

Historical Notes

The bushes yielding the resin do not grow more than 9 feet in height, but they are of sturdy build, with knotted branches, and branchlets that stand out at right-angles, ending in a sharp spine. The trifoliate leaves are scanty, small and very unequal, oval and entire. It was first recognized about 1822 at Ghizan on the Red Sea coast, a district so bare and dry that it is called 'Tehama,' meaning 'hell.'

Botanically, there is still uncertainty about the origin and identity of the various species.

There are ducts in the bark, and the tissue between them breaks down, forming large cavities, which, with the remaining ducts, becomes filled with a granular secretion which is freely discharged when the bark is wounded, or from natural fissures. It flows as a pale yellow liquid, but hardens to a reddish-brown mass, being found in commerce in tears of many sizes, the average being that of a walnut. The surface is rough and powdered, and the pieces are brittle, with a granular fracture, semi-transparent, oily, and often show whitish marks. The odour and taste are aromatic, the latter also acrid and bitter. It is inflammable, but burns feebly.

Several species are recognized in commerce. It is usually imported in chests weighing 1 or 2 cwts., and wherever produced comes chiefly from the East Indies.

Adulterations are not easily detected in the powder, so that it is better purchased in mass, when small stones, senegal gum, chestnuts, pieces of bdellium, or of a brownish resin called 'false myrrh,' may be sorted out with little difficulty.

It has been used from remote ages as an ingredient in incense, perfumes, etc., in the holy oil of the Jews and the Kyphi of the Egyptians for embalming and fumigations.

Little appears to be definitely known about the collection of myrrh. It seems probable that the best drug comes from Somaliland, is bought at the fairs of Berbera by the Banians of India, shipped to Bombay, and there sorted, the best coming to Europe and the worst being sent to China. The true myrrh is known in the markets as karam, formerly called Turkey myrrh, and the opaque bdellium as meena harma.

The gum makes a good mucilage and the insoluble residue from the tincture can be used in this way.

Constituents: Volatile oil, resin (myrrhin), gum, ash, salts, sulphates, benzoates, malates, and acetates of potassa.

It is partially soluble in water, alcohol, and ether. It may be tested by a characteristic violent reaction if nitric acid diluted with an equal volume of water is brought into contact with the residue resulting from the boiling of 0.1 gramme of coarsely powdered myrrh with 2 c.c. of 90 per cent alcohol, evaporated in a porcelain dish so as to leave a thin film.

The oil is thick, pale yellow, and contains myrrholic acid and heerabolene, a sesquiterpenene.

Historical Medicinal Uses - For Entertainment ONLY

Medicinal Action and Uses: Astringent, healing. Tonic and stimulant. A direct emmenagogue, a tonic in dyspepsia, an expectorant in the absence of feverish symptoms, a stimulant to the mucous tissues, a stomachic carminative, exciting appetite and the flow of gastric juice, and an astringent wash.

It is used in chronic catarrh, phthisis pulmonalis, chlorosis, and in amenorrhoea is often combined with aloes and iron. As a wash it is good for spongy gums, ulcerated throat and aphthous stomatitis, and the tincture is also applied to foul and indolentulcers. It has been found helpful in bronchorrhoea and leucorrhoea. It has also been used as a vermifuge.

When long-continued rubefacient effect is needed, a plaster may be made with 1 1/2 oz. each of camphor, myrrh, and balsam of Peru rubbed together and added to 32 oz. of melted lead plaster, the whole being stirred until cooling causes it to thicken.

Myrrh is a common ingredient of toothpowders, and is used with borax in tincture, with other ingredients, as a mouth-wash.

The Compound Tincture, or Horse Tincture, is used in veterinary practice for healing wounds.

Meetiga, the trade-name of Arabian Myrrh, is more brittle and gummy than that of Somaliland and has not its white markings.

The liquid Myrrh, or Stacte, spoken of by Pliny, and an ingredient of Jewish holy incense, was formerly obtainable and greatly valued, but cannot now be identified.

Dosages: 10 to 30 grains. Of fluid extract, 5 to 30 minims. Tincture, B.P. and U.S.P., 1/2 to 1 drachm. Of tincture of aloes and Myrrh, as purgative and emmenagogue, 30 minims. Of N.F. pills of aloes and Myrrh, 2 pills. Of Rufus's pills of aloes and Myrrh, as stimulant cathartic in debility and constipation, or in suppression of the menses, 4 to 8 grains of Br. mass.

Other Species:

Bissa Bôl, or perfumed bdellium of the Arabs, has an odour like mushrooms. Though it is sent from Arabian ports to India and China, it was formerly known as East Indian Myrrh. It is of a dark colour, and may be a product of Commiphora erythraea, var. glabrescens, of B. Kalaf, A. Kafal, B. Playfairii or Hemprichia erythraea.

B. Kua of Abyssinia has been found to yield Myrrh.

Mecca balsam, a product of B. or C. Opobalsamum, is said to be the Myrrh of the Bible, the Hebrew word mar having been confused with the modern Arabic morr or Myrrh in translation.

Bdellium, recognized as an inferior Myrrh and often mixed with or substituted for it, is a product of several species of Commiphora, according to American writers, or Balsamodendron according to English ones. Four kinds are collected in Somaliland, making sub-divisions of African Bdellium:

- Perfumed Bdellium or Habaghadi,
- African Bdellium,
- Opaque Bdellium,
- Hotai Bdellium.

These African bdelliums, said by some writers to be products of Balsamodendron (Heudelotia) Africanum, are in irregular, hard, roundish tears about an inch in diameter, pale yellow to red-brown, translucent, the fracture waxy, taste and odour slight.

The product of Ceradia furcata is also called African Bdellium.

The commercial Gugul, or Indian Bdellium, is said by some writers to be a product of Commiphora roxburghiana, by others of B. Mukul, and by others again of B. roxbhurghii or Amyris Bdellium. It is more moist than Myrrh; is found in irregular, dark reddishbrown masses, with a waxy fracture; softens with the heat of the hand; adheres to the teeth when chewed; and smells slightly of Myrrh.

It is used in the East Indies in leprosy, rheumatism and syphilis, and in Europe for plasters.

Dosage: 10 to 40 grains.

Oak Bark

Cupuliferae

Quercus sessiliflora Sm

Quick Facts

Latin/Linnaen:	*Quercus Robur*
Family:	*Fagaceae*
Old English :	Acrinde
Synonyms:	Tanner's Bark
Action:	Astringent, virustatic
Parts Used:	Bark
Indicated For:	External: Inflammatory skin diseases. Internal: Nonspecific, acute diarrhea, and local treatment of mild inflammation of the oral cavity and pharyngeal region, as well as genital and anal area.
Dosage:	Unless otherwise prescribed: Internal: Daily dosage: 3g of drug; equivalent preparations. For rinses, compresses and gargles: 20 g drug per 1 liter of water; equivalent preparations. For full and partial baths: 5 g drug per 1 liter of water; equivalent preparations.
Preparation:	Comminuted herb for decoctions and other galenical preparations for internal and topical use.
Cautions:	Not for more than 3-4 days of diarrhea or more than 2-3 weeks other applications. **Contraindications**: Internal: None known. External: skin damage over a large area. Baths: Full baths should not be taken, regardless of the active ingredients in the bath, under the following conditions: weeping eczema and skin damage covering large areas; febrile and infectious diseases, cardiac insufficiency; hypertonia. **Interactions with other drugs**: External: None known. Internal: The absorption of the alkaloids and other alkaline drugs may be reduced or inhibited.
Other Uses:	Tanning Leather

Description

Quercus robur (sometimes considered *Q. pedunculata* or "*Q. robur*") is commonly known as the English oak or pedunculate oak or French oak. It is native to most of Europe, and to Anatolia to the Caucasus, and also to parts of North Africa.

Quercus robur is a large deciduous tree 25–35 m (80–115 ') tall (exceptionally to 50 m (160 ')) and thick, with circumference of grand oaks from 4 m (13') to exceptional 12m (40'). Majesty Oak with the circumference of 12,2 m (40') is the thickest tree in Great Britain, but Kaive Oak in Latvia with the circumference of 10,2 m (33,5') is the thickest tree in Northern Europe. *Q. robur* has lobed and nearly sessile (very short-stalked) leaves 7–14 cm long. Flowering takes place in mid spring, and their fruit, called acorns, ripen by the following autumn. The acorns are 2–2.5 cm long, pedunculate (having a peduncle or acorn-stalk, 3–7 cm long) with one to four acorns on each peduncle.

It is a long-lived tree, with a large widespreading crown of rugged branches. While it may naturally live to an age of a few centuries, many of the oldest trees are pollarded or coppiced, both pruning techniques that extend the tree's potential lifespan, if not its health. Two individuals of notable longevity are the Stelmužė Oak in Lithuania and the Granit oak in Bulgaria, which are believed to be more than 1,500 years old, possibly making them the oldest oaks in Europe; another specimen, called the 'Kongeegen' ('Kings Oak'), estimated to be about 1,200 years old, grows in Jaegerspris, Denmark. Yet another can be found in Kvilleken, Sweden, that is over 1,000 years old and 14 meters around. Of maiden (not pollarded) specimens, one of the oldest is the great oak of Ivenack, Germany. Tree-ring research of this tree and other oaks nearby gives an estimated age of 700 to 800 years old. Also the Bowthorpe Oak in Lincolnshire, England is estimated to be 1,000 years old making it the oldest in the UK, although there is Knightwood Oak in the New Forest which is also said to be as old. Highest density of the *Q. robur* grand oaks with a circumference 4 meters and more is in Latvia.

Cultivation

Hardiness Zone:	4-10 depending on variety
Soil pH:	Dependant on the variety of oak
Soil type:	Dependant on the variety of oak
Cultivation:	Oaks are easily propagated from acorns.
Sunlight:	Full sun
Habitat:	Native to the northern hemisphere

There are hundreds of varieties of oak, but it is best to grow one that naturally occurs in your area. Take the time to seek out different varieties before deciding on what one you best like.

Historical Notes

In Celtic mythology, it is the tree of doors, believed to be a gateway between worlds, or a place where portals could be erected.

In Norse mythology, the oak was sacred to the thunder god, Thor. Some scholars speculate that this is because the oak, as the largest tree in northern Europe, was the one most often struck by lightning. Thor's Oak was a sacred tree of the Germanic Chatti tribe. Its destruction marked the Christianisation of the heathen tribes by the Franks.

The Common, or British Oak, for many centuries the chief forest tree of England, is intimately bound up with the history of these islands from Druid times. A spray of oak was for long engraved on one side of our sixpences and shillings, but is now superseded by the British lion. The Oak, although widely distributed over Europe, is regarded as peculiarly English.

The genus *Quercus* comprises numerous species, distributed widely over the Northern Hemisphere, and found also in Java, and the Mountains of Mexico and South America. One species from Guatemala, *Quercus Skinneri*, is remarkable for its resemblance to the Walnut (Juglans) in its lobed and wrinkled seed-leaves or cotyledons.

The Oak is subject to a good deal of variation; many species have been defined and many oaks of foreign origin are grown in our parks, the longest established being the Evergreen or Holm Oak (*Q. ilex*). There are two principal varieties of *Q. robur*, often regarded as separate species: *Q. pedunculata*, the Common Oak, which is distinguished by having acorns in ones and twos attached to the twigs by long stems, the leaves having scarcely any stalk at all; and *Q. sessiliflora*, the Durmast Oak, often included with the former, but distinct, the leaves being borne on long stalks, while the acorns 'sit' on the bough. This variety of oak is more generally found in the lower parts of Britain and in North Wales. It is not so long-lived as the Common Oak, and the wood, which has a straighter fibre and a finer grain, is generally thought less tough and less resisting.

Q. pedunculata and *Q. sessiliflora* make good timber, the latter being darker, heavier and more elastic. The wood of these trees when stained green by the growth of a peculiar fungus known as *Peziza oeriginosa* is much valued by cabinet-makers.

The shape of the oak leaves is too familiar to need description. The flowers are of two kinds; the male, or barren, in long drooping catkins, 1 to 3 inches long, appearing with the leaves, and the leaves and the fertile flowers in distant clusters, each with a cup-shaped, scaly involucre, producing, as fruit, an acorn 1/2 to 1 inch long.

The Oak is noted for the slowness of its growth, as well as for the large size to which it attains. In eighty years the trunk is said not to exceed 20 inches in diameter, but old trees reach a great girth. The famous Fairlop Oak in Hainault Forest measured 36 feet in girth, the spreading boughs extending above 300 feet in circumference. The Newland Oak in Gloucestershire measures 46 feet 4 inches at 1 foot from the ground, and is one of the largest and oldest in the kingdom, these measurements being exceeded, however, by those of the Courthorpe Oak in Yorkshire, which Hooker reports as attaining the extraordinary girth of 70 feet. King Arthur's Round Table was made from a single slice of oak, cut from an enormous bole, and is still shown at Winchester.

Humboldt refers to an oak in the Département de la Charente-Inférieure measuring nearly 90 feet in circumference near the base; near Breslau an oak fell in

1857 measuring 66 feet in circumference at the base. These large trees are for the most part decayed and hollow in the interior, and their age has been estimated at from one to two thousand years.

The famous Oak of Mamre, Abram's Oak, was illustrated formerly in the Transactions of the Linnean Society, by Dr. Hooker. It is a fine specimen of the species *Q. Coccifera*, the prickly evergreen or Kermes Oak, a native of the countries bordering on the Mediterranean; the insect (coccus) from which it derives its name yielding the dye known as 'Turkey red.' Abram's Oak is 22 feet in circumference; it is popularly supposed to represent the spot where the tree grew under which Abraham pitched his tent. There is a superstition that any person who cuts or maims this oak will lose his firstborn son.

The oak of Libbeiya in the Lebanon measures 37 feet in girth, and its branches cover an area whose circumference measured over 90 yards. The Arab name is Sindian.

The Greeks held the Oak sacred, the Romans dedicated it to Jupiter, and the Druids venerated it.

In England the name Gospel Oak is still retained in many counties, relating to the time when Psalms and Gospel truths were uttered beneath their shade. They were notable objects as resting-places in the 'beating of the parish bounds,' a practice supposed to have been derived from the feast to the god Terminus.

The following is a quotation from Withers:

'That every man might keep his own possessions,

Our fathers used, in reverent processions,

With zealous prayers, and with praiseful cheere,

To walk their parish limits once a year;

And well-known marks (which sacrilegious hands

Now cut or breake) so bordered out their lands,

That every one distinctly knew his owne,

And brawles now rife were then unknowne.'

The ceremony was performed by the clergyman and his parishioners going the boundaries of the parish and choosing the most remarkable sites (oak-trees being specially selected) to read passages from the Gospels, and ask blessings for the people.

'Dearest, bury me

Under that holy oke, or Gospel Tree;

Where, though thou see'st not, thou may'st think upon

Me, when you yearly go'st Procession.'

-----HERRICK

Many of these Gospel trees are still alive, five in different parts of England.

An old proverb relating to the oak is still a form of speculation on the weather in many country districts.

'If the Oak's before the Ash,

Then you'll only get a splash;

If the Ash before the Oak,

Then you may expect a soak.'

The technical name of the Oak is said to be derived from the Celtic quer (fine) and cuez (tree).

A curious custom in connexion with wearing an oak-leaf (or preferably an oak-apple) on May 29, still exists in some villages in South Wilts. Each one has the right to collect fallen branches in a certain large wood in the district. To claim this privilege each villager has to bring them home shouting 'Grovely, Grovely, and all Grovely!' (this being the name of the large wood).

After the Oak has passed its century, it increases by less than an inch a year, but the wood matured in this leisurely fashion is practically indestructible. Edward the Confessor's shrine in Westminster Abbey is of oak that has outlasted the changes of 800 years. Logs have been dug from peat bogs, in good preservation and fit for rough building purposes, that were submerged a thousand years ago. In the Severn, breakwaters are still used as casual landing-places, where piles of oak are said to have been driven by the Romans.

As timber, the particular and most valued qualities of the Oak are hardness and toughness; Box and Ebony are harder, Yew and Ash are tougher than Oak, but no timber is possessed of both these requisites in so great a degree as the British Oak. Its elasticity and strength made it particularly advantageous in shipbuilding, and the oaks of the Forest of Dean provided much material for the 'wooden walls of England.' We read that Philip of Spain gave special orders to the Armada to burn and destroy every oak in that forest, and a century later, during a period of twenty-five years, nearly 17,000 loads of oak timber, of the value of L. 30,000 (pounds sterling), were despatched to naval dockyards from this forest. Nelson drew up a special memorial to the Crown on the desirability of replanting this forest with oak trees, and at that time no forester dared to cut down a crooked tree before maturity, because its knees and twisted elbows were so desirable in shipbuilding. A tree should be winter felled, if perfection of grain is desired. Although not employed as of old, for building ships of war, it is in great request for peaceful land transit, sharing with Ash in the making of railway carriages and other rolling stock. The roots were formerly used to make hafts for daggers and knives.

Some of the American kinds also furnish valuable timber. Such are *Q. alba*, the White or Quebec Oak, the wood of which is used in shipbuilding, and by wheelwrights and coopers. *Q. virens*, the Live Oak, also yields excellent timber for naval purposes. The wood of *Q. ilex*, a Mediterranean species, is said to be as good as that of the Common Oak. *Q. cerris*, the Turkey Oak, supplies a wood much in favour with wheelwrights, cabinet-makers, turners, etc. There are also several Japanese oaks, used for their excellent timber.

The False Sandalwood of Crete is the produce of *Q. abelicea*. This wood is of a reddish colour, and has an agreeable perfume. The less valuable oaks furnish excellent charcoal and firewood.

The bark is universally used to tan leather, and for this purpose strips easily in April and May. An infusion of it, with a small quantity of copperas, yields a dye which was formerly used in the country to dye woollen of a purplish colour, which, though not very bright, was said to be durable. The Scotch Highlanders used it to dye their yarn. Oak sawdust used also to be the principal indigenous vegetable used in dyeing fustian, and may also be used for tanning, but is much inferior to the bark for that purpose. Oak apples have also been occasionally used in dyeing as a substitute for the imported Oriental galls, but the black obtained from them is not durable.

In Brittany, tan compressed into cakes is used as fuel. Oak-bark is employed for dyeing black, in conjunction with salts of iron. With alum, oak-bark yields a brown dye; with a salt of tin, a yellow colour; with a salt of zinc, Isabelia yellow. *Q. tinctoria*, a North American species, yields Quercitron Bark, employed for dyeing yellow; the American Indians are said to dye their skins red with the bark of *Q. prinus*. After the oakbark has been used for leather-tanning, it is still serviceable to gardeners for the-warmth it generates and is largely used by them under the name of Tan; it sometimes, however, favours the growth of certain fungi, which are harmful to plants. Refuse tan is also employed in the adulteration of chicory and coffee.

Acorns were of considerable importance formerly for feeding swine. About the end of the seventh century, special laws were made relating to the feeding of swine in woods, called pawnage, or pannage. In Saxon times of famine, the peasantry was thankful for a share of this nourishing, but somewhat indigestible food. The Board of Agriculture has lately issued a pamphlet, pointing out the use as fodder, which might be made both of the Acorn and of the Horse Chestnut. The analysis of the Acorn given by the Lancet is: water, 6.3 per cent; protein, 5.2 per cent; fat, 43 per cent; carbohydrates, 45 per cent. The most important constituent of both the Acorn and the Horse Chestnut is the carbohydrate in the form of starch, while the Acorn should have further value on account of the substantial proportion of fat which it contains. The flavour of Acorns is improved if they are dried, and a flour with nourishing properties can be obtained by grinding the dried kernels.

In many country districts acorns are still collected in sacks and given to pigs; but these must be mixed with other vegetable food to counteract their binding properties.

Oak trees are more persistently attacked by insects than any other trees.

Historical Medicinal Uses - For Entertainment ONLY

Medicinal Action and Uses: The astringent effects of the Oak were well known to the Ancients, by whom different parts of the tree were used, but it is the bark which is now employed in medicine. Its action is slightly tonic, strongly astringent and antiseptic. It has a strong astringent bitter taste, and its qualities are extracted both by water and spirit. The odour is slightly aromatic.

Like other astringents, it has been recommended in agues and haemorrhages, and is a good substitute for Quinine in intermittent fever, especially when given with Chamomile flowers.

It is useful in chronic diarrhoea and dysentery, either alone or in conjunction with aromatics. A decoction is made from 1 oz. of bark in a quart of water, boiled down to a pint and taken in wineglassful doses. Externally, this decoction has been advantageously employed as a gargle in chronic sore throat with relaxed uvula, and also as a fomentation. It is also serviceable as an injection for leucorrhoea, and applied locally to bleeding gums and piles.

Preparation and Dosage: Fluid extract, 1/2 to 1 drachm.

Oak bark when finely powdered and inhaled freely, has proved very beneficial in consumption in its early stages. Working tanners are well known to be particularly exempt from this disease. A remedial snuff is made from the freshly collected oak bark, dried and reduced to a fine powder.

The bark is collected in the spring from young trees, and dried in the sun. It is greyish, more or less polished externally and brownish internally. The fracture is fibrous and the inner surface rough, with projecting medullary rays.

The older herbalists considered the thin skin that covers the acorn effectual in staying spitting of blood, and the powder of the acorn taken in wine was considered a good diuretic. A decoction of acorns and oak bark, made with milk, was considered an antidote to poisonous herbs and medicines.

The distilled water of the oak bud was also thought 'to be good used either inwardly or outwardly to assuage inflammation.'

Galen applied the bruised leaves to heal wounds.

Galls are excrescences produced in plants by the presence of the larvae of different insects. The forms that they assume are many, and the changes produced in the tissues various. They occur in all parts of the plant and sometimes in great quantities.

The oak galls used in commerce and medicine are excrescences on the *Q. infectoria*, a small oak, indigenous to Asia Minor and Persia, and result from the puncture of the bark of the young twigs by the female Gallwasp, Cynips Gallae-tinctoriae, who lays its eggs inside. This species of oak seldom attains the height of 6 feet, the stem being crooked, with the habit of a shrub rather than a tree.

The Common Oaks of this country are much affected by galls. They occur sometimes on the leaves, where they form the socalled 'Oak-apples,' sometimes on the shoots, where they do great mischief by checking and distorting the growth of the tree.

The young larva that hatches from the eggs feeds upon the tissues of the plant and secretes in its mouth a peculiar fluid, which stimulates the cells of the tissues to a rapid division and abnormal development, resulting in the formation of a gall.

The larva thus becomes completely enclosed in a nearly spherical mass, which projects from the twig, furnishing it with a supply of starch and other nutritive material.

The growth of the gall continues only so long as the egg or larva lives or reaches maturity and passes into a chrysalis, from which the fully-developed gall-wasp emerges and escapes into the air through a hole bored with its mandibles in the side of the gall.

The best Aleppo galls, collected in Asiatic Turkey, principally in the province of Aleppo, are collected before the insects escape.

Galls are also largely imported from Persia and to a lesser extent from Greece.

Aleppo Galls of good quality are hard and heavy, without perforations, dark bluish-green or olive green, nearly spherical in shape, 12 to 18 mm. in diameter (about 2/5 to 4/5 inch), and known in commerce as blue or green galls.

The Aleppo galls (from *Q. infectoria*) sometimes also called 'Mecca Galls,' are supposed to be the Dead Sea or Sodom Apples, 'the fruit that never comes to ripeness' - the fruit so pleasant to the eye, so bitter to the taste.

If collected after the insects have escaped, galls are of a pale, yellowish-brown hue, spongy and lighter in weight, perforated near the centre with a small hole. These are known in commerce as white galls.

On breaking a gall, it appears yellowish or brownish-white within, with a small cavity containing the remains of a larva of the Gall-wasp.

Galls have no marked odour, but an intensely astringent taste, and slightly sweet after-taste.

Constituents: The chief constituents of Aleppo or Turkey Galls are 50 to 70 per cent of gallotannic acid, 2 to 4 per cent of gallic acid, mucilage, sugar, resin and an insoluble matter, chiefly lignin.

'White' galls contain less gallotannic acid than 'blue' or 'green.'

English Oak Galls, or Oak Apples, are smooth, globular, brown, usually perforated and much less astringent than Aleppo Galls, containing only 15 to 20 per cent of gallotannic acid. They have no commercial value.

China Galls - produced by a species of Aphis on Rhus semialata - are used mainly for the manufacture of tannic and gallic acids, pyrogallol, ink, etc. They are not spherical, but of extremely diverse and irregular form, with a thick, grey, velvety down, making them a reddish-brown colour. They contain about 70 per cent of gallotannic acid.

Mecca Galls, from Bassorah, known as 'mala nisana,' are spherical in shape and surrounded about the centre by a circle of horned protuberances. They are not official.

Medicinal Action and Uses: Galls are much used commercially in the preparation of gallic acid and tannic acid, and are extensively employed in tanning and dyeing, in the manufacture of ink, etc.

Medicinally, they are a powerful astringent, the most powerful of all vegetable astringents, used as a tincture internally, in cases of dysentery, diarrhoea, cholera, and as an injection in gonorrhoea, leucorrhoea, etc.

Preparations of gall are usually applied as a local astringent externally, mainly in Gall ointment (1 oz. powdered galls and 4 oz. benzoated lard), applied to painful haemorrhoids, and also to arrest haemorrhage from the nose and gums.

An infusion may be used also as a gargle in relaxed throat, inflamed tonsils, etc.

Preparations and Dosages: Powdered gall, 5 to 20 grains. Fluid extract, 5 to 20 drops. Tincture, U.S.P., 1 drachm. Ointment, B.P. Compound ointment, B.P.

Onion

Quick Facts

Latin/Linnaen:	*Allium Cepa*
Family:	*Amaryllidaceae*
Old English :	Hwit Leac
Synonyms:	Bulb Onion, Common Onion, Garden Onion, Potato Onion, The Underground Onion, Egyptian Onion.
Action:	Antibacterial, Lipid and blood pressure-lowering, Inhibition of thrombocyte aggregation.
Parts Used:	Root and shoots
Indicated For:	Loss of appetite, preventions of atherosclerosis.
Dosage:	Unless otherwise prescribed: Average daily dosage: 50g of fresh onions or 20g of dried drug; equivalent preparations.
Preparation:	Cut onions, pressed juice from fresh onions and other oral galenical preparations.
Cautions:	
Other Uses:	Culinary

Description

The onion (*Allium cepa*), which is also known as the bulb onion, common onion and garden onion, is the most widely cultivated species of the genus *Allium*. The genus *Allium* also contains a number of other species variously referred to as onions and cultivated for food, such as the Japanese bunching onion (*A. fistulosum*), Egyptian onion (*A. ×proliferum*), and Canada onion (*A. canadense*). The name "wild onion" is applied to a number of *Allium* species.

The vast majority of cultivars of *A. cepa* belong to the 'common onion group' (*A. cepa var. cepa*) and are usually referred to simply as 'onions'. The 'Aggregatum

Group' of cultivars (*A. cepa var. aggregatum*) includes both shallots and potato onions.

Allium cepa is known only in cultivation, but related wild species occur in Central Asia. The most closely related species include Allium *vavilovii* and *Allium asarense*

Cultivation

Hardiness Zone:	Annual crop
Soil pH:	6-7
Soil type:	Rich free draining soil
Cultivation:	Grow from seed or from sets (immature onion bulbs)
Sunlight:	Full sun
Habitat:	Native mainly to the Northern Hemisphere, but now cultivated in all temperate areas of the world.

Onions require weeding by hand as they do not like their roots disturbed. They should be watered only if the weather has been dry. Cut off flower parts as the plants energy should be concentrated on growing the bulb. The onion bulb is ready for harvest once the foliage turns yellow. Onions should be stored in a cool, dry, well ventilated place.

Historical Notes

The Potato Onion, also known as the Underground Onion, from its habit of increasing its bulbs beneath the surface, is very prolific. It is a valuable vegetable because it furnishes sound, tender, full-sized bulbs at midsummer, three months before the ordinary Onion crop is harvested. The bulbs are rather large, of irregular shape, from 2 to over 3 inches in diameter and about 2 inches thick. The flesh of the bulb is agreeable to the taste and of good quality. The skin is thickish and of a coppery yellow colour.

In Lindley's Treasury of Botany this Potato Onion is called the 'Egyptian Onion,' and is stated to have been introduced from Egypt about the beginning of the nineteenth century. It is much cultivated in the West of England, being quite hardy, productive, and as mild in quality as the Spanish Onion.

This variety of Onion produces no seeds and is propagated by the lateral bulbs, which it throws out underground in considerable numbers. It requires a well-worked, moderately rich soil, and is largely grown in Devonshire, where in view of the mildness of the climate, the rule is to plant it in warm, sheltered situations in mid-winter, generally on the shortest day, with the hope of taking up the crop at mid-summer. In colder parts, however, the planting must be deferred until late winter, or early spring, yet the earlier it can be effected the better. The bulbs should be planted almost on the surface, in ground that has been previously well prepared and manured, and in rows 15 inches apart, with 6 to 10 inches space between the bulbs in the rows.

Each bulb will throw out a number of offsets all round it, which grow and develop into full-sized bulbs, which are taken up and dried when ready for pulling, and then stored for use and for future propagation. If the plants attain full maturity each bulb will produce seven or eight bulbs of various sizes. The strongest of these will in their turn produce a number of bulbs, while the weaker ones generally grow into a single, large bulb. The largest bulbs do not always keep so well as the medium-sized ones.

Parsley

Gemeine Peterflie.

Quick Facts

Latin/Linnaen:	*Petroselinum crispum*, or *Petroselinum sativum*
Family:	*Apiaceae*
Old English :	Petresilige, Petorsilie
Synonyms:	Petersylinge, Persely, Persele.
Action:	Unknown
Parts Used:	Herb and root
Indicated For:	Used in flushing out the efferent urinary tract in disorders of the same and in prevention and treatment of kidney gravel.
Dosage:	Unless otherwise prescribed: Daily dose: 6g of the prepared drug.
Preparation:	The crushed drug for infusions as well as other galenical preparations with a comparably small proportion of essential oil to be taken orally.
Cautions:	The essential oil should not be used in isolation because of its toxicity. **Contraindications**: Pregnancy; inflammatory kidney conditions. **Precautions**: Irrigation therapy should not be carried out in the case of edema caused by impaired heart or kidney function. **Side effects**: Occasional allergic skin or mucous membrane reactions have been reported.
Other Uses:	

Description

Parsley (*Petroselinum hortense*) is a species of *Petroselinum* in the family *Apiaceae*, native to the central Mediterranean region (southern Italy, Algeria and Tunisia), naturalized elsewhere in Europe, and widely cultivated as an herb, a spice and a vegetable.

Garden parsley is a bright green hairless biennial herbaceous plant in temperate climates, an annual herb in sub-tropical and tropical areas.

Where it grows as a biennial; in the first year, it forms a rosette of tripinnate leaves 10–25 cm long with numerous 1–3 cm leaflets, and a taproot used as a food store over the winter. In the second year it grows a flowering stem to 75 cm tall with sparser leaves and flat-topped 3–10 cm diameter umbels with numerous 2 mm diameter yellow to yellowish-green flowers. The seeds are ovoid, 2–3mm long, with prominent style remnants at the apex. One of the compounds of the essential oil is apiol. The plant normally dies after seed maturation.

Cultivation

Hardiness Zone:	6-9 Parsley is a biennial and is best grown as an annual
Soil pH:	6.0-7.0
Soil type:	Rich, moist well drained soil
Cultivation:	Seed
Sunlight:	Full sun-partial shade
Habitat:	Native to the Mediterranean.

To preserve parsley it is best to freeze rather than dry it. When harvesting always leave at least 1/3 of the plant in order to keep it useful.

Historical Notes

The Garden Parsley is not indigenous to Britain: Linnaeus stated its wild habitat to be Sardinia, whence it was brought to England and apparently first cultivated here in 1548. Bentham considered it a native of the Eastern Mediterranean regions; De Candolle of Turkey, Algeria and the Lebanon. Since its introduction into these islands in the sixteenth century it has been completely naturalized in various parts of England and Scotland, on old walls and rocks.

Petroselinum, the specific name of the Parsley, from which our English name is derived, is of classic origin, and is said to have been assigned to it by Dioscorides. The Ancients distinguished between two plants Selinon, one being the Celery (*Apium graveolens*) and called heleioselinon - i.e. 'Marsh selinon,' and the other - our parsley - Oreoselinon, 'Mountain selinon'; or petroselinum, signifying 'Rock selinon.' This last name in the Middle Ages became corrupted into Petrocilium - this was anglicized into Petersylinge, Persele, Persely and finally Parsley.

There is an old superstition against transplanting parsley plants. The herb is said to have been dedicated to Persephone and to funeral rites by the Greeks. It was afterwards consecrated to St. Peter in his character of successor to Charon.

In the sixteenth century, Parsley was known as *A. hortense*, but herbalists retained the official name *petroselinum*. Linnaeus in 1764 named it *A. petroselinum*, but it is now assigned to the genus *Carum*.

The Greeks held Parsley in high esteem, crowning the victors with chaplets of Parsley at the Isthmian games, and making with it wreaths for adorning the tombs of their dead. The herb was never brought to table of old, being held sacred to oblivion and to the dead. It was reputed to have sprung from the blood of a Greek hero, Archemorus, the forerunner of death, and Homer relates that chariot horses were fed by warriors with the leaves. Greek gardens were often bordered with Parsley and Rue.

Several cultivated varieties exist, the principal being the common plain-leaved, the curled-leaved, the Hamburg or broadleaved and the celery-leaved. Of the variety crispum, or curled-leaved, there are no less than thirty-seven variations; the most valuable are those of a compact habit with close, perfectly curled leaves. The common sort bears close leaves, but is of a somewhat hardier nature than those of which the leaves are curled; the latter are, however, superior in every way. The variety crispum was grown in very early days, being even mentioned by Pliny.

Turner says, 'if parsley is thrown into fishponds it will heal the sick fishes therein.'

The Hamburg, or turnip-rooted Parsley, is grown only for the sake of its enlarged fleshy tap-root. No mention appears to have been made by the Ancients, or in the Middle Ages, of this variety, which Miller in his Gardeners' Dictionary (1771) calls 'the largerooted Parsley,' and which under cultivation develops both a parsnip-like as well as a turnip-shaped form. Miller says:

'This is now pretty commonly sold in the London markets, the roots being six times as large as the common Parsley. This sort was many years cultivated in Holland before the English gardeners could be prevailed upon to sow it. I brought the seeds of it from thence in 1727; but they refused to accept it, so that I cultivated it several years before it was known in the markets.'

At the present day, the 'long white' and the 'round sugar' forms are sold by seedgrowers and are in esteem for flavouring soups, stews, etc., the long variety being also cooked and eaten like parsnips.

Neapolitan, or celery-leaved, parsley is grown for the use of its leafstalks, which are blanched and eaten like those of celery.

The plain-leaved parsley was the first known in this country, but it is not now much cultivated, the leaves being less attractive than those of the curled, of a less brilliant green, and coarser in flavour. It also has too close a resemblance to Fool's Parsley (*Anthriscus cynapium*), a noxious weed of a poisonous nature infesting gardens and fields. The leaves of the latter, though similar, are, however, of a rather darker green and when bruised, emit an unpleasant odour, very different to that of Parsley. They are, also, more finely divided. When the two plants are in flower, they are easily distinguished, Anthriscus having three tiny, narrow, sharp-pointed leaflets hanging down under each little umbellule of the white umbel of flowers, whereas in the Garden Parsley there is usually only one leaflet under the main umbel, the leaflets or bracts at the base of the small umbellules only being short and as fine as hairs. Anthriscus leaves, also, are glossy beneath. Gerard called Anthriscus 'Dog's Parsley,' and says 'the whole plant is of a naughty smell.' It contains a peculiar alkaloid called Cynapium.

Stone Parsley (*Sison*), or Breakstone, is an allied plant, growing in chalky districts.

S. Amomum is a species well known in some parts of Britain, with cream-coloured flowers and aromatic seeds. The name is said to be derived from the Celtic sium (running stream), some of the species formerly included growing in moist localities.

Of our Garden Parsley (which he calls Parsele) Gerard says, 'It is delightful to the taste and agreeable to the stomache,' also 'the roots or seeds boiled in ale and drank, cast foorth strong venome or poyson; but the seed is the strongest part of the herbe.'

Though the medicinal virtues of Parsley are still fully recognized, in former times it was considered a remedy for more disorders than it is now used for. Its imagined quality of destroying poison, to which Gerard refers, was probably attributed to the plant from its remarkable power of overcoming strong scents, even the odour of garlic being rendered almost imperceptible when mingled with that of Parsley.

The plant is said to be fatal to small birds and a deadly poison to parrots, also very injurious to fowls, but hares and rabbits will come from a great distance to seek for it, so that it is scarcely possible to preserve it in gardens to which they have access. Sheep are also fond of it, and it is said to be a sovereign remedy to preserve them from footrot, provided it be given them in sufficient quantities.

Cultivation: Parsley requires an ordinary, good well-worked soil, but a moist one and a partially-shaded position is best. A little soot may be added to the soil.

The seed may be sown in drills, or broadcast, or, if only to be used for culinary purposes, as edging, or between dwarf or shortlived crops.

For a continuous supply, three sowings should be made: as early in February as the weather permits, in April or early in May, and in July and early August - the last being for the winter supply, in a sheltered position, with a southern exposure. Sow in February for the summer crop and for drying purposes. Seed sown then, however, takes several weeks to germinate, often as much as a full month. The principal sowing is generally done in April; it then germinates more quickly and provides useful material for cutting throughout the summer. A mid-August sowing will furnish good plants for placing in the cold frames for winter use.

An even broadcast sowing is preferable, if the ground is in the condition to be trodden which appears to fix the seed in its place, and after raking leaves a firm even surface.

The seed should be but slightly covered, not more than 1/2 inch deep and thinly distributed; if in drills, these should be 1 foot apart.

It is not necessary, however (though usual), to sow the seed where the plants are to be grown, as when large enough, the seedlings can be pricked out into rows.

When the seedlings are well out of the ground - about an inch high - adequate thinning is imperative, as the plants dislike being cramped, and about 8 inches from plant to plant must be allowed: a well-grown plant will cover nearly a square foot of ground.

The rows should be liberally watered in dry weather; a sheltered position is preferred, as the plants are liable to become burnt up in very hot and dry summers.

The rows should be kept clean of weeds, and frequent dressings may be applied with advantage.

If the growth becomes coarse in the summer, cut off all the leaves and water well. This will induce a new growth of fine leaves, and may always be done when the plants have grown to a good size, as it encourages a stocky growth.

Soon after the old or last year's plants begin to grow again in the spring, they run to flower, but if the flower stems are promptly removed, and the plants top dressed and watered, they will remain productive for some time longer. Renew the beds every two years, as the plant dies down at the end of the second season.

When sowing Parsley to stand the winter, a plain-leaved variety will often be found superior to the curled or mossy sorts, which are, perhaps, handsomer, but the leaves retain both snow and rain, and when frost follows, the plants soon succumb. A plainleaved Parsley is far hardier, and will survive even a severe winter and is equally good for cooking, though not so attractive for garnishing. Double the trouble is experienced in obtaining a supply of Parsley during the winter, when only the curled-leaved varieties are given.

Where curled Parsley is desired and is difficult to obtain, because there is no sufliciently sheltered spot in the garden for it, it may often be saved by placing a frame-light over the bed during severe weather to protect the plants, or they may be placed altogether in cold frames. Care must be taken with all Parsley plants grown thus in frames, to pick off all decaying leaves directly noticed, and the soil should be stirred occasionally with a pointed stick between the plants, to prevent its becoming sour. Abundance of air should be given on all favourable occasions, removing the light altogether on fine days.

Historical Medicinal Uses - For Entertainment ONLY

Medicinal Action and Uses: The uses of Parsley are many and are by no means restricted to the culinary sphere. The most familiar employment of the leaves in their fresh state is, of course, finely-chopped, as a flavouring to sauces, soups, stuffings, rissoles, minces, etc., and also sprinkled over vegetables or salads. The leaves are extensively cultivated, not only for sending to market fresh, but also for the purpose of being dried and powdered as a culinary flavouring in winter, when only a limited supply of fresh Parsley is obtainable.

In addition to the leaves, the stems are also dried and powdered, both as a culinary colouring and for dyeing purposes. There is a market for the seeds to supply nurserymen, etc., and the roots of the turnip-rooted variety are used as a vegetable and flavouring.

Medicinally, the two-year-old roots are employed, also the leaves, dried, for making Parsley Tea, and the seeds, for the extraction of an oil called Apiol, which is of considerable curative value. The best kind of seed for medicinal purposes is that obtained from the Triple Moss curled variety. The wholesale drug trade generally obtains its seeds from farmers on the East coast, each sample being tested separately before purchases are made. It has been the practice to buy secondyear seeds which are practically useless for growing purposes: it would probably hardly pay farmers to grow for Apiol producing purposes only, as the demand is not sufficiently great.

Constituents: Parsley Root is faintly aromatic and has a sweetish taste. It contains starch, mucilage, sugar, volatile oil and Apiin. The latter is white, inodorous, tasteless and soluble in boiling water.

Parsley fruit or 'seeds' contain the volatile oil in larger proportion than the root (2.6 per cent); it consists of terpenes and Apiol, to which the activity of the fruit is due. There are also present fixed oil, resin, Apiin, mucilage and ash. Apiol is an oily, nonnitrogenous allyl compound, insoluble in water, soluble in alcohol and crystallizable when pure into white needles. The British Pharmacopceia directs that Apiol be prepared by extracting the bruised fresh fruits with ether and distilling the solvent. The residue is the commercial liquid Apiol. It exercises all the virtues of the entire plant. Crystallized Apiol, or Parsley Camphor, is obtained by distilling the volatile oil to a low temperature. The value of the volatile oil depends on the amount of Apiol it contains. Oil obtained from German fruit contains this body in considerable quantity and becomes semi-solid at ordinary temperature, that from French fruit is much poorer in Apiol. In France, only the crystalline Apiol is official, but three different varieties, distinguished as green, yellow and white, are in use.

Apiol was first obtained in 1849 by Drs. Joret and Homolle, of Brittany, and proved an excellent remedy there for a prevailing ague. It is greatly used now in malarial disorders. The name Apiol has also been applied to an oleoresin prepared from the plant, which contains three closely-allied principles: apiol, apiolin and myristicin, the latter identical with the active principle of oil of Nutmeg. The term 'liquid Apiol' is frequently applied to the complete oleoresin. This occurs as a yellowish liquid with a characteristic odour and an acrid pungent taste. The physiological action of the oleoresin of Parsley has not been sufficiently investigated, it exercises a singular influence on the great nerve centres of the head and spine, and in large doses produces giddiness and deafness, fall of blood-pressure and some slowing of the pulse and paralysis. It is stated that the paralysis is followed by fatty degeneration of the liver and kidney, similar to that caused by myristicin.

Parsley has carminative, tonic and aperient action, but is chiefly used for its diuretic properties, a strong decoction of the root being of great service in gravel, stone, congestion of the kidneys, dropsy and jaundice. The dried leaves are also used for the same purpose. Parsley Tea proved useful in the trenches, where our men often got kidney complications, when suffering from dysentery.

A fluid extract is prepared from both root and seeds. The extract made from the root acts more readily on the kidneys than that from other parts of the herb. The oil extracted from the seeds, the Apiol, is considered a safe and efficient emmenagogue, the dose being 5 to 15 drops in capsules. A decoction of bruised Parsley seeds was at one time employed against plague and intermittent fever.

In France, a popular remedy for scrofulous swellings is green Parsley and snails, pounded in a mortar to an ointment, spread on linen and applied daily. The bruised leaves, applied externally, have been used in the same manner as Violet leaves (also Celandine, Clover and Comfrey), to dispel tumours suspected to be of a cancerous nature. A poultice of the leaves is said to be an efficacious remedy for the bites and stings of poisonous insects.

Culpepper tells us:

'It is very comfortable to the stomach . . . good for wind and to remove obstructions both of the liver and spleen . . . Galen commendeth it for the falling sickness . . . the seed is effectual to break the stone and ease the pains and torments thereof.... The leaves of parsley laid to the eyes that are inflamed with heat or swollen, relieves them if it be used with bread or meat.... The juice dropped into the ears with a little wine easeth the pains.'

Formerly the distilled water of Parsley was often given to children troubled with wind, as Dill water still is.

Preparations and Dosages: Fluid extract root, 1/2 to 1 drachm. Fluid extract seeds, 1/2 to 1 drachm. Apiol (oil), 5 to 15 drops in capsule.

Preparation for Market: The roots are collected for medicinal purposes in the second year, in autumn or late summer, when the plant has flowered.

To dry Parsley towards the close of the summer for culinary use, it may be put into the oven on muslin trays, when cooking is finished, this being repeated several times till thoroughly dry and crisp, when the leaves should be rubbed in the hands or through a coarse wire sieve and the powder then stored in tins, so that neither air nor light can reach it, or the good colour will not be preserved. In the trade, there is a special method of drying which preserves the colour.

The oil is extracted from the 'seeds' or rather fruits, when fresh, in which condition they are supplied to manufacturing druggists.

Plantain

MCLXIV.

E. B. 507.   Plantago lanceolata, var. vulgaris.   Common Rib-grass, var. α.

Quick Facts

Latin/Linnaen:	*Plantago Lanceolata*
Family:	*Plantaginaceae*
Old English :	Wegbraede
Synonyms:	Waybread, Greater Plantain, Dock, Snake Plantain, Black Plantain, Long Plantain, Ribble Grass, Ribwort, Black Jack, Jackstraw, Lamb's Tongue, Hen Plant, Wendles, Kemps, Cocks, Quinquenervia, Costa Canina.
Action:	Astringent, Antibacterial
Parts Used:	Above ground plant parts
Indicated For:	Catarrhs of the respiratory tract, inflammatory alterations of the oral and pharyngeal mucosa.
Dosage:	Unless otherwise prescribed: Average daily dosage: 3-6g of herb; equivalent preparations.
Preparation:	Comminuted herb and other galenical preparations for internal and external use.
Cautions:	
Other Uses:	

Description

Plantago lanceolata is a species of genus *Plantago* known by the common names ribwort plantain, English plantain, buckhorn plantain, and narrowleaf plantain. It is a common weed of cultivated land.

The plant is a rosette-forming perennial herb, with leafless, silky, hairy flower stems (10–40 cm/3.9–16 in). The basal leaves are lanceolate spreading or erect, scarcely toothed with 3-5 strong parallel veins narrowed to short petiole. Grouping leaf stalk deeply furrowed, ending in an oblong inflorescence of many small flowers each with a pointed bract. Each flower can produce up to two seeds. Flowers 4 mm (calyx green, corolla brownish), 4 bent back lobes with brown midribs, long white stamens. Found in British Isles, scarce on acidic soils (pH < 4.5). It is considered an invasive weed in North America. It is present and widespread in the Americas and Australia as an introduced species.

Cultivation

Hardiness Zone:	9-10
Soil pH:	5.5-7.0
Soil type:	Well drained rich soil
Cultivation:	Suckers/plant offshoots
Sunlight:	Can tolerate some shade, but will produce poor fruit. Best in full sun.
Habitat:	Native to Indo-Malesian, Asian and Australian tropics.

Historical Notes

Several of the wild Plantains have been used indiscriminately for *Plantago major*. Of these, the most important is *Plantago lanceolatus* (Linn.), the Ribwort Plantain.

This is a very dark green, slender perennial, growing much taller than *P. major*. Its leaf-blades rarely reach an inch in breadth, are three to five ribbed, gradually narrowed into the petioles, which are often more than a foot long. The flowerstalks are often more than 2 feet long, terminating in cylindrical blunt, dense spikes, 1/2 to 3 or 4 inches long and 1/3 to 1/2 inch thick. It has the same chemical constituents as *P. major*.

When this Plantain grows amongst the tall grasses of the meadow its leaves are longer, more erect and less harsh, than when we find it by the roadside, or on dry soil. The leaves are often slightly hairy and have at times a silvery appearance from this cause, especially in the roadside specimens. The flower-stalks are longer than the leaves, furrowed and angular and thrown boldly up. The flowerhead varies a good deal in size and form, sometimes being much smaller and more globular than others. The sepals are brown and paper-like in texture and give the head its peculiar rusty look. The corolla is very small and inconspicuous, tubed and having four spreading lobes. The stamens, four in number, are the most noticeable feature, their slender white filaments and pale yellow anthers forming a conspicuous ring around the flower-head.

In some old books we find this species called *Costa canina*, in allusion to the prominent veinings on the leaves that earned it the name of Ribwort, and it is this feature that caused it to receive also the mediaeval name of Quinquenervia. Another old popular name was 'Kemps,' a word that at first sight seems without meaning, but when fully understood has a peculiar interest. The stalks of this plant are particularly tough and wiry, and it is an old game with country children to strike the heads one against the other until the stalk breaks. The Anglo-Saxon word for a soldier was cempa, and we can thus see the allusion to 'kemps.'

This species of Plantain abounds in every meadow and was brought into notice at one time as a possible fodder plant. Curtis, in his Flora Londonensis, says:

'The farmers in general consider this species of plantain as a favourite food of sheep and hence it is frequently recommended in the laying down of meadow and pasture land, and the seed is for that purpose kept in the shops.'

But its cultivation was never seriously taken up, for though its mucilaginous leaves are relished by sheep and to a certain extent by cows and horses, it does not answer as a crop, except on very poor land, where nothing else will grow. Moreover, it is very bitter, and in pastures destroys the more delicate herbage around it by its coarse leaves.

The seeds are covered with a coat of mucilage, which separates readily when macerated in hot water. The gelatinous substance thus formed has been used at one time in France for stiffening some kinds of muslin and other woven fabrics.

The leaves contain a good fibre, which, it has been suggested, might be adapted to some manufacturing purpose.

Radish

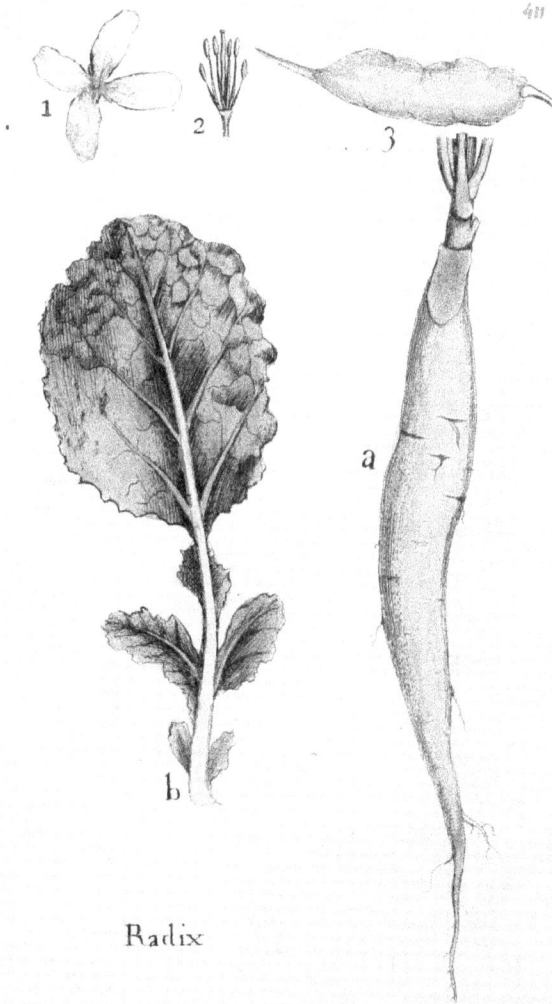

Radix

Quick Facts

Latin/Linnaen:	*Raphanus sativus*
Family:	*Brassicaceae*
Old English :	Rædic, Hrædic, Redic
Synonyms:	None known
Action:	Secretagogue for the upper gastrointestinal tract, Motility promoting, Antimicrobial.
Parts Used:	Root
Indicated For:	Peptic disorders, especially those related to dyskinesia of the bile ducts, catarrhs of the upper respiratory tract.
Dosage:	Unless otherwise prescribed: Average daily dosage: 50-100ml pressed juice.
Preparation:	Pressed juice for oral use.
Cautions:	
Other Uses:	**Culinary**
	Fuel: Wild radish seeds contain up to 48% oil content, and while not suitable for human consumption the oil is a potential source of biofuel.

Description

The radish (*Raphanus sativus*) is an edible root vegetable of the *Brassicaceae* family that was domesticated in Europe, in pre-Roman times. They are grown and consumed throughout the world. Radishes have numerous varieties, varying in size, color and duration of required cultivation time. There are some radishes that are grown for their seeds; oilseed radishes are grown, as the name implies, for oil production.

Cultivation

Hardiness Zone:	Annual crop
Soil pH:	6.5-7
Soil type:	Sandy loams
Cultivation:	By seed
Sunlight:	Full sun
Habitat:	Believed to be native to Asia, domesticated by early Egyptians

Radish requires a cool temperature to properly develop. It can be harvested in 20-30 days after planting, so you can do successive plantings to maintain a continual supply.

Historical Notes

Found in Europe, especially Britain, and temperate Asia. A native of China, and Japan.

The name of this familiar garden plant is suggested by its colour, being derived from the Saxon, rude, rudo, or reod (ruddy), or from the Sanskrit rudhira, meaning blood. The genus is distinguished by its elongated pod, which has no longitudinal partition when ripe, but contains several seeds separated by a pithy substance filling the pod. The actual plant is unknown in a wild state, but is supposed to have come from Southern Asia, and may be descended from the wild Raphanus raphanistrum of the Mediterranean shores, the long roots developing seeds sown in a loose soil, and the turniprooted kinds in a stiff soil. In the days of the Pharaohs, the Radish was extensively cultivated in Egypt, but apparently it did not reach Britain until A.D. 1548. Gerard mentions four varieties as being recognized in 1597. The leaves are rough and partly divided into segments, the outer one being larger and broader than the rest. The flower stem grows to about 3 feet in height, bearing medium-sized flowers that vary in colour from white to pale violet, with strongly marked, dark veins. Structurally, it resembles the turnip, as the swollen, fleshy portion is really a stem which gradually passes downwards into the real root. Many kinds are named, the best known being (1) turnip-rooted, both red and white, including the white and black Spanish kinds; (2) oliveshaped, including the white, scarlet, and French breakfast forms; (3) the long, tapering varieties, like Long Red and Lady's Finger. The flesh is white, crisp, and tender, not specially nourishing, but valued as an antiscorbutic because of its quantity of nitrous juice. When too large for eating raw, they can be steamed for half an hour and served like asparagus. They should be well washed, but never peeled except when preparing the juice for medicinal purposes; in dry weather the bed should be watered the day before they are pulled. The young, green, seed-pods may be used for pickling, alone or with other vegetables, and are considered a fair substitute for capers.

Constituents: Phenyl-ethyl isothiocyanite, a pungent, volatile oil, and an amylclytic enzyme.

Other Species:

- R. Raphanistrum (Wild Radish, or Jointedpodded Charlock). It was stated by Linnaeus that in wet seasons this abounds as a weed among barley, in Sweden, and being ground with the corn, it is eaten in barley bread, causing violent convulsive complaints, or an epidemic, spasmodic disease. Other authorities say that it is harmless, liked by domestic animals and bees. It is bristly, and has rather large, straw-coloured flowers.
- R. Sibiricus, or Siberian Radish, has cylindrical pods.
- R. caudatus, the Java, or Rat's Tail Radish, a native of Final, furnishes long, edible pods, purple or violet in colour. They should be used half-grown. The root of this species is not used.
- R. maritimus is an indigenous, seaside variety.
- R. Erucoides, of Italy, has pods with a beak of their own length, and a simple, biennial root, scarcely thicker than the stem.
- R. Tenellus, another native of Siberia, flowers in Britain in June and July, having awl-shaped, jointed, two-celled, smooth pods.

Historical Medicinal Uses - For Entertainment ONLY

Medicinal Action and Uses: Radishes are an excellent food remedy for stone, gravel and scorbutic conditions. The juice has been used in the treatment of cholelithiasis as an aid in preventing the formation of biliary calculi. The expressed juice of white or black Spanish radishes is given in increasing doses of from 1/2 to

2 cupfuls daily. The 2 cupfuls are continued for two or three weeks then the dose is decreased until 1/2 cupful is taken three times a week for three or four more weeks. The treatment may be repeated by taking 1 cupful at the beginning, then 1/2 daily, and later, 1/2 every second day.

The colouring matter is recommended as a sensitive indicator in alkalimetry.

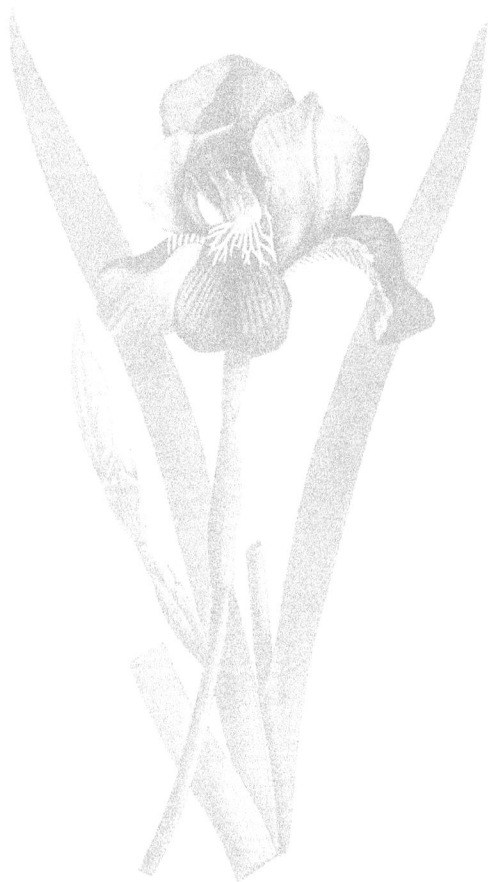

Rose

Rosa Gallica Pontiana.   *Rosier du Pont.*

Quick Facts

Latin/Linnaen:	*Rosa centifolia syn. Rosa Gallica*
Family:	*Rosaceae*
Old English :	
Synonyms:	Rose
Action:	Astringent
Parts Used:	Dried petals (collected prior to fully unfolding)
Indicated For:	Mild inflammations of the oral and pharyngeal mucosa.
Dosage:	Unless otherwise prescribed: 1-2g of drug per cup of water for tea
Preparation:	Comminuted herb for teas and other galenical preparations for mouth rinses.
Cautions:	
Other Uses:	**Culinary:** Used to flavour butter, as well as eaten in sandwiches
	Decoration: Used in potpouris

Description

Rosaceae (the rose family) are a medium-sized family of flowering plants, including about 2830 species in 95 genera. The name is derived from the type genus *Rosa*. The largest genus by far is *Prunus* (plums, cherries, peaches, apricots and almonds) with about 430 species.

Roses can be herbs, shrubs or trees. Most species are deciduous, but some are evergreen. They have a worldwide range, but are most diverse in the northern hemisphere.

Several economically important products come from *Rosaceae*, including many edible fruits (such as apples, apricots, plums, cherries, peaches, pears, raspberries, and strawberries), almonds, and ornamental trees and shrubs (such as roses, meadowsweets, photinias, firethorns, rowans, and hawthorns).

Rosaceae centifolia (lit. hundred leaved/petaled rose; syn. *R. gallica var. centifolia* (L.) Regel), the provence rose or cabbage rose or Rose de Mai is a hybrid rose developed by Dutch rose breeders in the period between the 17th century and the 19th century, possibly earlier. It is a complex hybrid bred from *Rosa gallica*, *Rosa moschata*, *Rosa canina*, and *Rosa damascena* its exact hereditary history is not well documented.

Individual plants are shrubby in appearance, growing to 1.5–2 m tall, with long drooping canes and greyish green pinnate leaves with 5-7 leaflets. The flowers are round and globular, with numerous thin overlapping petals that are highly scented; they are usually pink, less often white to dark red-purple.

Rosaceae centifolia is particular to the French city of Grasse, known as the perfume capital of the world. It is widely cultivated for its singular fragrance--clear and sweet, with light notes of honey. The flowers are commercially harvested for the production of rose oil, which is commonly used in perfumery.

Sylvia Plath mentions the cabbage rose in many of her earlier poems, such as The Thin People.

Rosa gallica (Gallic Rose, French Rose, or Rose of Provins) is a species of rose native to southern and central Europe eastwards to Turkey and the Caucasus.

Cultivars of the species *R. gallica* and hybrids close in appearance are considered as a Cultivar Group, the Gallica Group roses. Their exact ancestry is usually unknown and other species may be involved. The Gallica Group roses share the vegetative characters of the species, forming low suckering shrubs. The flowers can be single, but most commonly are double or semidouble. The colours range from white (rare) to pink and deep purple. All Gallica Group roses are once flowering. They are easily cultivated.

Plants with semidouble deep pink flowers have been treated as either a variety, under the name *R. gallica var. officinalis*, or as a cultivar, *R. gallica 'Officinalis'*. It is also called the Apothecary's Rose or the "Red Rose of Lancaster". It is the county flower of Lancashire.

The names *Rosa gallica f. trigintipetala* or Rosa 'Trigintipetala' are considered to be synonyms of *Rosa × damascena*.

Rosa gallica is a deciduous shrub forming large patches of shrubbery, the stems with prickles and glandular bristles. The leaves are pinnate, with three to seven bluish-green leaflets. The flowers are clustered one to four together, single with five petals, fragrant, deep pink. The hips are globose to ovoid, 10–13 mm diameter, orange to brownish.

Cultivation

Hardiness Zone:	Some varieties are hardy to zone 3
Soil pH:	6.0-6.9
Soil type:	High in organic material
Cultivation:	Generally by rooting a cutting
Sunlight:	Full sun
Habitat:	Native to most of the world

Historical Notes

The birthplace of the cultivated Rose was probably Northern Persia, on the Caspian, or Faristan on the Gulf of Persia. Thence it spread across Mesopotamia to Palestine and across Asia Minor to Greece. And thus it was that Greek colonists brought it to Southern Italy. It is beyond doubt that the Roses used in ancient days were cultivated varieties. Horace, who writes at length on horticulture, gives us an interesting account of the growing of Roses in beds. Pliny advises the deep digging of the soil for their better cultivation. In order to force their growth, it was the practice to dig a ditch round the plants and to pour warm water into the ditch just as the rose-buds had formed. The varieties were then very limited in number, but it would appear that the Romans, at all events, knew and cultivated the red Provins Rose (*Rosa gallica*), often mistakenly called the Provence Rose. The word rosa comes from the Greek word rodon (red), and the rose of the Ancients was of a deep crimson colour, which probably suggested the fable of its springing from the blood of Adonis.

The voluptuous Romans of the later Empire made lavish use of the blossoms of the Rose. Horace enjoins their unsparing use at banquets, when they were used not only as a means of decoration, but also to strew the floors, and even in winter the luxurious Romans expected to have petals of roses floating in their Falernian wine. Roman brides and bridegrooms were crowned with roses, so too were the images of Cupid and Venus and Bacchus. Roses were scattered at feasts of Flora and Hymen, in the paths of victors, or beneath their chariot-wheels, or adorned the prows of their war-vessels. Nor did the self-indulgent Romans disdain to wear rose garlands at their feasts, as a preventive against drunkenness. To them, the Rose was a sign of pleasure, the companion of mirth and wine, but it was also used at their funerals.

As soon as the Rose had become known to nations with a wide literature of their own, it was not only the theme of poets, but gave rise to many legends. Homer's allusions to it in the Iliad and Odyssey are the earliest records, and Sappho, the Greek poetess, writing about 600 B.C., selects the Rose as the Queen of Flowers. (The 'Rose of Sharon' of the Old Testament is considered to be a kind of Narcissus, and the 'Rose of Jericho' is a small woody annual, also not allied to the Rose.)

It was once the custom to suspend a Rose over the dinner-table as a sign that all confidences were to be held sacred. Even now the plaster ornament in the centre of a ceiling is known as 'the rose.' It has been suggested that because the Pretender could only be helped secretly, sub rosa, that the Jacobites took the white rose as his symbol. Although we have no British 'Order of the Rose,' British national flower figures largely in the insignia of other orders, such as the Garter, the order of the Bath, etc.

Constituents: The essential oil to which the perfume of the Rose is due is found in both flowers and leaves, sometimes in one, sometimes in both, and sometimes in neither, for there are also scentless roses. In the flower, the petals are the chief secreting part of the blossom, though a certain amount of essential oil resides in the epidermal layers of cells, both surfaces of the petals being equally odorous and secretive. An examination of the stamens, which are transformed into petals in the cultivated roses, shows that the epidermal cells also contain essential oil.

More than 10,000 roses are known in cultivation and three types of odours are recognized, viz. those of the Cabbage Rose (*R. centifolia*), the Damask Rose (*R. damascena*) and the Tea Rose (*R. indica*), but there are many roses of intermediate character as regards perfume, notably the 'perpetual hybrid' and 'hybrid tea' classes, which exhibit every gradation between the three types and no precise classification of roses by their odour is possible.

The flowers adapted for the preparation of essence of roses are produced by several species of rose trees. The varieties cultivated on a large scale for perfumery purposes are *R. damascena* and *R. centifolia*. *R. damascena* is cultivated chiefly in Bulgaria, Persia and India: it is a native of the Orient and was introduced into Europe at the period of the Crusades. *R. centifolia* is cultivated in Provence, Turkey and Tunis; it has been found wild in the forests of the Caucasus, where double-flowered specimens are often met with.

Although the Rose was highly esteemed in the dawn of history, it does not appear that it was then submitted to the still, the method of preserving the aroma being to steep the petals in oil, or possibly to extract it in the form of a pomade. The Oleum Rosarum, *Ol. rosatum* or *Ol. rosacetum* of the Ancients was not a volatile oil, but a fatty oil perfumed with rose petals. The first preparation of rosewater by Avicenna was in the tenth century. It was between 1582 and 1612 that the oil or OTTO OF ROSES was discovered, as recorded in two separate histories of the Grand Moguls. At the wedding feast of the princess Nour-Djihan with the Emperor Djihanguyr, son of Akbar, a canal circling the whole gardens was dug and filled with rose-water. The heat of the sun separating the water from the essential oil of the Rose, was observed by the bridal pair when rowing on the fragrant water. It was skimmed off and found to be an exquisite perfume. The discovery was immediately turned to account and the manufacture of Otto of Roses was commenced in Persia about 1612 and long before the end of the seventeenth century the distilleries of Shiraz were working on a large scale. The first mention of Persian Otto or Attar of Roses is by Kampfer (1683), who alludes to the export to India. Persia no longer exports Attar of Roses to any extent, and the production in Kashmir and elsewhere in India - probably as ancient as that of Persia - practically serves for local consumption only.

Through the Turks, the manufacture was introduced into Europe, by way of Asia Minor, where it has long been produced. It is probable that the first otto was distilled in Bulgaria, then part of the Turkish Empire, about 1690 - its sale in Europe, at a high cost, is first alluded to in 1694.

It is necessary to distil about 10,000 lb. of roses to obtain 1 lb. of oil. Oil of Rose is light yellow in colour, sometimes possessing a green tint. It has a strong odour of fresh roses. When cooled, it congeals to a translucent soft mass, which is again liquefied by the warmth of the hand. The congealing point lies between 15 degrees and 22 degrees C., mostly between 17 degrees and 21 degrees C.

Apart from French Otto of Roses, the world's supply is mainly drawn from Bulgaria, the greater part being distilled by small peasant growers. The Bulgarian rose industry is confined to one special mountain district, having for its centre the town of Kazanlik.

The Bulgarian rose industry has developed steadily since 1885, though the Great War seriously handicapped it. In 1919 the entire Bulgarian crop of Otto of Roses was taken over by the Government of that country in consequence of an agreement between the Bulgarian Government and the United States Food Administration, by which payment for food supplied to Bulgaria from America was to be made out of the proceeds of the Bulgarian otto crop.

Recipes

POT-POURRI OF ROSES

All varieties of both R. *gallica* and R. *centifolia* are used in the making of pot-pourri, the dried petals of all scented roses being valuable for the purpose as they retain their scent for a considerable time. Nearly every fragrant flower and scented leaf can be used as an ingredient of pot-pourri, blending with suitable spices to give charm to this favourite, old-fashioned sweet mixture, which in winter recalls so delightfully the vanished summer days. It must be understood that rose-petals should preponderate, and that the other component parts ought to be added in such proportions that the scent of one cannot kill the perfume of another.

There are two principal methods of making pot-pourri, the dry and the moist.

For the dry kind, the bulk of the rosepetals is fully dried and everything else - Sweet Geranium and Sweet Verbena leaves, Bay leaves and Lavender is also dried.

The best way of drying is to spread out on sheets of paper in an airy room. Anything of lasting scent, such as cedar or sandalwood sawdust, or shavings, can be added. When all is ready, the spices and sweet gums, all in powder, are put together and the whole is thoroughly mixed. For two-thirds of a bushel of dried petals and leaves, the spice mixture is 2 oz. each of Cloves, Mace and Cinnamon, 1/2 oz. each of Coriander, Allspice, Gum Storax and Gum Benzoin, and 4 oz. Violet Powder.

The moist method of preparation takes more time and needs greater care. The rose leaves are not fully, but only partly dried, so that they lose a good half of their bulk and acquire a kind of tough, leathery consistency. To preserve them and to maintain them in this state, a certain proportion of salt is added. The salt is a mixture of half Bay salt and half common salt. Bay Salt is sold in lumps, these are roughly pounded, so that some of it is quite small and the larger pieces are about the size of a small hazel nut, and then mixed with the common salt. The roses must be absolutely dry when picked. The petals are stripped off and carefully separated and laid out to partially dry. The length of time depends on the temperature and atmospheric conditions, but they are usually ready the second day after picking. Large jars of glazed earthenware should be employed for storing the rose leaves, the most convenient being cylindrical, with lids of the same glazed ware and with flat leaded disks (supplied with handles), for pressing down the contents. Put two good handsful of the rose leaves in at a time and press them down with the handled rammer. Then sprinkle a small handful of the salt mixture, then more rose leaves and so on. Then weight down till the next batch is put in. Besides rose leaves, the other chief ingredient is leaves of the Sweet Geranium, torn into shreds, dried like the Roses and put into the jars in the same way, rammed, salted and pressed. Bay leaves, Sweet Verbena and Lavender are all of a drier nature and can be put into the jars and salted just as they are. When all is ready, the contents of the preparation jars are taken out and broken up small; the mass, especially of the rose-petals, will come out in thick flakes, closely compacted. It is then mixed with the spices and sweet powders. If the freshly made mixture be rammed rather tightly into a jar or wooden barrel and left for six months, or better still for a year, the quality is much improved by being thus matured.

Mr. Donald McDonald, in Sweet-scented Flowers and Fragrant Leaves, gives the following pot-pourri recipe.

I. Gather early in the day and when perfectly dry, a peck of Roses, pick off the petals and strew over them 3/4 lb. common salt. Let them remain two or three days and if fresh flowers are added, some more salt must be sprinkled over them. Mix with the roses 1/2 lb. of finely powdered Bay salt, the same quantity of allspice, cloves and brown sugar, 1/4 lb. gum benzoin, and 2 oz. Orris root. Add 1 gill of brandy and any sort of fragrant flowers, such as Orange and Lemon flowers, Lavender and lemon-scented Verbena leaves and any other sweet-scented flowers. They should be perfectly dry when added. The mixture must be occasionally stirred and kept in close-covered jars, the covers to be raised only when the perfume is desired in the room. If after a time the mixture seems to dry, moisten with brandy only, as essences too soon lose their quality and injure the perfume.

This mixture is said to retain its fragrance for fifty years.

Lady Rosalind Northcote in The Book of Herbs gives:

A Devonshire Recipe

'Gather flowers in the morning when dry and lay them in the sun till the evening:

Roses, Orange flowers, Jasmine, Lavender.

In smaller quantities: Thyme, Sage, Marjoram, Bay.

'Put them into an earthen wide jar or hand basin in layers. Add the following ingredients:

- 6 lb. Bay Salt
- 4 oz. Yellow Sandal Wood
- 4 oz. Acorus Calamus Root
- 4 oz. Cassia Buds
- 2 oz. Cinnamon
- 2 oz. Cloves
- 4 oz. Gum Benzoin
- 1 oz. Storax Calamite
- 1 oz. Otto of Rose
- 1 drachm Musk
- 1/2 oz. Powdered Cardamine Seeds.

'Place the rose leaves, etc., in layers in the jar. Sprinkle the Bay salt and other ingredients on each layer, press it tightly down and keep for two or three months before taking it out.'

Another recipe (which was used by an old fashioned Scottish chemist for some fifty years) was purely a liquid one, the essences consisting of Musk, Vanilla, Sandalwood, Patchouli, Verbena, Neroli and Otto of Roses. The mixture was bottled and sold under the all-bracing and appropriate title, 'A' the floers o' th' gairden in a wee bit bottle.'

Recipe for Crystallized Roses

Choose a dry day for gathering the roses and wait until the dew evaporates, so that the petals are dry. Before gathering the roses, dissolve 2 oz. of gum-arabic in 1/2 pint of water. Separate the petals and spread them on dishes. Sprinkle them with the gumarabic solution, using as many petals as the solution will cover. Spread them on sheets of white paper and sprinkle with castor sugar, then let them dry for 24 hours. Put 1 lb. of sugar (loaf) and 1/2 pint of cold water into a pan, stir until the sugar has melted, then boil fast to 250 degrees F., or to the thread degree. This is ascertained by dipping a stick into cold water, then into the syrup and back into the water. Pinch the syrup adhering to the stick between the thumb and finger and draw them apart, when a thread should be formed. Keep the syrup well skimmed. Put the rosepetals into shallow dishes and pour the syrup over. Leave them to soak for 24 hours, then spread them on wire trays and dry in a cool oven with the door ajar. The syrup should be coloured with cochineal or carmine, in order to give more colour to the rose-petals.

Rose-petals have also been employed to flavour butter, for which the following recipe may be of interest:

Rose-Petal Sandwiches

Put a layer of Red Rose-petals in the bottom of a jar or covered dish, put in 4 oz. of fresh butter wrapped in waxed paper. Cover with a thick layer of rose-petals. Cover closely and leave in a cool place overnight. The more fragrant the roses, the finer the flavour imparted. Cut bread in thin strips or circles, spread each with the perfumed butter and place several petals from fresh Red Roses between the slices, allowing edges to show. Violets or Clover blossoms may be used in place of Roses.

Historical Medicinal Uses - For Entertainment ONLY

The petals of the dark red Rose, R. *gallica*, known as the Provins Rose, are employed medicinally for the preparation of an infusion and a confection. In this country (UK) it is specially grown for medicinal purposes in Oxfordshire and Derbyshire.

The petals of this rose are of a deep, purplish-red, velvety in texture, paler towards the base. They have the delicate fragrance of the Damask Rose and a slightly astringent taste.

The British Pharmacopoeia directs that Red Rose petals are to be obtained only from R. *gallica*, of which, however, there are many variations, in fact there are practically no pure R. *gallica* now to be had, only hybrids, so that the exact requirements of the British Pharmacopoeia are difficult to follow. Those used in medicine and generally appearing in commerce are actually any scented roses of a deep red colour, or when dried of a deep rose tint. The main point is that the petals suitable for medicinal purposes must yield a deep rose-coloured and somewhat astringent and fragrant infusion when boiling water is poured upon them. The most suitable are the so-called Hybrid Perpetuals, flowering from June to October, among which may be specially recommended the varieties:

- Eugène Furst, deep dark red, sweet-scented.
- General Jacqueminot, a fine, rich crimson, scented rose.
- Hugh Dickson, rather a large petalled one, but of a fine, deep red colour and sweetscented.
- Ulrich Brunner, bright-red.
- Richmond, deep crimson-red.
- Liberty, scarlet-red.

Collection and Preparation: When employed for the preparation of the drug, only flower-buds just about to open are collected, no fully-expanded flowers. They must only be gathered in dry weather and no petals of any roses that have suffered from effects of damp weather must be taken. The whole of the unexpanded petals are plucked from the calyx so that they remain united in small conical masses, leaving the stamens behind. Any stamens that may have come away with the petals should be shaken out. The lighter-coloured, lower portion is then cut off from the deep purplish-red upper part. The little masses, kept as entire as possible, are used in the fresh state for preparation of the 'confection,' but for making the infusion, they are dried carefully and quickly on trays in a good current of warm air. They are dried until crisp and while crisp packed in tins that the colour and crispness may be retained. If exposed to the air, they will re-absorb moisture and lose colour.

Constituents, Red Rose Pedals: The important constituent of Red Rose petals is the red colouring matter of an acid nature. There have also been isolated two yellow crystalline substances, the glucoside Quercitrin, which has been found in many other plants and Quercetin, yielded when Quercitrin is boiled with a dilute mineral acid. The astringency is due to a little gallic acid, but it has not yet been definitely proved whether quercitannic acid, the tannin of oak bark, is also a constituent. The odour is due to a very small amount of volatile oil, not identical with the official *Ol. Rosae.* A considerable amount of sugar, gum. fat, etc., are also present.

Preparations: Red Rose petals are official in nearly all Pharmacopoeias. Though formerly employed for their mild astringency and tonic value, they are to-day used almost solely to impart their pleasant odour to pharmaceutical preparations. The British Pharmacopceia preparations are a Confection, Acid Infusion and a Fluid Extract. The Confection is directed to be made by beating 1 lb. of fresh Red Rose petals in a stone mortar with 3 lb. of sugar. It is mostly used in pill making. Formerly this was prescribed for haemorrhage of the lungs and for coughs. The United States official confection is made by rubbing Red Rose petals, powdered, with heated rose-water, adding gradually fine, white sugar and heating the whole together till thoroughly mixed. The Fluid Extract is made from powdered Red Rose petals with glycerine and dilute alcohol. It is of a deep red colour, an agreeable odour of rose and of a pleasant, mildly astringent taste. The Acid Infusion is made from dried, broken-up, Red Rose petals, diluted with sulphuric acid, sugar and boiling water, infused in a covered vessel for 15 minutes and strained. It has a fine red colour and agreeable flavour and has been employed for its astringent effects in the treatment of stomatitis and pharyngitis. Its virtue is principally due to the aromatic sulphuric acid which it contains and the latter ingredient renders it a useful preparation, in the treatment of nightsweats resulting from depression. A Simple (non-acid) Infusion is mainly used as a flavouring for other medicines. It is also used as a lotion for ophthalmia, etc.

Syrup of Red Rose, official in the United States Pharmacopceia, is used to impart an agreeable flavour and odour to other syrups and mixtures. The syrup is of a fine red colour and has an agreeable, acidulous, somewhat astringent taste. Honey of Roses, also official in the United States Pharmacopoeia, is prepared from clarified honey and fluid extract of roses. It is considered more agreeable than ordinary honey and somewhat astringent. In olden days, Honey of Roses was popular for sore throats and ulcerated mouth and was made by pounding fresh petals in a small quantity of boiling water, filtering the mass and boiling the liquid with honey. Rose Vinegar, a specific on the Continent for headache caused by hot sun, is prepared by steeping dried rose petals in best distilled vinegar, which should not be boiled. Cloths or linen rags are soaked in the liquid and are then applied to the head.

Two liqueurs made by the French also have rose petals as one of the chief ingredients. A small quantity of spirits of wine is distilled with the petals to produce 'Spirit of Roses.' The fragrant spirit, when mixed with sugar, undergoes certain preparatory processes and makes the liqueur called 'L' Huile de Rose.' It is likewise the base of another liqueur, called 'Parfait Amour.'

The pale petals of the Hundred-leaved Rose or Cabbage Rose are also used in commerce. On account of its fragrance, the petals of this variety of rose are much used in France for distillation of rosewater. Though possessing aperient properties, they are seldom now used internally and preparations of them are not official in the British Pharmacopoeia.

The roses grouped as varieties of R. *centifolia* have all less scent than R. *gallica.*

The best of them is the old Cabbage Rose. It is a large rose, sweet-scented, of a pink or pale rose-purple colour, the petals whitish towards the base. Its branches are covered with numerous nearly straight spines: the petioles and peduncles are nearly unarmed, but more or less clothed with glandular bristles and the leaves have five or sometimes seven ovate, glandular leaflets, softly hairy beneath. This species and its varieties have given rise to innumerable handsome garden roses.

The flowers are collected and deprived of the calyx and ovaries, the petals alone being employed. In drying, they become brownish and lose some of their delicious rose odour.

The Constituents of the Pink Rose are closely similar to those of the Red. The very little colouring matter is apparently identical with that of the Red Rose. A little tannin is present.

Rosewater. The British Pharmacopceia directs that it shall be prepared by mixing the distilled rosewater of commerce, obtained mostly from R. *damascena*, but also from R. *centifolia* and other species, with twice its volume of distilled water immediately before use. It is used as a vehicle for other medicines and as an eye lotion. Triple rosewater is water saturated with volatile oil of Rose petals, obtained as a by-product in the distillation of oil of Roses. The finest rose-water is obtained by distillation of the fresh petals. It should be clear and colourless, not mucilaginous, and to be of value medicinally must be free from all metallic impurities, which may be detected by hydrogen sulphide and ammonium sulphide, neither of which should produce turbidity in the water.

Ointment of rose-water, commonly known as Cold Cream, enjoys deserved popularity as a soothing, cooling application for chapping of the hands, face, abrasions and other superficial lesions of the skin. For its preparation, the British Pharmacopceia directs that 1 1/2 oz. each of spermaceti and white wax be melted with 9 oz. of Almond oil, the mixture poured into a warmed mortar and 7 fluid ounces of rose-water and 8 minims of oil of Rose then incorporated with it.

Medicinal Action and Uses: The old herbalists considered the Red Rose to be more binding and more astringent than any of the other species:

'it strengtheneth the heart, the stomach, the liver and the retentive faculty; is good against all kinds of fluxes, prevents vomiting, stops tickling coughs and is of service in consumption. '

Culpepper gives many uses for the Rose, both white and red and damask.

'Of the Red Roses are usually made many compositions, all serving to sundry good uses, viz. electuary of roses, conserve both moist and dry, which is usually called sugar of roses, syrup of dry roses and honey of roses; the cordial powder called aromatic rosarum, the distilled water of roses, vinegar of roses, ointment and oil of roses and the rose leaves dried are of very great use and effect.'

'The electuary,' he tells us, 'is purging and is good in hot fevers, jaundice and jointaches. The moist conserve is of much use both binding and cordial, the old conserve mixed with aromaticum rosarum is a very good preservative in the time of infection. The dry conserve called the sugar of roses is a very good cordial against faintings, swoonings, weakness and trembling of the heart, strengthens a weak stomach, promotes digestion and is a very good preservative in the time of infection. The dry conserve called the sugar of roses is a very good cordial to strengthen the heart and spirit. The syrup of roses cooleth an over-heated liver and the blood in agues, comforteth the heart and resisteth putrefaction and infection. Honey of roses is used in gargles and lotions to wash sores, either in the mouth, throat or other parts, both to cleanse and heal them. Red rose-water is well known, it is cooling, cordial, refreshing, quickening the weak and faint spirits, used either in meats or broths to smell at the nose, or to smell the sweet vapours out of a perfume pot, or cast into a hot fire-shovel. It is of much use against the redness and inflammation of the eyes to bathe therewith and the temples of the head. The ointment of roses is much used against heat and inflammation of the head, to anoint the forehead and temples and to cool and heal red pimples. Oil of roses is used to cool hot inflammation or swellings and to bind and stay fluxes of humours to sores and is also put into ointments and plasters that are cooling and binding. The dried leaves of the red roses are used both outwardly and inwardly; they cool, bind and are cordial. Rose-leaves and mint, heated and applied outwardly to the stomach, stay castings, strengthen a weak stomach and applied as a fomentation to the region of the liver and heart, greatly cool and temper them, quiet the over-heated spirits and cause rest and sleep. The decoction of red roses made with white wine and used is very good for head-ache and pains in the eyes, ears, throat and gums.'

Preparations: Rose-water, B.P., 1 to 2 oz. Fluid extract, 1/2 to 1 drachm. Confec., B.P. and U.S.P., 2 to 4 drachms. Infusion acid, B.P., 1/2 to 1 oz. Syrup U.S.P. Oil, B.P.

In modern herbal medicine the flowers of the common Red Rose dried are given in infusions and sometimes in powder for haemorrhage. A tincture is made from them by pouring 1 pint of boiling water on 1 oz. of the dried petals, adding 15 drops of oil of Vitriol and 3 or 4 drachms of white sugar. The tincture when strained is of a beautiful red colour. Three or four spoonsful of the tincture taken two or three times a day are considered good for strengthening the stomach and a pleasant remedy in all haemorrhages.

Culpepper mentions a syrup made of the pale red petals of the Damask Rose by infusing them 24 hours in boiling water, then straining off the liquor and adding twice the weight of refined sugar to it, stating that this syrup is an excellent purge for children and adults of a costive habit, a small quantity to be taken every night. A conserve of the buds has the same properties as the syrup.

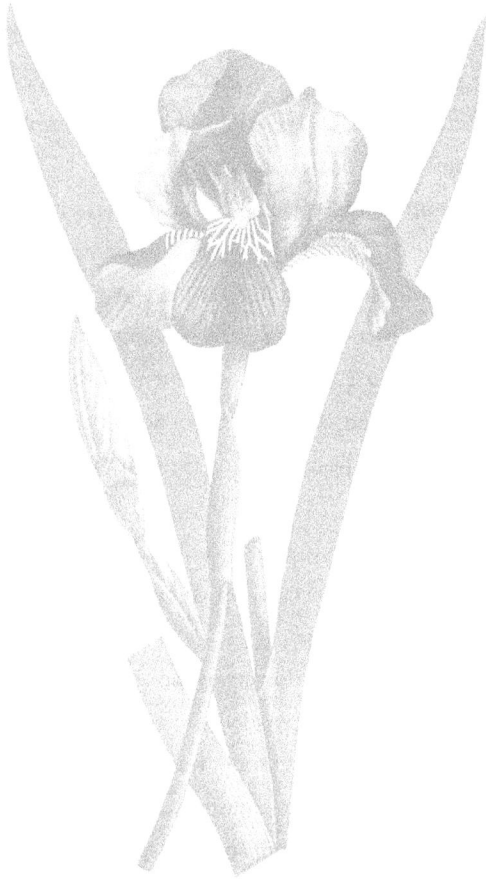

Rosemary

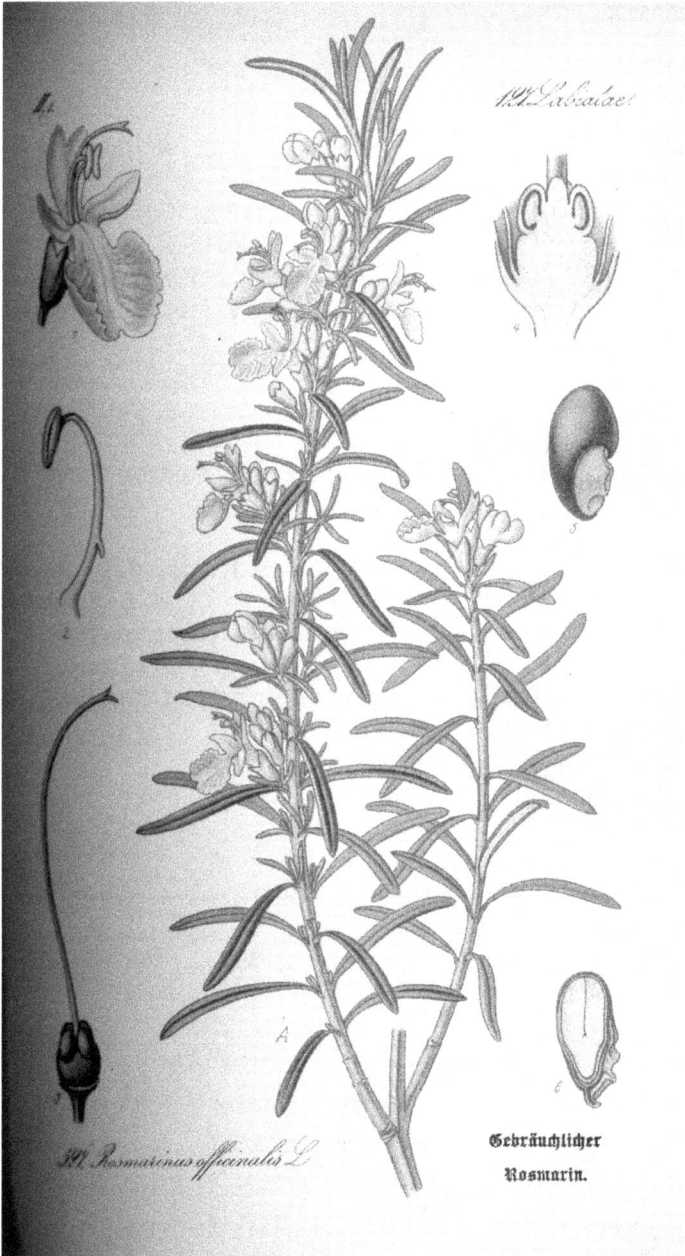

Gebräuchlicher
Rosmarin.

Quick Facts

Latin/Linnaen:	*Rosmarinus officinalis*
Family:	*Lamiaceae*
Old English :	
Synonyms:	Polar Plant, Compass-weed, Compass Plant, (Old French) Incensier.
Action:	Antispasmodic on gall passages and small intestines, Positive inotropic, Increases flow through the coronary artery, Skin irritating, Stimuates increased blood supply (external).
Parts Used:	Leaf
Indicated For:	Internal: Dyspeptic complaints. External: Supportive therapy for rheumatic diseases, circulatory problems.
Dosage:	Internal: Daily dosage: 4-6g of herb; 1-2 drops of essential oil; equivalent preparations. External 50g of herb for one full bath; 6-10 percent essential oil in semi solid and liquid preparations; equivalent preparations.
Preparation:	Cut drug for infusions, powder, dry extracts and other galenical preparations for internal and external use.
Cautions:	
Other Uses:	

Description

Rosemary, *Rosmarinus officinalis*, is a woody, perennial herb with fragrant, evergreen, needle-like leaves and white, pink, purple or blue flowers, native to the Mediterranean region. It is a member of the mint family *Lamiaceae*, which includes many other herbs, and is one of two species in the genus *Rosmarinus*. The name "rosemary" derives from the Latin name rosmarinus, derived from "dew" (ros) and "sea" (marinus), or "dew of the sea" because in many locations it needs no water other than the humidity carried by the sea breeze to live. The plant is also sometimes called Anthos, from the ancient Greek word, meaning "flower".

Rosemary is used as a decorative plant in gardens and has many culinary and medical uses. The plant is said to improve the memory and is used as a symbol of remembrance, especially in Australia and New Zealand to commemorate ANZAC Day. The leaves are used to flavor various foods, like stuffings and roast meats. Rosemary contains the antioxidants carnosic acid and rosmarinic acid, and other bioactive compounds including camphor, caffeic acid, ursolic acid, betulinic acid, rosmaridiphenol, and rosmanol. Some of these may be useful in preventing or treating cancers, strokes and Alzheimer's disease.

Cultivation

Hardiness Zone:	6-10
Soil pH:	6.0-7.5
Soil type:	Well drained soil
Cultivation:	Best by cuttings
Sunlight:	Full sun
Habitat:	Native to the Mediterranean but now cultivated worldwide

Rosemary can be planted outdoors and transplanted to a pot brought indoors to overwinter in colder zones. Rosemary does not like to be over watered, but should never dry out completely.

Historical Notes

The evergreen leaves of this shrubby herb are about 1 inch long, linear, revolute, dark green above and paler and glandular beneath, with an odour pungently aromatic and somewhat camphoraceous. The flowers are small and pale blue. Much of the active volatile principle resides in their calyces. There are silver and goldstriped varieties, but the green-leaved variety is the kind used medicinally.

The Ancients were well acquainted with the shrub, which had a reputation for strengthening the memory. On this account it became the emblem of fidelity for lovers. It holds a special position among herbs from the symbolism attached to it. Not only was it used at weddings, but also at funerals, for decking churches and banqueting halls at festivals, as incense in religious ceremonies, and in magical spells.

At weddings, it was entwined in the wreath worn by the bride, being first dipped into scented water. Anne of Cleves, we are told, wore such a wreath at her wedding. A Rosemary branch, richly gilded and tied with silken ribands of all colours, was also presented to wedding guests, as a symbol of love and loyalty. Together with an orange stuck with cloves it was given as a New Year's gift - allusions to this custom are to be found in Ben Jonson's plays.

Miss Anne Pratt (Flowers and their Associations) says:

'But it was not among the herbalists and apothecaries merely that Rosemary had its reputation for peculiar virtues. The celebrated Doctor of Divinity, Roger Hacket, did not disdain to expatiate on its excellencies in the pulpit. In a sermon which he entitles "A Marriage Present," which was published in 1607, he says: "Speaking of the powers of rosemary, it overtoppeth all the flowers in the garden, boasting man's rule. It helpeth the brain, strengtheneth the memorie, and is very medicinable for the head. Another property of the rosemary is, it affects the heart. Let this rosmarinus, this flower of men ensigne of your wisdom, love and loyaltie, be carried not only in your hands, but in your hearts and heads."

Sir Thomas More writes:

'As for Rosmarine, I lett it runne all over my garden walls, not onlie because my bees love it, but because it is the herb sacred to remembrance, and, therefore, to friendship; whence a sprig of it hath a dumb language that maketh it the chosen emblem of our funeral wakes and in our buriall grounds.'

In early times, Rosemary was freely cultivated in kitchen gardens and came to represent the dominant influence of the house mistress 'Where Rosemary flourished, the woman ruled.'

The Treasury of Botany says:

'There is a vulgar belief in Gloucestershire and other counties, that Rosemary will not grow well unless where the mistress is "master"; and so touchy are some of the lords of creation upon this point, that we have more than once had reason to suspect them of privately injuring a growing rosemary in order to destroy this evidence of their want of authority.'

Rosemary was one of the cordial herbs used to flavour ale and wine. It was also used in Christmas decoration.

'Down with the rosemary and so,

Down with the baies and mistletoe,

Down with the holly, ivie all

Wherewith ye deck the Christmas Hall.'

---HERRICK.

In place of more costly incense, the ancients used Rosemary in their religious ceremonies. An old French name for it was Incensier.

The Spaniards revere it as one of the bushes that gave shelter to the Virgin Mary in the flight into Egypt and call it Romero, the Pilgrim's Flower. Both in Spain and Italy, it has been considered a safeguard from witches and evil influences generally. The Sicilians believe that young fairies, taking the form of snakes, lie amongst the branches.

It was an old custom to burn Rosemary in sick chambers, and in French hospitals it is customary to burn Rosemary with Juniper berries to purify the air and prevent infection. Like Rue, it was placed in the dock of courts of justice, as a preventative from the contagion of gaol-fever. A sprig of Rosemary was carried in the hand at funerals, being distributed to the mourners before they left the house, to be cast on to the coffin when it had been lowered into the grave. In many parts of Wales it is still a custom.

One old legend compares the growth of the plant with the height of the Saviour and declares that after thirty-three years it increases in breadth, but never in height.

There is a tradition that Queen Philippa's mother (Countess of Hainault) sent the first plants of Rosemary to England, and in a copy of an old manuscript in the library of Trinity College, Cambridge, the translator, 'danyel bain,' says that Rosemary was unknown in England until this Countess sent some to her daughter.

Miss Rohde gives the following quotation from **Banckes' Herbal:**

'Take the flowers thereof and make powder thereof and binde it to thy right arme in a linnen cloath and it shale make theee light and merrie.

'Take the flowers and put them in thy chest among thy clothes or among thy Bookes and Mothes shall not destroy them.

'Boyle the leaves in white wine and washe thy face therewith and thy browes, and thou shalt have a faire face.

'Also put the leaves under thy bedde and thou shalt be delivered of all evill dreames.

'Take the leaves and put them into wine and it shall keep the wine from all sourness and evill savours, and if thou wilt sell thy wine thou shalt have goode speede.

'Also if thou be feeble boyle the leaves in cleane water and washe thyself and thou shalt wax shiny.

'Also if thou have lost appetite of eating boyle well these leaves in cleane water and when the water is colde put thereunto as much of white wine and then make sops, eat them thereof wel and thou shalt restore thy appetite againe.

'If thy legges be blowen with gowte, boyle the leaves in water and binde them in a linnen cloath and winde it about thy legges and it shall do thee much good.

'If thou have a cough drink the water of the leaves boyld in white wine and ye shall be whole.

'Take the Timber thereof and burn it to coales and make powder thereof and rubbe thy teeth thereof and it shall keep thy teeth from all evils. Smell it oft and it shall keep thee youngly.

'Also if a man have lost his smellyng of the ayre that he may not draw his breath, make a fire of the wood, and bake his bread therewith, eate it and it shall keepe him well.

'Make thee a box of the wood of rosemary and smell to it and it shall preserve thy youth.'

From the Grete Herbal:

'ROSEMARY. - For weyknesse of ye brayne. Against weyknesse of the brayne and coldenesse thereof, sethe rosemaria in wyne and lete the pacyent receye the smoke at his nose and keep his heed warme.'

Parts Used: The oil of Rosemary, distilled from the flowering tops, as directed in the British Pharmacopceia, is a superior oil to that obtained from the stem and leaves, but nearly all the commercial oil is distilled from the stem and leaves of the wild plant before it is in flower. (Rosemary is one of the plants like lavender which grows better in England than anywhere, else, and English oil of Rosemary, though it is infinitely superior to what of other countries, is hardly found in commerce to-day. The bulk of the commercial oil comes from France, Dalamatia, Spain and Japan.)

The upper portions of the shoots are taken, with the leaves on and the leaves are stripped off the portions of the shoots that are very wooden.

Constituents: The plant contains some tannic acid, together with a resin and a bitter principle and a volatile oil. The chief constituents of the oil are Borneol, bornyl acetate and other esters, a special camphor similar to that possessed by the myrtle, cineol, pinene and camphene. It is colourless, with the odour of Rosemary and a warm camphoraceous taste. The chief adulterants of oil of Rosemary are oil of turpentine and petroleum. Rosemary yields its virtues partly to water and entirely to rectified spirits of wine.

From 100 lb. of the flowering tops, 8 oz. of the oil are usually obtained.

Historical Medicinal Uses - For Entertainment ONLY

Medicinal Action and Uses: Tonic, astringent, diaphoretic, stimulant. Oil of Rosemary has the carminative properties of other volatile oils and is an excellent stomachic and nervine, curing many cases of headache.

It is employed principally, externally, as spiritus Rosmarini, in hair-lotions, for its odour and effect in stimulating the hair-bulbs to renewed activity and preventing premature baldness. An infusion of the dried plant (both leaves and flowers) combined with borax and used when cold, makes one of the best hairwashes known. It forms an effectual remedy for the prevention of scurf and dandruff.

The oil is also used externally as a rubefacient and is added to liniments as a fragrant stimulant. Hungary water, for outward application to renovate the vitality of paralysed limbs, was first invented for a Queen of Hungary, who was said to have been completely cured by its continued use. It was prepared by putting 1 1/2 lb. of fresh Rosemary tops in full flower into 1 gallon of spirits of wine, this was allowed to stand for four days and then distilled. Hungary water was also considered very efficacious against gout in the hands and feet, being rubbed into them vigorously.

A formula dated 1235, said to be in the handwriting of Elizabeth, Queen of Hungary, is said to be preserved in Vienna.

Rosemary Wine when taken in small quantities acts as a quieting cordial to a weak heart subject to palpitation, and relieves accompanying dropsy by stimulating the kidneys. It is made by chopping up sprigs of green Rosemary and pouring on them white wine, which is strained off after a few days and is then ready for use. By stimulating the brain and nervous system, it is a good remedy for headaches caused by feeble circulation.

The young tops, leaves and flowers can be made into an infusion, called Rosemary Tea, which, taken warm, is a good remedy for removing headache, colic, colds and nervous diseases, care being taken to prevent the escape of steam during its preparation. It will relieve nervous depression. A conserve, made by beating up the freshly gathered tops with three times their weight of sugar, is said to have the same effect.

A spirit of Rosemary may be used, in doses of 30 drops in water or on sugar, as an antispasmodic.

Rosemary and Coltsfoot leaves are considered good when rubbed together and smoked for asthma and other affections of the throat and lungs.

Rosemary is also one of the ingredients used in the preparation of Eau-de-Cologne.

Preparations: Oil, 1/2 to 3 drops. Spirit, B.P., 5 to 20 drops.

Sage

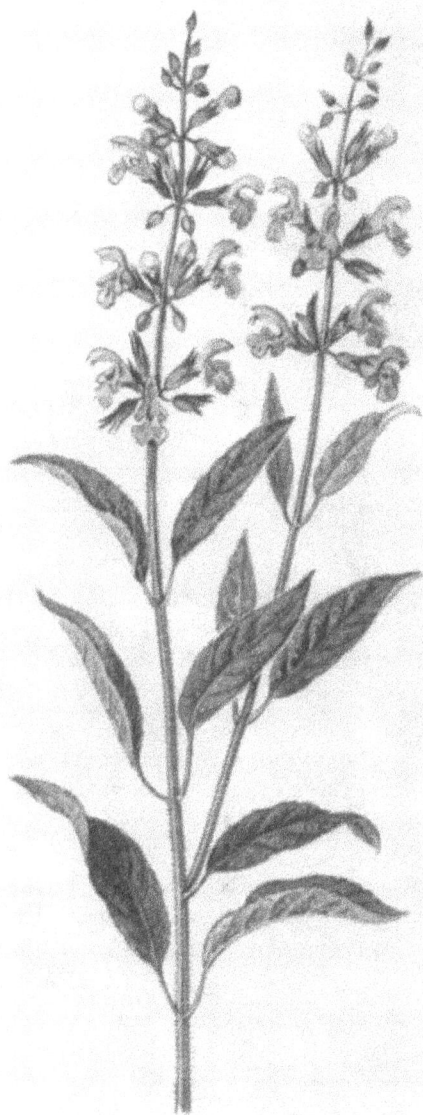

48

Прил. 48. Градински чай — Salvia officinalis L.

Quick Facts

Latin/Linnaen:	*Salvia Officinalis*
Family:	*Lamiaceae*
Old English :	Saluie, Salfie
Synonyms:	(Old English) Sawge. Garden Sage. Red Sage. Broad-leaved White Sage. Narrow-leaved White Sage. Salvia salvatrix.
Action:	Antibacterial, Fungistatic, Virustatic, Astringent, Secretion promoting, Perspiration inhibiting
Parts Used:	Leaf
Indicated For:	External: Inflammations of the mucous membranes of the nose and throat. Internal: Dyspeptic symptoms, excessive perspiration.
Dosage:	Unless otherwise prescribed: Internal: Daily dosage: 4-6g of herb; 0.1-0.3 g of essential oil; 2.5-7.5g of tincture, 1.5-3g of fluidextract. For gargles and rinses: 2.5g of herb or 2-3 drops of essential oil in 100ml of water as infusion or 5g of alcoholic extract in 1 glass of water. External: Undiluted alcohol extract.
Preparation:	Cut herb for infusions, alcoholic extracts and distillates for gargles, rinses and other topical applications, as well as for internal use. Also pressed juice of fresh plants.
Cautions:	**Contraindications:** The pure essential oil and alcoholic extracts should not be used internally during pregnancy. **Side Effects:** After prolonged ingestion of alcohol extracts or of the pure essential oil, epileptiform convulsions can occur.
Other Uses:	

Description

Salvia officinalis (garden sage, common sage) is a perennial, evergreen subshrub, with woody stems, grayish leaves, and blue to purplish flowers. It is a member of the family *Lamiaceae* and is native to the Mediterranean region, though it has naturalized in many places throughout the world. It has a long history of medicinal and culinary use, and in modern times as an ornamental garden plant. The common name "sage" is also used for a number of related and unrelated species.

Cultivars are quite variable in size, leaf and flower color, and foliage pattern, with many variegated leaf types. The Old World type grows to approximately 2 ft (0.61 m) tall and wide, with lavender flowers most common, though they can also be white, pink, or purple. The plant flowers in late spring or summer. The leaves are oblong, ranging in size up to 2.5 in (6.4 cm) long by 1 in (2.5 cm) wide. Leaves are grey-green, rugose on the upper side, and nearly white underneath due to the many short soft hairs. Modern cultivars include leaves with purple, rose, cream, and yellow in many variegated combinations.

Cultivation

Hardiness Zone:	4-8
Soil pH:	6.0-6.5
Soil type:	Rich well drained soil
Cultivation:	By seed, cutting, or dividing.
Sunlight:	Full sun
Habitat:	Native to the Mediterranean, now cultivated worldwide

Sage should be harvested before blooming, and dried in a well ventilated area away from sunlight.

Historical Notes

Salvia officinalis was described by Carl Linnaeus in 1753. It has been grown for centuries in the Old World for its food and healing properties, and was often described in old herbals for the many miraculous properties attributed to it. The specific epithet, officinalis, refers to the plant's medicinal use--the officina was the traditional storeroom of a monastery where herbs and medicines were stored. S.

officinalis has been classified under many other scientific names over the years, including six different names since 1940 alone.

Salvia officinalis has been used since ancient times for warding off evil, snakebites, increasing women's fertility, and more. The Romans likely introduced it to Europe from Egypt as a medicinal herb. Theophrastus wrote about two different sages, a wild undershrub he called sphakos, and a similar cultivated plant he called elelisphakos. Pliny the Elder said the latter plant was called salvia by the Romans, and used as a diuretic, a local anesthetic for the skin, a styptic, and for other uses. Charlemagne recommended the plant for cultivation in the early Middle Ages, and during the Carolingian Empire, it was cultivated in monastery gardens. Walafrid Strabo described it in his poem Hortulus as having a sweet scent and being useful for many human ailments--he went back to the Greek root for the name and called it lelifagus.

The plant had a high reputation throughout the Middle Ages, with many sayings referring to its healing properties and value. It was sometimes called *S. salvatrix* (sage the savior), and was one of the ingredients of Four Thieves Vinegar, a blend of herbs which was supposed to ward off the plague. Dioscorides, Pliny, and Galen all recommended sage as a diuretic, hemostatic, emmenagogue, and tonic.

The Common Sage, the familiar plant of the kitchen garden, is an evergreen undershrub, not a native of these islands, its natural habitat being the northern shores of the Mediterranean. It has been cultivated for culinary and medicinal purposes for many centuries in England, France and Germany, being sufficiently hardy to stand any ordinary winter outside. Gerard mentions it as being in 1597 a well-known herb in English gardens, several varieties growing in his own garden at Holborn.

Sage generally grows about a foot or more high, with wiry stems. The leaves are set in pairs on the stem and are 1 1/2 to 2 inches long, stalked, oblong, rounded at the ends, finely wrinkled by a strongly-marked network of veins on both sides, greyish-green in colour, softly hairy and beneath glandular. The flowers are in whorls, purplish and the corollas lipped. They blossom in August. All parts of the plant have a strong, scented odour and a warm, bitter, somewhat astringent taste, due to the volatile oil contained in the tissues.

Habitat: Sage is found in its natural wild condition from Spain along the Mediterranean coast up to and including the east side of the Adriatic; it grows in profusion on the mountains and hills in Croatia and Dalmatia, and on the islands of Veglia and Cherso in Quarnero Gulf, being found mostly where there is a limestone formation with very little soil. When wild it is much like the common garden Sage, though more shrubby in appearance and has a more penetrating odour, being more spicy and astringent than the cultivated plant. The best kind, it is stated, grows on the islands of Veglia and Cherso, near Fiume, where the surrounding district is known as the Sage region. The collection of Sage forms an important cottage industry in Dalmatia. During its blooming season, moreover, the bees gather the nectar and genuine Sage honey commands there the highest price, owing to its flavour.

In cultivation, Sage is a very variable species, and in gardens varieties may be found with narrower leaves, crisped, red, or variegated leaves and smaller or white flowers. The form of the calyx teeth also varies, and the tube of the corolla is sometimes much longer. The two usually absent upper stamens are sometimes present in very small-sterile hooks. The Red Sage and the Broad-leaved variety of the White (or Green) Sage - both of which are used and have been proved to be the best for medical purposes - and the narrow-leaved White Sage, which is best for culinary purposes as a seasoning, are classed merely as varieties of *Salvia officinalis*, not as separate species. There is a variety called Spanish, or Lavender-leaved Sage and another called Wormwood Sage, which is very frequent.

A Spanish variety, called *S. Candelabrum*, is a hardy perennial, the upper lip of its flower greenish yellow, the lower a rich violet, thus presenting a fine contrast.

S. Lyrala and *S. urticifolia* are well known in North America.

S. hians, a native of Simla, is hardy, and also desirable on account of its showy violet-and-white flowers.

The name of the genus, *Salvia*, is derived from the Latin salvere, to be saved, in reference to the curative properties of the plant, which was in olden times celebrated as a medicinal herb. This name was corrupted popularly to Sauja and Sauge (the French form), in Old English, 'Sawge,' which has become our present-day name of Sage.

In the United States Pharmacopceia, the leaves are still officially prescribed, as they were formerly in the London Pharrnacopceia, but in Europe generally, Sage is now neglected by the regular medical practitioner, though is still used in domestic medicine. Among the Ancients and throughout the Middle Ages it was in high repute: Cur moriatur homo cui Salvia crescit in horto? ('Why should a man die whilst sage grows in his garden?') has a corresponding English proverb:

'He that would live for aye,

Must eat Sage in May.'

An old tradition recommends that Rue shall be planted among the Sage, so as to keep away noxious toads from the valued and cherished plants. It was held that this plant would thrive or wither, just as the owner's business prospered or failed, and in Bucks, another tradition maintained that the wife rules when Sage grows vigorously in the garden.

In the Jura district of France, in Franche-Comte, the herb is supposed to mitigate grief, mental and bodily, and Pepys in his Diary says: 'Between Gosport and Southampton we observed a little churchyard where it was customary to sow all the graves with Sage.'

The following is a translation of an old French saying:

'Sage helps the nerves and by its powerful might

Palsy is cured and fever put to flight,'

and Gerard says:

'Sage is singularly good for the head and brain, it quickeneth the senses and memory, strengtheneth the sinews, restoreth health to those that have the palsy, and taketh away shakey trembling of the members.'

He shared the popular belief that it was efficacious against the bitings of serpents, and says:

'No man need to doubt of the wholesomeness of Sage Ale, being brewed as it should be with Sage, Betony, Scabious, Spikenard, Squinnette (Squinancywort) and Fennell Seed.'

Many kinds of Sage have been used as substitutes for tea, the Chinese having been said to prefer Sage Tea to their own native product, at one time bartering for it with the Dutch and giving thrice the quantity of their choicest tea in exchange. It is recorded that George Whitfield, when at Oxford in 1733, lived wholesomely, if sparingly, on a diet of Sage Tea, sugar and coarse bread. Balsamic Sage, *S. grandiflora*, a broad-leaved Sage with many-flowered whorls of blossoms, used to be preferred to all others for making tea. An infusion of Speedwell (*Veronica officinalis*), Sage and Wood Betony is said to make an excellent beverage for breakfast, as a substitute for tea, Speedwell having somewhat the flavour of Chinese green tea. In Holland the leaves of *S. glutinosa*, the yellow-flowered Hardy Sage, both flowers and foliage of which exhale a pleasant odour, are used to give flavour to country wines, and a good wine is made by boiling with sugar, the leaves and flowers of another Sage, *S. sclarea*, the Garden Clary. The latter is known in France as 'Toute bonne' - for its medicinal virtues.

It was formerly thought that Sage used in the making of Cheese improved its flavour, and Gay refers to this in a poem:

'Marbled with Sage, the hardening cheese she pressed.'

Italian peasants eat Sage as a preservative of health, and many other country people eat the leaves with bread and butter, than which, it has been said, there is no better and more wholesome way of taking it.

A species of Sage, *S. pomifera*, the Applebearing Sage, of a very peculiar growth, is common on some of the Greek islands. It has firm, fleshy protuberances of about 3/4 inch thickness, swelling out from the branches of the plant and supposed to be produced in the same manner as oak apples, by the puncture of an insect of the Cynips genus. These excrescences are semi-transparent like jelly. They are called Sage Apples, and under that name are to be met with in the markets. They are candied with sugar and made into a kind of sweetmeat and conserve which is regarded by the Greeks as a great delicacy, and is said to possess healing and salutary qualities. It has an agreeable and astringent flavour. This plant is considerably larger than the common Sage of our gardens and its flavour and smell are much more powerful, being more like a mixture of Lavender and Sage. It grows very abundantly in Candia, Syros and Crete, where it attains to the size of a small shrub. The leaves are collected annually, dried and used medicinally as an infusion, the Greeks being particular as to the time and manner in which they are collected, the date being May 1, before sunrise. The infusion produces profuse perspiration, languor, and even faintness if used to excess. There is a smaller Salvia in Greece, the *S. Candica*, without excrescences.

Another south European species, an annual, *S. Horminum*, the Red-Topped Sage, has its whorls of flowers terminated by clusters of small purple or red leaves, being for this peculiarity often grown in gardens as an ornamental plant. The leaves and seed of this species, put into the vat, while fermenting, greatly increase the inebriating quality of the liquor. An infusion of the leaves has been considered a good gargle for sore gums, and powdered makes a good snuff.

Certain varieties of Sage seeds are mucilaginous and nutritive, and are used in Mexico by the Indians as food, under the name of Chia.

It is a hardy plant, but though a perennial, does not last above three or four years without degenerating, so that the plantation should be renewed at least every four years. It is propagated occasionally by seed, but more frequently by cuttings. New plantations are readily made by pulling off the young shoots from three-year-old plants in spring, generally in the latter end of April, as soon as they attain a sufficiency of hardness to enable them to maintain themselves on the moisture of the ground and atmosphere, while the lower extremities are preparing roots. If advantage be taken of any showery weather that may occur, there is little trouble in obtaining any number of plants, which may either be struck in the bed where they are to grow, inserting a foot apart each way, or in some other shady spot whence they may be removed to permanent quarters when rooted. The latter plan is the best when the weather is too bright and sunny to expect Sage to strike well in its ordinary quarters. See the young plants do not suffer from want of water during their first summer, and hoe the rows regularly to induce a bushy growth, nipping off the growing tips if shooting up too tall. Treat the ground with soot and mulch in winter with old manure. Cuttings may also be taken in the autumn, as soon as the plants have ceased flowering.

Sage is also often propagated by layers, in the spring and autumn, the branches of old plants being pegged down on the ground and covered with 1/2 inch of earth. The plant, being like other of the woody-stemmed garden herbs, a 'stem rooter,' each of the stems thus covered will produce quantities of rootlets by just lying in contact with the ground, and can after a time be cut away from the old plant and transplanted to other quarters as a separate plant.

Red Sage is always propagated by layering or by cuttings, as the seed does not produce a red-leaved plant, but reverts back to the original green-leaved type, though efforts are being made to insure the production of a Red Sage that shall set seed and remain true and develop into the red-leaved plant.

Sages backed by late-flowering Orange Lilies go very well together, and being in flower at the same time make an effective grouping. The calyces of Sage flowers remain on the plants well into late summer and give a lovely haze of reddish spikes; the smell of these seeding spikes is very distinct from the smell of the leaves, and much more like that of the Lemon-scented Verbena, pungent, aromatic and most refreshing.

At the present day, by far the largest demand for Sage is for culinary use, and it should pay to grow it in quantity for this purpose as it is little trouble. For this, the White variety, with somewhat pale green leaves should be taken.

In Dalmatia, where the collection of Sage in its wild condition forms an important cottage industry, it is gathered before blooming, the leaves being harvested from May to September, those plucked in midsummer being considered the best. The general opinion is that it should be gathered before the bloom opens, but the Austrian Pharmacopoeia states that it is best when gathered during bloom.

Chemical Constituents: The chief constituent of Sage and its active principle is a yellow or greenish-yellow volatile oil (sp. gr. 0.910 to 0.930) with a penetrating odour. Tannin and resin are also present in the leaves, 0.5 to 1.0 per cent of the oil is yielded from the leaves and twigs when fresh, and about three times this quantity when dry.

The Sage oil of commerce is obtained from the herb *S. officinalis*, and distilled to a considerable extent in Dalmatia and recently in Spain, but from a different species of Salvia. A certain amount of oil is also distilled in Germany. The oil distilled in Dalmatia and in Germany is of typically Sage odour, and is used for flavouring purposes. The botanical origin of Spanish Sage oil is now identified as *S. triloba,* closely allied to *S. officinalis*, though probably other species may also be employed. The odour of the Spanish oil more closely resembles that of Spike Lavender than the Sage oil distilled in Germany for flavouring purposes, and is as a rule derived from the wild Dalmatian herb, *S. officinalis*. The resemblance of the Spanish oil to Spike Lavender oil suggests the possibility of its use for adulterative purposes, and it is an open secret that admixture of the Spanish Sage oil with

Spanish Spike Lavender oil does take place to a considerable extent, though this can be detected by chemical analysis. It is closer in character to the oil of *S. sclarea*, Clary oil, which has a decided lavender odour, although in the oil of *S. triloba*, the ester percentage does not appear to be as high as in the oil of the *S. sclarea* variety.

Pure Dalmatian or German Sage oil is soluble in two volumes of 80 per cent alcohol, Spanish Sage oil is soluble in six volumes of 70 per cent alcohol.

Sage oil contains a hydrocarbon called Salvene; pinene and cineol are probably present in small amount, together with borneol, a small quantity of esters, and the ketone thujone, the active principle which confers the power of resisting putrefaction in animal substances. Dextro-camphor is also present in traces. A body has been isolated by certain chemists called Salviol, which is now known to be identical with Thujone.

English distilled Sage oil has been said to contain Cedrene.

S. cypria, a native of the island of Cyprus, yields an essential oil, having a camphoraceous odour and containing about 75 per cent of Eucalyptol.

S. mellifer (syn. Ramona stachyoides) is a labiate plant found in South California, known as Black Sage, with similar constituents, and also traces of formic acid.

CULINARY RECIPES

Sage and Onion stuffing for ducks, geese and pork enables the stomach to digest the rich food.

From Warner's Ancient Cookery, 1791, for 'Sawgeat,' Sawge. Sawgeat

'Take Pork and seeth (boil) it wel and grinde it smale and medle (mingle) it with ayren (eggs) and ygrated (grated) brede (bread). Do thereto salt sprinkled and saffron. Take a close litull ball of it in foiles (leaves) of Sawge. Wet it with a bator (batter) of ayren, fry and serve forth.'

From The Cook's Oracle, 1821:

'Sage and Onion Sauce

'Chop very fine an ounce of onion and 1/2 oz. of green Sage leaves, put them in a stamper with 4 spoonsful of water, simmer gently for 10 minutes, then put in a teaspoonful of pepper and salt and 1 oz. of fine breadcrumbs. Mix well together, then pour to it 1/4 pint of Broth, Gravy or Melted Butter, stir well together and simmer a few minutes longer. This is a relishing sauce for Roast Pork, Geese or Duck, or with Green Peas on Maigre Days.'

The same book gives:

'A Relish for Roast Pork. or Goose

'2 oz. of leaves of Green Sage, an ounce of fresh lemon peel, pared thin, same of salt, minced shallot and 1/2 drachm of Cayenne pepper, ditto of citric acid, steeped for a fortnight in a pint of claret. Shake it well every day; let it stand a day to settle and decant the clear liquid. Bottle it and cork it close. Use a tablespoonful or more in 1/4 pint of gravy or melted butter.'

Another modern Sage Sauce, excellent with Roast Pork is:

Sagina Sauce

Take 6 large Sage leaves, 2 onions, 1 teaspoonful of flour, 1 teaspoonful of vinegar, butter the size of a walnut, salt, pepper, and 1/2 pint of good, brown gravy. Scald the Sage leaves and chop them with the onions to a mincemeat. Put them in a stewpan with the butter, sprinkle in the flour, cover close and steam 10 minutes. Then add the vinegar, gravy and seasoning and simmer half an hour.

From Walsh's Manual of Domestic Economy, 1857:

'Sage Cheese

'Bruise the tops of young red Sage in a mortar with some leaves of spinach and squeeze the juice; mix it with the rennet in the milk, more or less, according to the preferred colour and taste. When the curd is come, break it gently and put it in with the skimmer till it is pressed two inches above the vat. Press it 8 or 10 hours. Salt it and turn every day.'

Historical Medicinal Uses - For Entertainment ONLY

Medicinal Action and Uses: Stimulant, astringent, tonic and carminative. Has been used in dyspepsia, but is now mostly employed as a condiment. In the United States, where it is still an official medicine, it is in some repute, especially in the form of an infusion, the principal and most valued application of which is as a wash for the cure of affections of the mouth and as a gargle in inflamed sore throat, being excellent for relaxed throat and tonsils, and also for ulcerated throat. The gargle is useful for bleeding gums and to prevent an excessive flow of saliva.

When a more stimulating effect to the throat is desirable, the gargle may be made of equal quantities of vinegar and water, 1/2 pint of hot malt vinegar being poured on 1 oz. of leaves, adding 1/2 pint of cold water.

The infusion when made for internal use is termed Sage Tea, and can be made simply by pouring 1 pint of boiling water on to 1 oz. of the dried herb, the dose being from a wineglassful to half a teacupful, as often as required, but the old-fashioned way of making it is more elaborate and the result is a pleasant drink, cooling in fevers, and also a cleanser and purifier of the blood. Half an ounce of fresh Sage leaves, 1 oz. of sugar, the juice of 1 lemon, or 1/4 oz. of grated rind, are infused in a quart of boiling water and strained off after half an hour. (In Jamaica the [natives] sweeten Sage Tea with lime-juice instead of lemon.)

Sage Tea or infusion of Sage is a valuable agent in the delirium of fevers and in the nervous excitement frequently accompanying brain and nervous diseases and has considerable reputation as a remedy, given in small and oft-repeated doses. It is highly serviceable as a stimulant tonic in debility of the stomach and nervous system and weakness of digestion generally. It was for this reason that the Chinese valued it, giving it the preference to their own tea. It is considered a useful medicine in typhoid fever and beneficial in biliousness and liver complaints, kidney troubles, haemorrhage from the lungs or stomach, for colds in the head as well as sore throat and quinsy and measles, for pains in the joints, lethargy and palsy. It will check excessive perspiration in phthisis cases, and is useful as an emmenagogue. A cup of the strong infusion will be found good to relieve nervous headache.

The infusion made strong, without the lemons and sugar, is an excellent lotion for ulcers and to heal raw abrasions of the skin. It has also been popularly used as an application to the scalp, to darken the hair.

The fresh leaves, rubbed on the teeth, will cleanse them and strengthen the gums. Sage is a common ingredient in tooth-powders.

The volatile oil is said to be a violent epileptiform convulsant, resembling the essential oils of absinthe and nutmeg. When smelt for some time it is said to cause a sort of intoxication and giddiness. It is sometimes prescribed in doses of 1 to 3 drops, and used for removing heavy collections of mucus from the respiratory organs. It is a useful ingredient in embrocations for rheumatism.

In cases where heat is required, Sage has been considered valuable when applied externally in bags, as a poultice and fomentation.

In Sussex, at one time, to munch Sage leaves on nine consecutive mornings, whilst fasting, was a country cure for ague, and the dried leaves have been smoked in pipes as a remedy for asthma.

In the region where Sage grows wild, its leaves are boiled in vinegar and used as a tonic.

Among many uses of the herb, **Culpepper says** that it is:

'Good for diseases of the liver and to make blood. A decoction of the leaves and branches of Sage made and drunk, saith Dioscorides, provokes urine and causeth the hair to become black. It stayeth the bleeding of wounds and cleaneth ulcers and sores. Three spoonsful of the juice of Sage taken fasting with a little honey arrests spitting or vomiting of blood in consumption. It is profitable for all pains in the head coming of cold rheumatic humours, as also for all pains in the joints, whether inwardly or outwardly. The juice of Sage in warm water cureth hoarseness and cough. Pliny saith it cureth stinging and biting serpents. Sage is of excellent use to help the memory, warming and quickening the senses. The juice of Sage drunk with vinegar hath been of use in the time of the plague at all times. Gargles are made with Sage, Rosemary, Honeysuckles and Plantains, boiled in wine or water with some honey or alum put thereto, to wash sore mouths and throats, as need requireth. It is very good for stitch or pains in the sides coming of wind, if the place be fomented warm with the decoction in wine and the herb also, after boiling, be laid warm thereto.'

MEDICINAL RECIPES

A Gargle for a Sore Throat

A small glass of port wine, a tablespoonful of Chile vinegar, 6 Sage leaves, and a dessertspoonful of honey; simmer together on the fire for 5 minutes.

A Cure for Sprains

Bruise a handful of Sage leaves and boil them in a gill of vinegar for 5 minutes; apply this in a folded napkin as hot as it can be borne to the part affected.

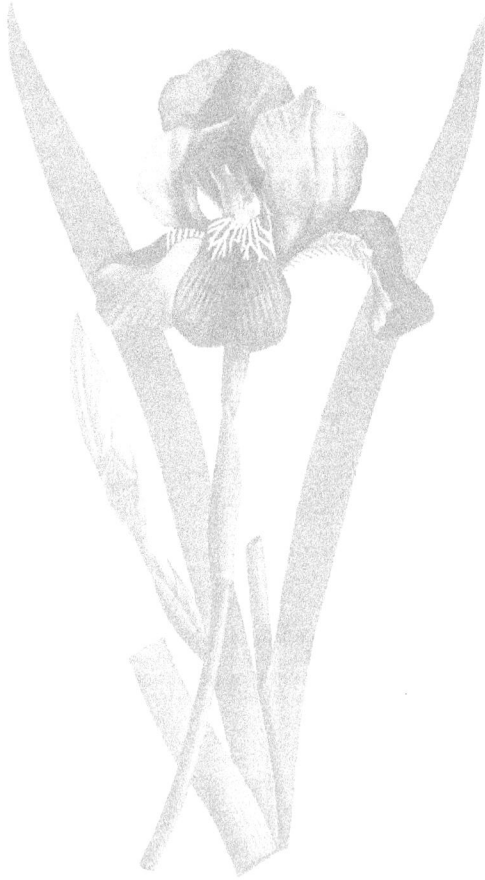

Soapwort, Red

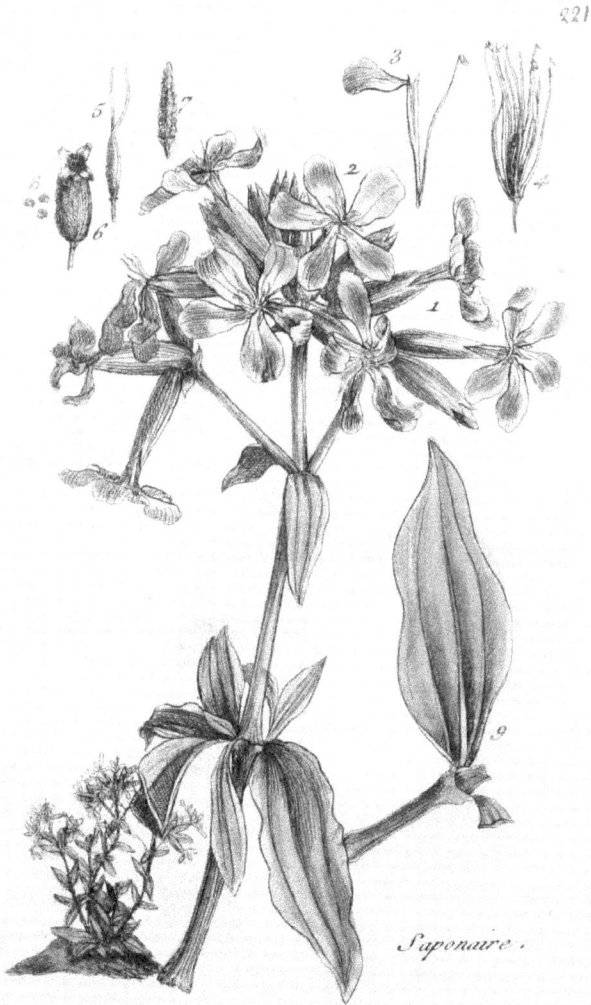

Saponaire.

Quick Facts

Latin/Linnaen:	*Saponaria Officinalis*
Family:	*Caryophyllaceae*
Old English :	
Synonyms:	Soapwort, Bruisewort, Soaproot, Bouncing Bet, Latherwort, Fuller's Herb, Crow Soap, Sweet Betty, Wild Sweet William.
Action:	Expectorant by irritation of the gastric mucosa. Cytotoxic in high concentrations
Parts Used:	Root
Indicated For:	Catarrhs of the upper respiratory tract.
Dosage:	Unless otherwise prescribed: Daily dosage: 1.5g root or equivalent preparations.
Preparation:	Comminuted herb for teas and other galenical preparations for internal use.
Cautions:	Can be poisonous. Side effects: In rare cases, stomach irritation.
Other Uses:	As a gentle cleanser.

Description

Common Soapwort (*Saponaria officinalis*) is a vespertine flower, and a common perennial plant from the carnation family (*Caryophyllaceae*). Other common names are Bouncing Bet and Sweet William; locally it is simply "the Soapwort" although there are about 20 species of soapworts altogether.

The scientific name Saponaria is derived from the Latin sapo (stem sapon-) meaning "soap," which, like its common name, refers to its utility in cleaning. From this same Latin word is derived the name of the toxic substance saponin, contained in the roots at levels up to 20 percent when the plant is flowering (Indian soapnuts contain only 15 percent). It produces a lather when in contact with water. The epithet officinalis indicates its medicinal functions.

Soapwort's native range extends throughout Europe to western Siberia. It grows in cool places at low or moderate elevations under hedgerows and along the shoulders of roadways.

The plants possesses leafy, unbranched stems (often tinged with red). It grows in patches, attaining a height of 70 cm. The broad, lanceolate, sessile leaves are opposite and between 4 and 12 cm long. Its sweetly scented flowers are radially symmetrical and pink, or sometimes white. Each of the five flat petals have two small scales in the throat of the corolla. They are about 2.5 cm wide. They are arranged in dense, terminal clusters on the main stem and its branches. The long tubular calyx has five pointed red teeth.

In the northern hemisphere soapwort blooms from May to September, and in the southern hemisphere October to March.

Cultivation

Hardiness Zone:	3-9
Soil pH:	Neutral-alkaline
Soil type:	Well drained rich soil.
Cultivation:	By seeds or plant division.
Sunlight:	Full sun
Habitat:	Native to Europe, naturalized in the US.

Soapwort can be invasive if given the right environment.

Historical Notes

A stout herbaceous perennial with a stem growing in the writer's garden (M. Grieve's) to 4 or 5 feet high. Leaves lanceolate, slightly elliptical, acute, smooth, 2 or 3 inches long and 1/3 inch wide. Large pink flowers, often double in paniculate fascicles; calyx cylindrical, slightly downy; five petals, unguiculate; top of petals linear, ten stamens, two styles; capsule oblong, one-celled, flowering from July till September (in England). No odour, with a bitter and slightly sweet taste, followed by a persistent pungency and a numbing sensation in the mouth.

Constituents: Constituents of the root, Saponin, also extractive, resin, gum, woody fibre, mucilage, etc.

Soapwort root dried in commerce is found in pieces 10 and 12 inches long, 1/12 inch thick, cylindrical, longitudinally wrinkled, outside light brown, inside whitish with a thick bark. Contains number of small white crystals and a pale yellow wood.

Historical Medicinal Uses - For Entertainment ONLY

A decoction cures the itch. Has proved very useful in jaundice and other visceral obstructions. For old venereal complaints it is a good cure specially where mercury has failed. It is a tonic, diaphoretic and alterative, a valuable remedy for rheumatism or cutaneous troubles resulting from any form of syphilis. It is also sternutatory. Should be very cautiously used owing to its saponin content.

Dose: Decoction, 2 to 4 fluid ounces three or four times daily. Extract or the inspissated juice will be found equally efficacious: dose, 10 to 20 grains. As a sternutatory 2 to 6 grains. Fluid extract, 1/4 to 1 drachm.

St. John's Wort

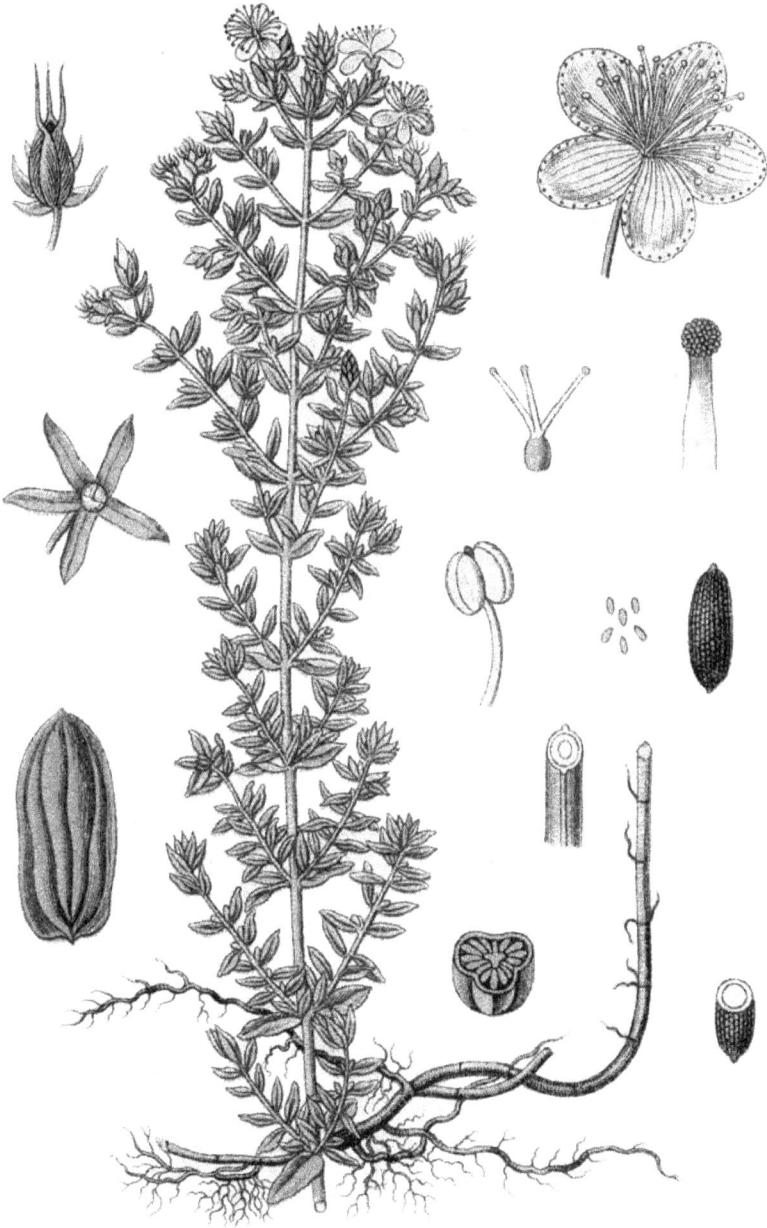

Quick Facts

Latin/Linnaen:	*Hypericum Perforatum*
Family:	*Hypericaceae*
Old English :	
Synonyms:	Hypericon, Corion, Tipton's weed, Chase-devil, or Klamath weed.
Action:	A mild antidepressant action of the herb and its preparations has been observed and reported by numerous physicians. According to experimental observation, hypericin can be categorized among the MAO inhibitors. Oily hypericum preparations demonstrate an anti-inflammatory action
Parts Used:	Herb gathered during flowering season.
Indicated For:	Internal: Psychovegetative disturbances, depressive moods, anxiety and/or nervous unrest. Oily hypericum preparations for dyspeptic complaints. External: Oily hyericum preparations for treatment and post-therapy of acute and contused injuries, myalgia and first degree burns.
Dosage:	Unless otherwise prescribed: Average daily dosage for internal use: 2-4g drug or 0.2-1.0mg of total hypericin in other forms of drug application.
Preparation:	Chopped herb, herb powder, liquid and solid preparations for internal use. Liquid and semi solid preparations for external use. Preparations made with fatty oils for external and internal use.
Cautions:	Photosensitivity is possible, especially in fair skinned people.
Other Uses:	

Description

Saint John's wort is the plant species *Hypericum perforatum*, and is also known as Tipton's weed, chase-devil, or Klamath weed.

With qualifiers, St John's wort is used to refer to any species of the genus *Hypericum*. Therefore, *H. perforatum* is sometimes called common St John's wort to differentiate it. The species of *Hypericum* are classified in the *Hypericaceae* family, having previously been classified as *Guttiferae* or *Clusiaceae*. Approximately 370 species of the genus *Hypericum* exist worldwide with a native geographical distribution including temperate and subtropical regions of North America, Europe, Turkey, Russia, India, China and Brazil.

St John's wort is widely known as an herbal treatment for depression.

Cultivation

Hardiness Zone:	3-10
Soil pH	6.8-7.2
Soil type	Prefers dry rocky soils, but is tolerant of most soil conditions.
Cultivation:	By seed or root division.
Sunlight:	Full sun
Habitat:	Native to Europe and North Africa

Best time to harvest St. John's Wort is when half the flowers are in bud and half are open. Some governments classify St. John's Wort as a noxious weed, therefore check your local regulations regarding propagation of this plant.

Historical Notes

A herbaceous perennial growing freely wild to a height of 1 to 3 feet in uncultivated ground, woods, hedges, roadsides, and meadows; short, decumbent, barren shoots and erect stems branching in upper part, glabrous; leaves pale green, sessile, oblong, with pellucid dots or oil glands which may be seen on holding leaf to light. Flowers are bright cheery yellow in terminal corymb. Calyx and corolla marked with black dots and lines; sepals and petals five in number; ovary pear-shaped with three long styles. Stamens are in three bundles joined by their bases only. Blooms June to August, followed by numerous small round blackish seeds which have a resinous smell and are contained in a three-celled capsule; odour peculiar, terebenthic; taste bitter, astringent and balsamic.

There are many ancient superstitions regarding this herb. Its name Hyperieum is derived from the Greek and means 'over an apparition,' a reference to the belief that the herb was so obnoxious to evil spirits that a whiff of it would cause them to fly.

Historical Medicinal Uses - For Entertainment ONLY

Medicinal Action and Uses: Aromatic, astringent, resolvent, expectorant and nervine. Used in all pulmonary complaints, bladder troubles, in suppression of urine, dysentery, worms, diarrhoea, hysteria and nervous depression, haemoptysis and other haemorrhages and jaundice. For children troubled with incontinence of urine at night an infusion or tea given before retiring will be found effectual; it is also useful in pulmonary consumption, chronic catarrh of the lungs, bowels or urinary passages. Externally for fomentations to dispel hard tumours, caked breasts, ecchymosis, etc.

Preparations and Dosages: 1 oz. of the herb should be infused in a pint of water and 1 to 2 tablespoonsful taken as a dose. Fluid extract, 1/2 to 1 drachm.

The oil of St. John's Wort is made from the flowers infused in olive oil.

Stinging Nettle

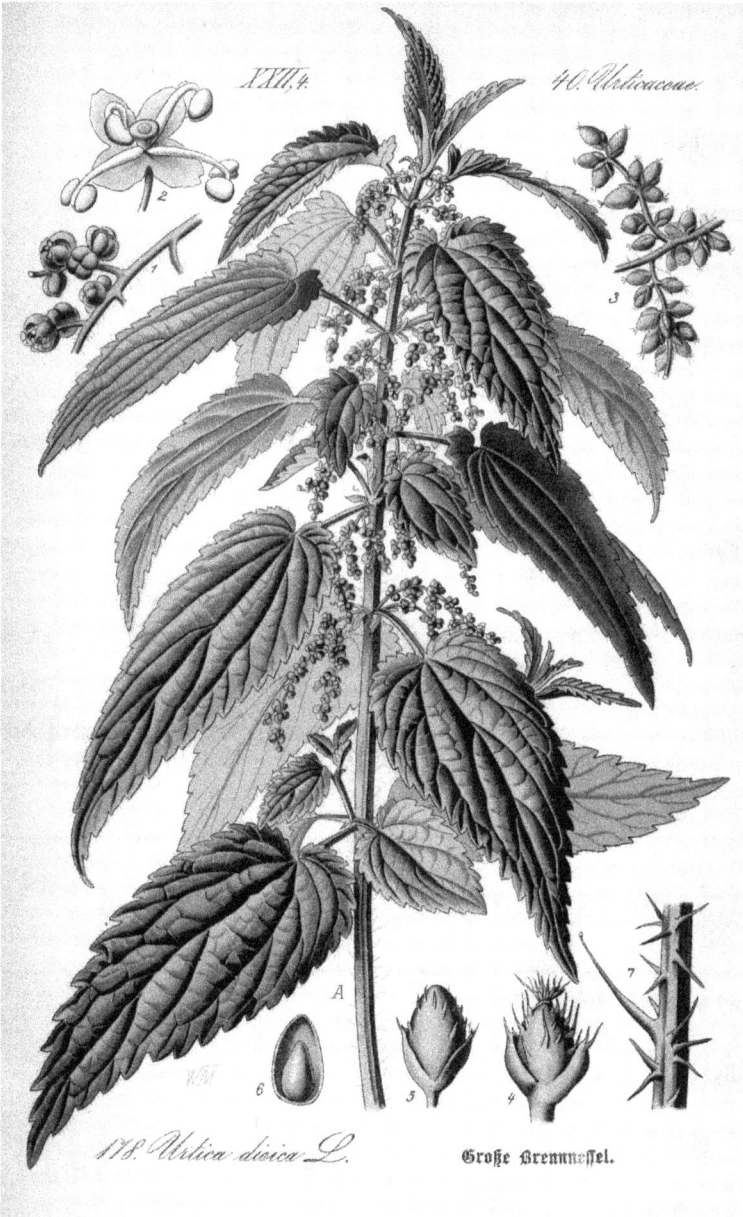

178. Urtica dioica L.   Große Brennessel.

Quick Facts (Herb & Leaf)

Latin/Linnaen:	*Urtica dioica*
Family:	*Urticaceae*
Old English :	Netele
Synonyms:	
Action:	Unknown
Parts Used:	Above ground parts
Indicated For:	Internal and external application: As supportive therapy for rheumatic ailments. Internal: As irrigation therapy for inflammatory diseases of the lower urinary tract and prevention and treatment of kidney gravel.
Dosage:	Unless otherwise prescribed: Average daily dosage: 8-12g of drug; equivalent preparations.
Preparation:	Comminuted herb for teas and other galenical preparations for internal use, as stinging nettle spirit for external applications.
Cautions:	In irrigation therapy, intake of copious amounts of fluids must be observed.
Other Uses:	

Quick Facts (Root)

Latin/Linnaen:	*Urtica dioica*
Family:	*Urticaceae*
Old English :	Netele
Synonyms:	
Action:	Increase of urinary volume, Increase of maximum urinary flow, Reduction of

	residual urine
Parts Used:	Root
Indicated For:	Difficulty in urination in benign prostatic hyperplasia stages 1 and 2.
Dosage:	Unless otherwise prescribed: Daily dosage: 4-6g of drug; equivalent preparations.
Preparation:	Comminuted drug for infusions as well as other galenical preparations for oral use.
Cautions:	This drug only relieves the symptoms of an enlarged prostate without reducing the enlargement. Please consult a physician at regular intervals. Side Effect: Occasionally, mild gastrointestinal upsets.
Other Uses:	

Description

Stinging nettle or common nettle, *Urtica dioica*, is a herbaceous perennial flowering plant, native to Europe, Asia, northern Africa, and North America, and is the best-known member of the nettle genus *Urtica*. The plant has many hollow stinging hairs called trichomes on its leaves and stems, which act like hypodermic needles that inject histamine and other chemicals that produce a stinging sensation when contacted by humans and other animals. The plant has a long history of use as a medicine and as a food source.

Stinging nettle is 1 to 2 m (3 to 7 ft) tall in the summer and dies down to the ground in winter. It has widely spreading rhizomes and stolons, which are bright yellow as are the roots. The soft green leaves are 3 to 15 cm (1 to 6 in) long and are borne oppositely on an erect wiry green stem. The leaves have a strongly serrated margin, a cordate base and an acuminate tip with a terminal leaf tooth longer than adjacent laterals. It bears small greenish or brownish numerous flowers in dense axillary inflorescences. The leaves and stems are very hairy with non-stinging hairs and also bear many stinging hairs (trichomes), whose tips come off when touched, transforming the hair into a needle that will inject several chemicals: acetylcholine, histamine, 5-HT (serotonin), moroidin, leukotrienes, and possibly formic acid. This mixture of chemical compounds cause a painful sting or paresthesia from which the species derives its common name, as well as the colloquial names burn nettle, burn weed, burn hazel.

Cultivation

Hardiness Zone:	7-10
Soil pH:	5.0-8.0
Soil type:	Loose soil high in nitrogen
Cultivation:	By seed or rhizome
Sunlight:	Full sun-part sun
Habitat:	Native to Europe, Asia, North Africa and North America

Stinging nettle is best planted away from the main garden and kept under control by removing flowers before they seed.

Historical Notes

The Nettle tribe, *Urticaceae*, is widely spread over the world and contains about 500 species, mainly tropical, though several, like our common Stinging Nettle, occur widely in temperate climates. Many of the species have stinging hairs on their stems and leaves. Two genera are represented in the British Isles, *Urtica*, the Stinging Nettles, and *Parietaria*, the Pellitory. Formerly botanists included in the order *Urticaceae* the Elm family, *Ulmaceae*; the Mulberry, Fig and Bread Fruit family, *Moraceae*; and that of the Hemp and Hop, *Cannabinacece*; but these are now generally regarded as separate groups.

The British species of Stinging Nettle, belonging to the genus *Urtica* (the name derived from the Latin, uro, to burn), are well known for the burning properties of the fluid contained in the stinging hairs with which the leaves are so well armed. Painful as are the consequences of touching one of our common Nettles, they are far exceeded by the effects of handling some of the East Indian species: a burning heat follows the sensation of pricking, just as if hot irons had been applied, the pain extending and continuing for many hours or even days, attended by symptoms similar to those which accompany lockjaw. A Java species, *U. urentissima*, produces effects which last for a whole year, and are even said to cause death. *U. crenulato* and *U. heterophylla*, both of India, are also most virulent. Another Indian species, *U. tuberosa*, on the other hand, has edible tubers, which are eaten either raw, boiled or roasted, and considered nutritious.

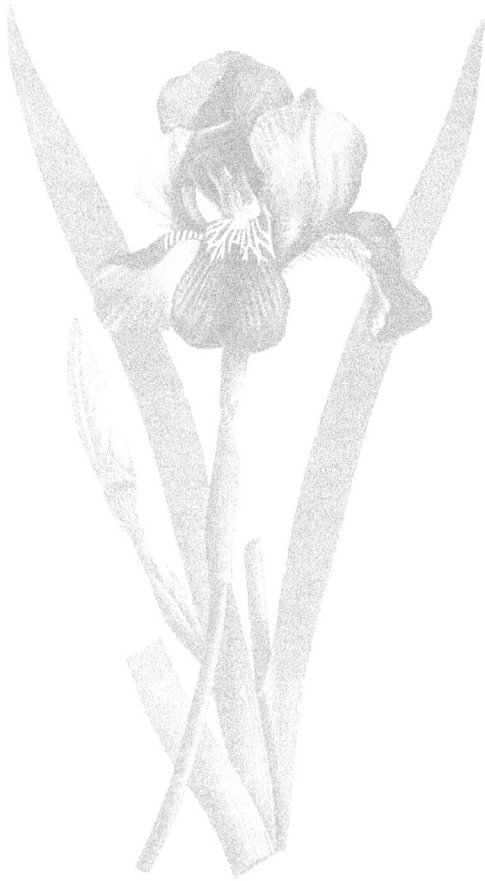

Thyme

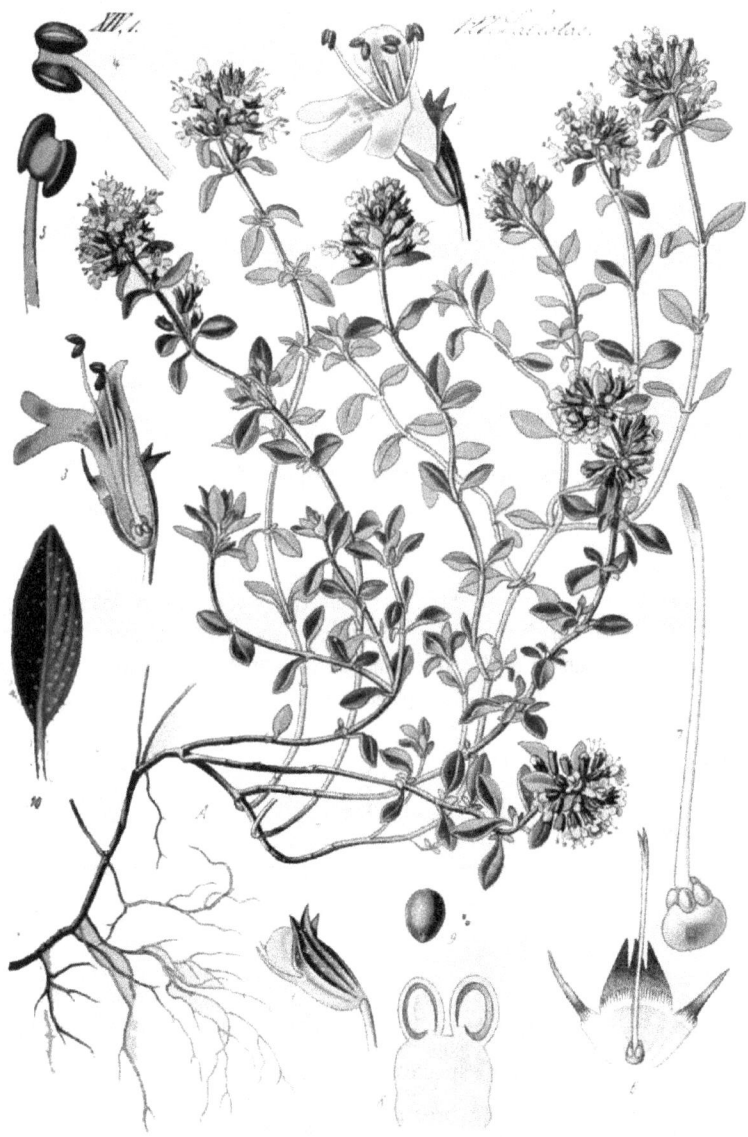

516. Thymus Serpyllum L. Feld-Quendel.

Quick Facts

Latin/Linnaen:	*Thymus Serpillum*
Family:	*Lamiaceae*
Old English :	Wuducunelle
Synonyms:	Thymus serpyllum,
Action:	Bronchoantispasmodic, Expectorant, Antibacterial
Parts Used:	Leaves and flowers
Indicated For:	Symptoms of bronchitis and whooping cough. Catarrhs of the upper respiratory tracts.
Dosage:	Unless otherwise prescribed: 1-2g of herb for 1 cup of tea, several times a day as needed; 1-2g fluid extract 1-3 times daily; 5 percent infusion for compresses.
Preparation:	Cut herb, powder, liquid extract or dry extract for infusions and other galenical preparations. Liquid and solid medicinal forms for internal and external application. Combinations with other herbs with have expectorant action could be appropriate.
Cautions:	
Other Uses:	Culinary & For Beverage, Tea

Description

Thymus serpyllum, known by the common names of Breckland Thyme, Wild Thyme or Creeping Thyme is a species of thyme native to most of Europe and North Africa. It is a low, usually prostrate subshrub growing to 2 cm tall with creeping stems up to 10 cm long, with oval evergreen leaves 3–8 mm long. The strongly scented flowers are either lilac, pink-purple, magenta, or a rare white, all 4–6 mm long and produced in clusters. The hardy plant tolerates some pedestrian traffic and produces odors ranging from heavily herbal to lightly lemon, depending on the plant.

It is part of the *Lamiaceae* family, and is related to the mint and Dead Nettle plants.

Cultivation

Hardiness Zone:	4-8
Soil pH:	6.5-7.0
Soil type:	Light sandy soil
Cultivation:	By cuttings or seed
Sunlight:	Full sun
Habitat:	Native to the Mediterranean, Balkans, and Causasus.

Thyme makes a good companion plant to eggplant, tomatoes and potatoes. Do not make a second harvest before winter if you wish to keep as a perennial.

Propagate by seeds, cuttings, or division of roots. Care must be taken to weed. Manure with farmyard manure in autumn or winter and nitrates in spring.

Cut when in full flower, in July and August, and dry.

Historical Notes

The Wild Thyme is indigenous to the greater part of the dry land of Europe, though is a great deal less abundant than the Common Thyme so widely cultivated. It is found up to a certain height on the Alps, on high plateaux, and in valleys, along ditches and roads, on rocks, in barren and dry soil, and also in damp clay soil destitute of chalk. It is seen in old stony, abandoned fields, dried-up lawns and on clearings. In England it is found chiefly on heaths and in mountainous situations, and is also often cultivated as a border in gardens or on rockeries and sunny banks. It was a great favourite of Francis Bacon, who in giving us his plan for the perfect garden, directs that alleys should be planted with fragrant flowers: 'burnet, wild thyme and watermints, which perfume the air most delightfully being trodden upon and crushed,' so that you may 'have pleasure when you walk or tread.'

The herb wherever it grows wild denotes a pure atmosphere, and was thought to enliven the spirits by the fragrance which it diffuses into the air around. The Romans gave Thyme as a sovereign remedy to melancholy persons.

Wild Thyme is a perennial, more thickset than the Garden Thyme, though subject to many varieties, according to the surroundings in which it grows. In its most natural state, when found on dry exposed downs, it is small and procumbent, often forming dense cushions; when growing among furze or other plants which afford it shelter, it runs up a slender stalk to a foot or more in height, which gives it a totally different appearance. The specific name, serpyllum, is derived from a Greek word meaning to creep, and has been given it from its usually procumbent and trailing habit.

The root is woody and fibrous, the stems numerous, hard, branched, procumbent, rising from 4 inches to 1 foot high, ordinarily reddish-brown in colour. The bright green oval leaves 1/8 inch broad, tapering below into very short foot-stalks, are smooth and beset with numerous small glands. They are fringed with hairs towards the base and have the veins prominent on the under surfaces. Their margins are entire and not recurved as in Garden Thyme. As with all other members of the important order *Labiatae*, to which the Thymes belong, the leaves are set in pairs on the stem. The plant flowers from the end of May or early June to the beginning of autumn, the flowers, which are very similar to those of the Garden Thyme, being purplish and in whorls at the top of the stems.

Bees are especially fond of the Thyme blossoms, from which they extract much honey. Spenser speaks of the 'bees-alluring time,' and everyone is familiar with Shakespeare's the 'bank whereon the wild thyme blows,' the abode of the queen of the Fairies. It was looked upon as one of the fairies' flowers, tufts of Thyme forming one of their favourite playgrounds.

In some parts it was a custom for girls to wear sprigs of Thyme, with mint and lavender, to bring them sweethearts!

It is much picked in France, chiefly in the fields of the Aisne, for the extraction of its essential oil.

Thyme has also been associated with death. It is one of the fragrant flowers planted on graves (in Wales, particularly), and the Order of Oddfellows still carry sprigs of Thyme at funerals and throw them into the grave of a dead brother. An old tradition says that Thyme was one of the herbs that formed the fragrant bed of the Virgin Mary.

Wild Thyme is the badge of the Drummond clan.

Constituents: When distilled, 100 kilos (about 225 lb.) of dried material yield 150 grams of essence (about 5 or 6 oz.). It is a yellow liquid, with a weaker scent than that of oil of Thyme extracted from *T. vulgaris*, and is called oil of Serpolet. It contains 30 to 70 per cent of phenols: Thymol, Carvacrol, etc. It is made into an artificial oil, together with the oil of Common Thyme. In perfumery, oil of Serpolet is chiefly used for soap.

The flowering tops, macerated for 24 hours or so in salt and water, are made into perfumed water.

Historical Medicinal Uses - For Entertainment ONLY

Medicinal Action and Uses: In medicine, Wild Thyme or Serpolet has the same properties as Common Thyme, but to an inferior degree. It is aromatic, antiseptic, stimulant, antispasmodic, diuretic and emmenagogue.

The infusion is used for chest maladies and for weak digestion, being a good remedy for flatulence, and favourable results have been obtained in convulsive coughs, especially in whooping cough, catarrh and sore throat. The infusion, prepared with 1 oz. of the dried herb to a pint of boiling water, is usually sweetened with sugar or honey and made demulcent by linseed or acacia. It is given in doses of 1 or more tablespoonfuls several times daily.

The infusion is also useful in cases of drunkenness, and Culpepper recommends it as a certain remedy taken on going to bed for 'that troublesome complaint the nightmare,' and says:

'if you make a vinegar of the herb as vinegar of roses is made and annoint the head with it, it presently stops the pains thereof. It is very good to be given either in phrenzy or lethargy.'

Wild Thyme Tea, either drunk by itself or mixed with other plants such as rosemary, etc., is an excellent remedy for headache and other nervous affections.

Formerly several preparations of this plant were kept in shops, and a distilled spirit and water, which were both very fragrant.

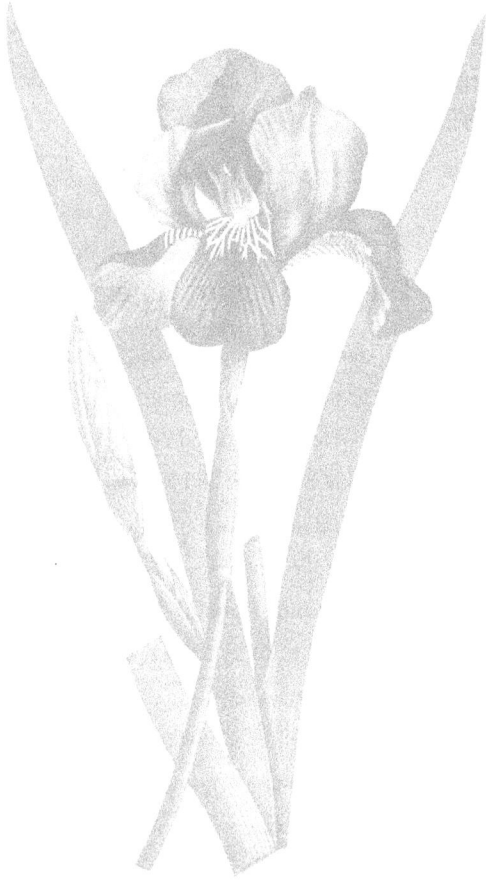

Tormentil

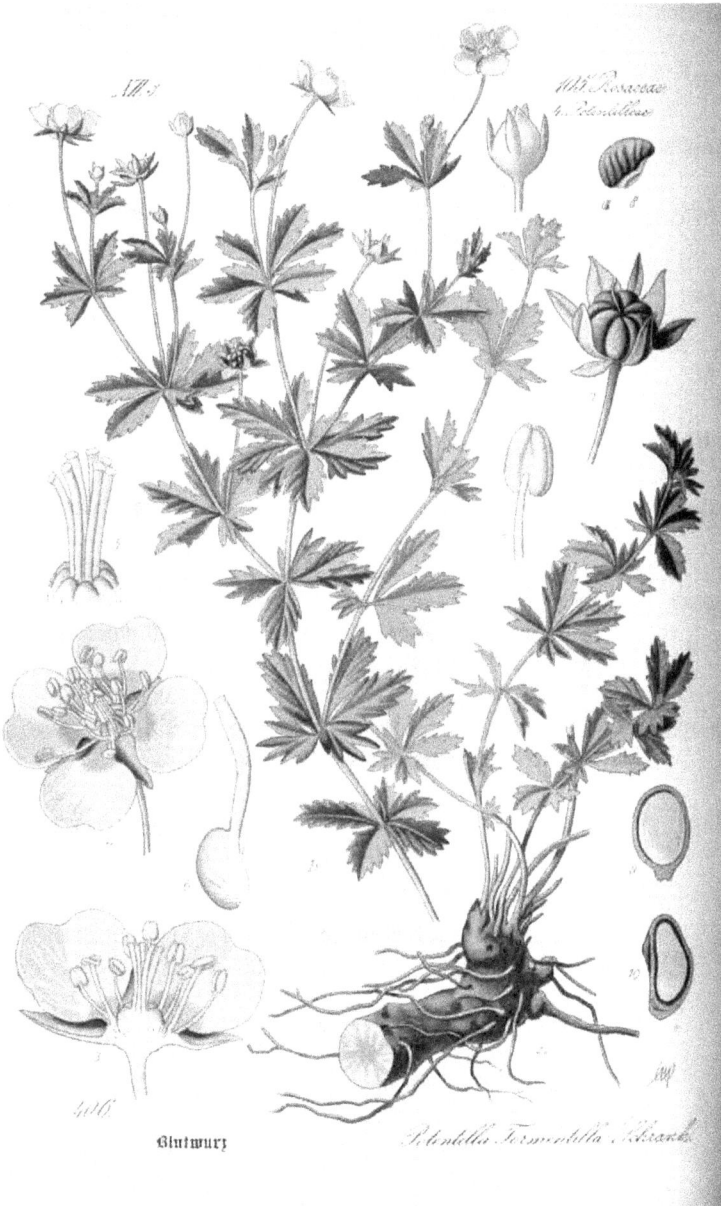

Glutwurz

Potentilla Tormentilla Schrank

Quick Facts

Latin/Linnaen:	*Potentilla tormentilla*
Family:	*Rosaceae*
Old English :	Seofenleafe
Synonyms:	Common Tormentil (Potentilla erecta syn. Tormentilla erecta, Potentilla tormentilla), Eptifilon, Septifolium, Septfoil. Thormantle, Biscuits, Bloodroot, Earthbank, Ewe Daisy, Five Fingers, Flesh and Blood, Shepherd's Knapperty, Shepherd's Knot, English Sarsaparilla.
Action:	Unknown
Parts Used:	Root
Indicated For:	Unspecified diarrhea disorders; mild mucous membrane inflammations of the mouth and pharynx.
Dosage:	When not otherwise prescribed: Average daily dosage; 4-6g of the drug; equivalent preparations. Tormentil tincture: 10-20 drops to one glass of water daily to rinse out the mouth and throat.
Preparation:	Crushed drug for boiling and infusing, as well as in other galenical preparations to be taken orally and applied locally.
Cautions:	Side Effects: Stomach complaints in sensitive subjects. Duration: Should the diarrhea last more than 3-4 days, a physician should be consulted.
Other Uses:	**Culinary:** The rhizomatous root is thick. It can be used for food in times of need.
	Dye: The root produces a red dye suitable for leather.
	Beverage: The roots are a main ingredient of a bitter liqueur from Bavaria and the Black Forest area, called Blutwurz.

Description

Common Tormentil (*Potentilla erecta syn. Tormentilla erecta, Potentilla tormentilla*) is an herbaceous perennial belonging to the rose family (*Rosaceae*), also known as Septfoil or simply as "tormentil" (which may also refer to similar species of Potentilla however).

It is a low, clumb-forming plant with slender, procumbent to arcuately upright stalks, growing 10–30 cm. tall and with non-rooting runners. It grows wild all over Asia and northern Europe, mostly in a wide variety of habitats, such as clearings, meadows, sandy soils and dunes.

This plant is flowering from May to August/September. There is one yellow, 7–11 mm wide flower, growing at the tip of a long stalk. There are almost always four notched petals, each with a length between 3 and 6 mm. Four petals are rather uncommon in the rose family. The petals are somewhat longer than the sepals. There are 20-25 stamens.

The glossy leaves are pinnately compound. The radical leaves have a long petiole, while the leaves on the stalks are usually sessile and have sometimes shorter petioles. Each leaf consists of three obovate leaflets with serrate leaf margins. The stipules are leaflike and palmately lobed.

There are 2-8 dry, inedible fruits.

Cultivation

Hardiness Zone:	5-8
Soil pH:	Prefers an acidic soil.
Soil type:	Well drained light rocky soil.
Cultivation:	By seed or rhizomes
Sunlight:	Full sun-part shade
Habitat:	Native to Europe and temperate Asia.

Historical Notes

In *Potentilla Tormentilla* the flowers are yellow as in *P. reptans*, but smaller, and have four petals instead of five, and eight sepals, not ten so separated as to form a Maltese cross when regarded from above.

From the root-stock come leaves on long stalks, divided into three or five oval leaflets (occasionally, but rarely, seven, hence the names Septfoil and Seven Leaves), toothed towards their tips. The stem-leaves, in this species, are stalkless with three leaflets.

A small-flowered form is very frequent on heaths and in dry pastures, a larger-flowered, in which the slender stems do not rise, but trail on the ground, is more general in woods, and on hedge-banks. From the ascending form, 6 to 12 inches high, this species has been called *P. erecta*, but even in this case the long stems are more often creeping and ascending rather than actually erect.

The name Tormentil is said to be derived from the Latin tormentum, which signifies such gripings of the intestines as the herb will serve to relieve, likewise the twinges of toothache.

The plant is very astringent, and has been used in some places for tanning.

It has been official in various Pharmacopoeias and was formerly in the Secondary List of the United States Pharmacopoeia.

It is considered one of the safest and most powerful of our native aromatic astringents, and for its tonic properties has been termed 'English Sarsaparilla.'

All parts of the plant are astringent, especially the red, woody rhizome.

The rhizome is 1 to 2 inches long, as thick as the finger, or smaller, tapering to one end, usually with one to three short branches near the larger end, ridged, with several strong, longitudinal wrinkles between them, bearing numerous blunt indentations. It is brown or blackish externally; internally, light brownish red; the fracture short and somewhat resinous, showing a thin bark, one or two circles of small, yellowish wood-wedges, broad medullary rays and a large pith. It has a peculiar faint, slightly aromatic odour and a strongly astringent taste.

Chemical Constituents: It contains 18 to 30 per cent of tannin, 18 per cent of a red colouring principle - Tormentil Red, a product of the tannin and yielding with potassium hydroxide, protocatechuic acid and phloroglucin. It is soluble in alcohol, but insoluble in water. Also some resin and ellagic and kinovic acids have been reported.

Historical Medicinal Uses - For Entertainment ONLY

There is a great demand for the rhizome, which in modern herbal medicine is used extensively as an astringent in diarrhoea and other discharges, operating without producing any stimulant effects. It also imparts nourishment and support to the bowels.

It is employed as a gargle in sore, relaxed and ulcerated throat and also as an injection in leucorrhoea.

It may be given in substance, decoction or extract. The dose of the powdered root or fluid extract is 1/2 to 1 drachm.

The fluid extract acts as a styptic to cuts, wounds, etc.

A strongly-made decoction is recommended as a good wash for piles and inflamed eyes. The decoction is made by boiling 2 oz. of the bruised root in 50 oz. of water till it is reduced one-third. It is then strained and taken in doses of 1 1/2 oz. It may be used as an astringent gargle.

If a piece of lint be soaked in the decoction and kept applied to warts, they will disappear.

The decoction for internal use should be made with 4 drachms to 1/2 pint of water, boiled for 10 minutes, adding 1/2 drachm of cinnamon stick at the end of boiling. Dose, 1 or 2 tablespoonsful.

Compound Powder of Tormentil. (A very reliable medicine in diarrhoea and dysentery.) Powdered Tormentil, 1 OZ; Powdered Galangal, 1 OZ.; Powdered Marshmallow root, 1 OZ.; Powdered Ginger, 4 drachms.

An infusion is made of the powdered ingredients by pouring 1 pint of boiling water upon them, allowing to cool and then straining the liquid. Dose, 1 or 2 fluid drachms, every 15 minutes, till the pain is relieved - then take three or four times a day.

A simple infusion is made by scalding 1 oz. of the powdered Tormentil with 1 pint of water and taking as required in wineglassful doses for chronic diarrhcea, fluxes, etc.

A continental recipe for an astringent decoction is equal parts of Tormentilla, Bistort and Pomegranate.

Dr. Thornton declared that in fluxes of blood, 1 drachm of Tormentil given four times a day in an infusion of Hops did wonders.

Thornton tells of a poor old man who made wonderful cures of ague, smallpox, whooping cough, etc., from an infusion of this herb and became so celebrated locally that Lord William Russell gave him a piece of ground in which to cultivate it, which he did, keeping it a secret for long.

It was much given for cholera, and also sometimes in intermittent fevers, and used in a lotion for ulcers and long-standing sores. The juice of the fresh root, or the powder of the dried, was used in compounding ointments and plasters for application to wounds and sores.

The fresh root, bruised, and applied to the throat and jaws was held to heal the King's Evil.

Culpepper says:

'Tormentil is most excellent to stay all fluxes of blood or humours, whether at nose, mouth or belly. The juice of the herb and root, or the decoction thereof, taken with some Venice treacle and the person laid to sweat, expels any venom or poison, or the plague, fever or other contagious disease, as the pox, measles, etc., for it is an ingredient in all antidotes or counterpoisons.'. . . 'It resisteth putrefaction.' . . . 'The root taken inwardly is most effectual to help any flux of the belly, stomach, spleen or blood and the juice wonderfully opens obstructions of the spleen and lungs and cureth yellow jaundice. Tormentil is no less effectual and powerful a remedy against outward wounds, sores and hurts than for inward and is therefore a special ingredient to be used in wound drinks, lotions and injections. . . . It is also effectual for the piles. . . . The juice or powder of the root, put into ointments, plasters and such things that are applied to wounds or sores is very effectual.'

In the Western Isles of Scotland and in the Orkneys the roots were used for tanning leather and considered superior even to oak bark, being first boiled in water and the leather steeped in the cold liquor. The Laplanders employed the thickened red juice of the root for staining leather red.

The Americans use the name Tormentil for Geranium maculatum, the Spotted Cranesbill, which has similar properties. Many of the 150 species of Potentilla have been similarly used in medicine.

Valerian

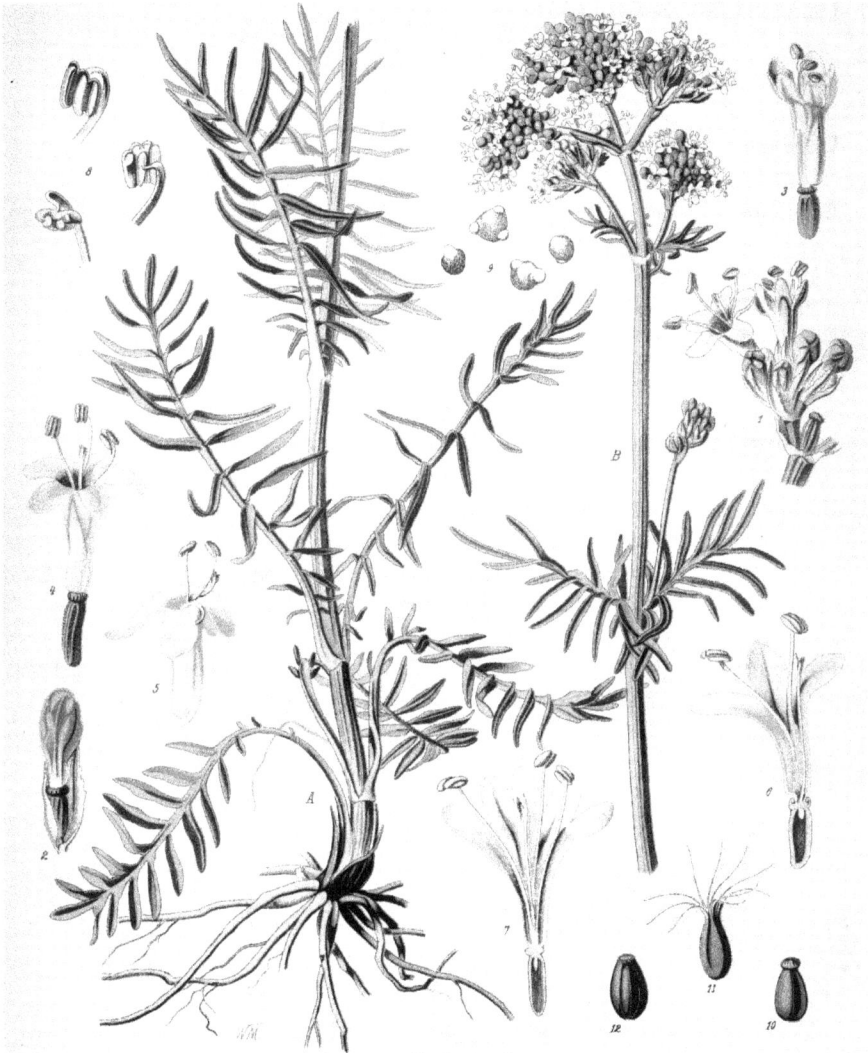

Valeriana officinalis L

Quick Facts

Latin/Linnaen:	*Valeriana Officinalis*
Family:	*Valerianaceae*
Old English :	Ualeriane
Synonyms:	Phu (Galen), All-Heal, Great Wild Valerian, Amantilla, Setwall, Setewale, Capon's Tail.
Action:	Sedative, Sleep promoting
Parts Used:	Root
Indicated For:	Restlessness, sleeping disorders based on nervous conditions.
Dosage:	Unless otherwise prescribed: Infusions: 2-3g of drug per cup, once to several times per day. Tincture: ½-1 teaspoon (1-3ml), once to several times per day. Extracts: Amount equivalent to 2-3g of drug, once to several times per day. External Use: 100g for one full bath; equivalent preparations.
Preparation:	Internal: As expressed juice from fresh plants, tincture, extracts, and other galenical preparations. External: As a bath additive.
Cautions:	
Other Uses:	

Description

Valerian (*Valeriana officinalis*, *Valerianaceae*) is a hardy perennial flowering plant, with heads of sweetly scented pink or white flowers which bloom in the summer months. Valerian flower extracts were used as a perfume in the sixteenth century.

Native to Europe and parts of Asia, valerian has been introduced into North America. It is consumed as food by the larvae of some Lepidoptera (butterfly and moth) species including Grey Pug.

Other names used for this plant include garden valerian (to distinguish it from other Valeriana species), garden heliotrope (although not related to Heliotropium) and all-heal. The garden flower red valerian is also sometimes referred to as "valerian", but is a different species from the same family and not very closely related.

Valerian, in pharmacology and phytotherapic medicine, is the name of an herb or dietary supplement prepared from roots of the plant, which, after maceration, trituration and dehydration processes, are packaged, usually into capsules. Based on its pharmacological mode of action, valerian root has been demonstrated to possess sedative and anxiolytic effects. The amino acid valine is named after this plant.

Cultivation

Hardiness Zone:	3-9
Soil pH:	6.6-7.5
Soil type:	Moisture retentive rich soil.
Cultivation:	By seed or by root division.
Sunlight:	Full sun-Semi shade
Habitat:	Native to Europe and parts of Asia.

Valerian needs at least 2 years to establish a good root system before harvesting the roots. Removing flowers as they appear will result in better root growth.

Valerian does well in all ordinary soils, but prefers rich, heavy loam, well supplied with moisture.

In Derbyshire, cultivation is from wild plants collected in local woods and transplanted to the prepared land. Preference is given in collecting to root offsets - daughter plants and young flowering plants, which develop towards the close of summer, at the end of slender runners given off by the perennial rhizomes of old plants. These should be set 1 foot apart in rows, 2 or 3 feet apart. The soil should first be treated with farmyard manure, and after planting it is well to give liquid manure from time to time, as well as plenty of water. The soil must be well manured to secure a good crop. Weeding requires considerable attention.

Propagation may also be by seed, either sown when ripe in cold frames, or in March in gentle heat, or in the open in April. In the first two cases, transplant in May to permanent quarters. But to ensure the best alkaloidal percentage, it is best to transplant and cultivate the daughter plants of the wild Valerian.

Historical Notes

Two species of Valerian, *Valeriana officinalis* and *V. dioica*, are indigenous in Britain, while a third, *V. pyrenaica*, is naturalized in some parts. The genus comprises about 150 species, which are widely distributed in the temperate parts of the world.

In medicine, the root of *V. officinalis* is intended when Valerian is mentioned. It is supposed to be the Phu (an expression of aversion from its offensive odour) of Dioscorides and Galen, by whom it is extolled as an aromatic and diuretic.

It was afterwards found to be useful in certain kinds of epilepsy. The plant was in such esteem in mediaeval times as a remedy, that it received the name of All Heal, which is still given it in some parts of the country.

The plant is found throughout Europe and Northern Asia, and is common in England in marshy thickets and on the borders of ditches and rivers, where its tall stems may generally be seen in the summer towering above the usual herbage, the erect, sturdy growth of the plant, the rich, dark green of the leaves, their beautiful form, and the crowning masses of light-coloured flowers, making the plant conspicuous.

The roots tend to merge into a short, conical root-stock or erect rhizome, the development of which often proceeds for several years before a flowering stem is sent up, but slender horizontal branches which terminate in buds are given off earlier, and from these buds proceed aerial shoots or stolons, which produce fresh plants where they take root. Only one stem arises from the root, which attains a height of 3 or 4 feet. It is round, but grooved and hollow, more or less hairy, especially near the base. It terminates in two or more pairs of flowering stems, each pair being placed at right angles to those above and below it. The lower flowering stems lengthen so as to place their flowers nearly or often quite on a level with the flowers borne by the upper branches, forming a broad and flattened cluster at the summit, called a cyme. The leaves are arranged in pairs and are united at their bases. Each leaf is made up of a series of lance-shaped segments, more or less opposite to one another on each side of the leaf (pinnate). The leaflets vary very much in number, from six to ten pairs as a rule, and vary also in breadth, being broad when few in number and narrower when more numerous; they are usually 2 to 3 inches long. The margins are indented by a few coarsely-cut teeth. The upper surface is strongly veined, the under surface is paler and frequently more or less covered with short, soft hairs. The leaves on the stem are attached by short, broad sheaths, the radical leaves are larger and long-stemmed and the margins more toothed.

The flowers are in bloom from June to September. They are small, tinged with pink and flesh colour, with a somewhat peculiar, but not exactly unpleasant smell. The corolla is tubular, and from the midst of its lobes rise the stamens, only three in number, though there are five lobes to the corolla. The limb of the calyx is remarkable for being at first inrolled and afterwards expanding in the form of a feathery pappus, which aids the dissemination of the fruit. The fruit is a capsule containing one oblong compressed seed. Apart from the flowers, the whole plant has a foetid smell, much accentuated when bruised.

Although more often growing in damp situations, Valerian is also met with on dry, elevated ground. It is found throughout Britain, but in the northern counties is more often found on higher and dryer ground - dry heaths and hilly pastures - than in the south, and then is usually smaller, not more than 2 feet high, with narrow leaves and hairy, and is often named sylvestris. The medicinal qualities of this form are considered to be especially strong.

Though none of the varieties differ greatly from the typical form, Valerian is more subject than many plants to deviations, which has caused several more or less permanent varieties to be named by various botanists. One of the chief is *V. sambucifolia* (Mikan), the name signifying 'Elder-leaved,' from the form of its foliage, the segments being fewer (only four to six pairs) and broader than in the type form, and having somewhat of the character of the elder.

V. celtica is supposed to be the Saliunca of ancient writers. It is used by Eastern nations to aromatize their baths. The roots are collected by the Styrian peasants, and are exported by way of Trieste to Turkey and Egypt, whence they are conveyed to India and Ethiopia. *V. sitchensis*, a native of northwestern America, is considered by the Russians the most powerful of all species.

The derivation of the name of this genus of plants is differently given. It is said by some authors to have been named after Valerius, who first used it in medicine; while others derive the name from the Latin word valere (to be in health), on account of its medicinal qualities. The word Valeriana is not found in the classical authors; we first meet with it in the ninth or tenth century, at which period and for long afterwards it was used as synonymous with Phu or Fu; Fu, id est valeriana, we find it described in ancient medical works of that period. The word Valerian occurs in the recipes of the AngloSaxon leeches (eleventh century). Valeriana, Amantilla and Fu are used as synonymous in the Alphita, a mediaeval vocabulary of the important medical school of Salernum. Saladinus of Ascoli (about 1450) directs the collection in the month of August of radices fu, id est Valerianae. Referring to the name Amantilla, by which it was known in the fourteenth century, Professor Henslow quotes a curious recipe of that period, a translation of which runs as follows: 'Men who begin to fight and when you wish to stop them, give to them the juice of Amantilla id est Valeriana and peace will be made immediately.' Theriacaria, Marinella, Genicularis and Terdina are other old names by which Valerian has been known in former days. Another old name met with in Chaucer and other old writers is 'Setwall' or 'Setewale,' the derivation of which is uncertain. Mediaeval herbalists also called the plant 'Capon's Tail,' which has rather fantastically been explained as a reference to its spreading head of whitish flowers.

Drayton (Polyolbion) mentions the use of Valerian for cramp; and a tea was made from its roots.

Harvesting and Preparation for Market: The flowering tops must be cut off as they appear, thus enabling the better development of the rhizome. Many of the young plants do not flower in the first year, but produce a luxuriant crop of leaves, and yield rhizome of good quality in the autumn.

In September or early October, all the tops are cut off with a scythe and the rhizomes are harvested, the clinging character of the Derbyshire soil not allowing them to be left in the ground longer.

The drug as found in commerce consists usually of the entire or sliced erect rhizome, which is dark yellowish-brown externally, about 1 inch long and 1/2 inch thick, and gives off numerous slender brittle roots from 2 1/2 to 4 inches long, whilst short, slender, lateral branches (stolons) are also occasionally present. The root-stock, which is sometimes crowned with the remains of flowering stems and leaf-scales is usually firm, horny and whitish or yellowish internally, but old specimens may be hollow. A transverse section is irregular in outline and exhibits a comparatively narrow bark, separated by a dark line from an irregular circle of wood bundles of varying size.

The drug may also consist of small, undeveloped rhizomes about 1/4 inch long, crowned with the remains of leaves and bearing short slender roots, the young rhizome having been formed where the stolons given off from mature root-stocks have taken root and produced independent plants.

The roots of Valerian are of similar colour to the erect rhizome, about 1/10 inch thick, striated longitudinally and usually not shrivelled to any great extent; a transverse section shows a thick bark and small wood.

The drug has a camphoraceous, slightly bitter taste and a characteristic, powerful, disagreeable odour, which gradually develops during the process of drying, owing to a change which occurs in the composition of the volatile oil contained in the sub-epidermal layer of cells: the odour of the fresh root, though not very agreeable, is devoid of the unpleasant valerianaceous odour.

The colour and odour of Valerian rhizome distinguish it readily from other drugs. The rhizome somewhat resembles Serpentary rhizome (*Aristolochia Serpentaria*, Virginian Snakeroot), but may be distinguished therefrom by its odour, erect method of growth, and by the roots being thicker, shorter and less brittle.

Chemical Constituents: The chief constituent of Valerian is a yellowish-green to brownish-yellow oil, which is present in the dried root to the extent of 0.5 to 2 per cent though an average yield rarely exceeds 0.8 per cent. This variation in quantity is partly explained by the influence of locality, a dry, stony soil, yielding a root richer in oil than one that is moist and fertile.

Lindley's Treasury of Botany states: 'What is known to chemists as volatile oil of Valerian seems not to exist naturally in the plant, but to be developed by the agency of water.'

The oil is contained in the sub-epidermal layer of cells in the root, not in isolated cells or glands. It is of complex composition, containing valerianic, formic and acetic acids, the alcohol known as borneol, and pinene. The valerianic acid present in the oil is not the normal acid, but isovalerianic acid, an oily liquid to which the characteristically unpleasant odour of Valerian is due. It is gradually liberated during the process of drying, being yielded by the decomposition of the chief constituent, bornyl-isovalerianate, by the ferment present. It is strongly acid, burning to the palate and with the odour of the plant. The oil is soluble in 30 parts of water and readily in alcohol and ether. It is found in nature in the oil of several plants, also in small proportion in train oil and the oil of Cetacea (whales, porpoises, etc.), which owe their smell to it. It is also one of the products of oxidation of animal matters and of fat oils, and is secreted in certain portions of animal bodies. Its salts are soluble and have a sweetish taste and fatty aspect.

The root also contains two alkaloids - Chatarine and Valerianine - which are still under investigation and concerning which little is known, except that they form crystalline salts. There are also a glucoside, alkaloid and resin all physiologically active, discovered in the fresh rhizome by Chevalier as recently as 1907. He claims that the fresh root is of greater medicinal value than the dry on this account.

On incineration, the drug, if free from adherent earthy matter, yields about 8 or 9 per cent of ash.

The chief preparation of the British Pharmacopoeia is the Tinctura Valerianae Ammoniata, containing Valerian, oil of Nutmeg, oil of Lemon and Ammonia: it is an extremely nauseous and offensive preparation. An etherial tincture and the volatile oil are official in some of the Continental Pharmacopceias, and a distilled water and syrup in the French Codex.

Valerianate of oxide of ethyl, or valerianic ether is a fragrant compound occurring in some vegetable products. The valerianic acid in use is not prepared from the root, but synthetically from amyl alcohol. Valerianic acid combines with various bases (the oxides of metals) to form salts called Valerianates. Valerianate of zinc, prepared by double decomposition, is used as an antispasmodic and is official in the British Pharmacopoeia.

Historical Medicinal Uses - For Entertainment ONLY

Valerian is a powerful nervine, stimulant, carminative and antispasmodic.

It has a remarkable influence on the cerebro-spinal system, and is used as a sedative to the higher nerve centres in conditions of nervous unrest, St. Vitus's dance, hypochrondriasis, neuralgic pains and the like.

The drug allays pain and promotes sleep. It is of especial use and benefit to those suffering from nervous overstrain, as it possesses none of the after-effects produced by narcotics.

During the recent War (WWI), when air-raids were a serious strain on the overwrought nerves of civilian men and women, Valerian, prescribed with other simple ingredients, taken in a single dose, or repeated according to the need, proved wonderfully efficacious, preventing or minimizing serious results.

Though in ordinary doses, it exerts an influence quieting and soothing in its nature upon the brain and nervous system, large doses, too often repeated, have a tendency to produce pain in the head, heaviness and stupor.

It is commonly administered as Tinctura Valerianae Ammoniata, and often in association with the alkali bromides, and is sometimes given in combination with quinine, the tonic powers of which it appreciably increases.

Oil of Valerian is employed to a considerable extent on the Continent as a popular remedy for cholera, in the form of cholera drops, and also to a certain extent in soap perfumery.

Ettmuller writes of its virtues in strengthening the eyesight, especially when this is weakened by want of energy in the optic nerve.

The juice of the fresh root, under the name of Energetene of Valerian, has of late been recommended as more certain in its effects, and of value as a narcotic in insomnia, and as an anti-convulsant in epilepsy. Having also some slight influence upon the circulation, slowing the heart and increasing its force, it has been used in the treatment of cardiac palpitations.

Valerian was first brought to notice as a specific for epilepsy by Fabius Calumna in 1592, he having cured himself of the disease with it.

Preparations and Dosages: Fluid extract, 1/2 to 1 drachm. Solid extract, 5 to 10 grains. Tincture, B.P. and U.S.P., 1885, 1 to 2 drachms. Ammoniated tincture, B.P. and U.S.P. 1898, 1/2 to 1 drachm.

Culpepper (1649) joins with many old writers to recommend the use both of herb and root, and praises the herb for its longevity and many comforting virtues, reminding us that it is 'under the influence of Mercury, and therefore hath a warming faculty.' Among other uses, he adds:

'The root boiled with liquorice, raisons and aniseed is good for those troubled with cough. Also, it is of special value against the plague, the decoction thereof being drunk and the root smelled. The green herb being bruised and applied to the head taketh away pain and pricking thereof.'

Gerard tells us that herbalists of his time thought it 'excellent for those burdened and for such as be troubled with croup and other like convulsions, and also for those that are bruised with falls.' He relates that the dried root was held in such esteem as a medicine among the poorer classes in the northern counties and the south of Scotland, that 'no broth or pottage or physicall meats be worth anything if Setewale (the old name for Valerian) be not there.'

Sutherland describes many varieties of Valerian, and himself grew the Indian Valerian which is still sent to Mincing Lane, and offered on the British market. Hanbury states that, according to its habitat, it has many variations which some botanists take as separate species. In the south of England, when once it obtains a hold of the ground, nothing will eradicate it. It was well known to the Anglo-Saxons, who used it as a salad.

Valerian has an effect on the nervous system of many animals, especially cats, which seem to be thrown into a kind of intoxication by its scent. It is scarcely possible to keep a plant of Valerian in a garden after the leaves or root have been bruised or disturbed in any way, for cats are at once attracted and roll on the unfortunate plant. It is equally attractive to rats and is often used by rat-catchers to bait their traps. It has been suggested that the famous Pied Piper of Hamelin owed his irresistible power over rats to the fact that he secreted Valerian roots about his person.

In the Middle Ages, the root was used not only as a medicine but also as a spice, and even as a perfume. It was the custom to lay the roots among clothes as a perfume (vide Turner, Herbal, 1568, Pt. III, p. 56), just as some of the Himalayan Valerians are still used in the East, especially *V. Jatamansi*, the Nard of the Ancients, believed to be the Spikenard referred to in the Scriptures. It is still much used in ointments. Its odour is not so unpleasant as that of our native Valerians, and this and other species of Valerian are used by Asiatic nations in the manufacture of precious scents. Several aromatic roots were known to the Ancients under the name of Nardus, distinguished according to their origin or place of growth by the names of *Nardus indica*, *N. celtica*, *N. montana*, etc., and supposed to have been derived from different valerianaceous plants. Thus the *N. indica* is referred to *V. Jatamansi* (Roxb.), of Bengal, the *N. celtica* to *V. celtica* (Linn.), inhabiting the Alps and the N. *montana* to *V. tuberosa*, which grows in the mountains of the south of Europe.

Other Species: Japanese Valerian, or Kesso Root, was formerly believed to be the product of *Patrinia scabiosaefolia* (Link.), but is now known to be obtained from a Japanese variety of *V. officinalis*. It yields a volatile oil. By the absence of a well-marked, upright rhizome, it widely differs from true Valerian, though at first sight agrees to some extent with it. In colour and taste it is almost identical.

The roots of *V. Mexicana* (D.C.), Mexican Valerian, which occurs in Mexican commerce in slices, or fleshy disks, contain a large percentage of valerianic acid, which they yield readily and economically. As much as 3.3 per cent of oil has been extracted from the roots of this species.

V. pyrenaica (Linn.), the Heart-Leaved Valerian, a native of the Pyrenees, is occasionally found in Great Britain naturalized in plantations. It is a large, coarse herb, the stem 2 to 4 feet high, the radical leaves sometimes very large, often a foot in diameter, heart-shaped, the upper ones smaller, with a few basal leaflets, the flowers much as in *V. officinalis*. It is not employed medicinally.

V. montana and *V. angustifolia* are Alpine varieties, but can be grown in this country with a little care. They are almost entirely grown for decorative purposes, flowering from May to August, and possessing none of the unpleasant smell of Valerian.

Culpepper describes a plant which he calls 'Water Valerian' (*V. Aquatica*), with 'much larger' flowers than the garden Valerian, which, however, they resemble, and of a 'pale purple colour.' He states it grows 'promiscuously in marshy grounds and moist meadows' and flowers in May.

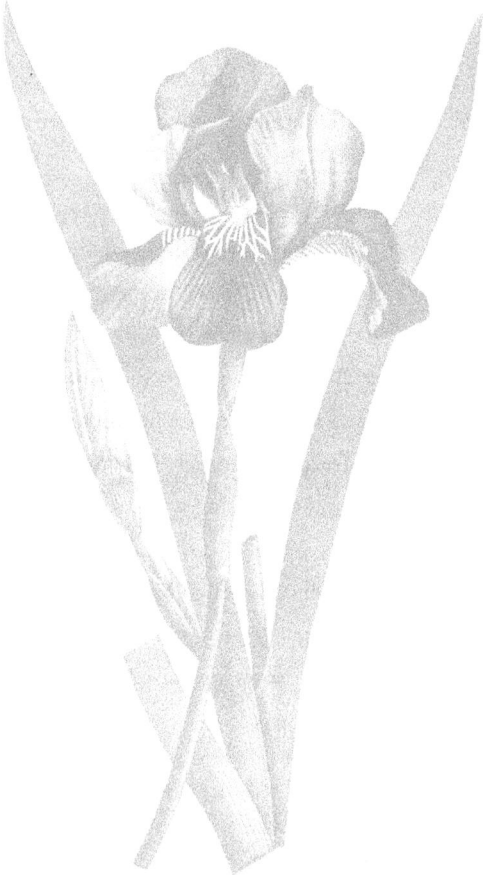

Watercress

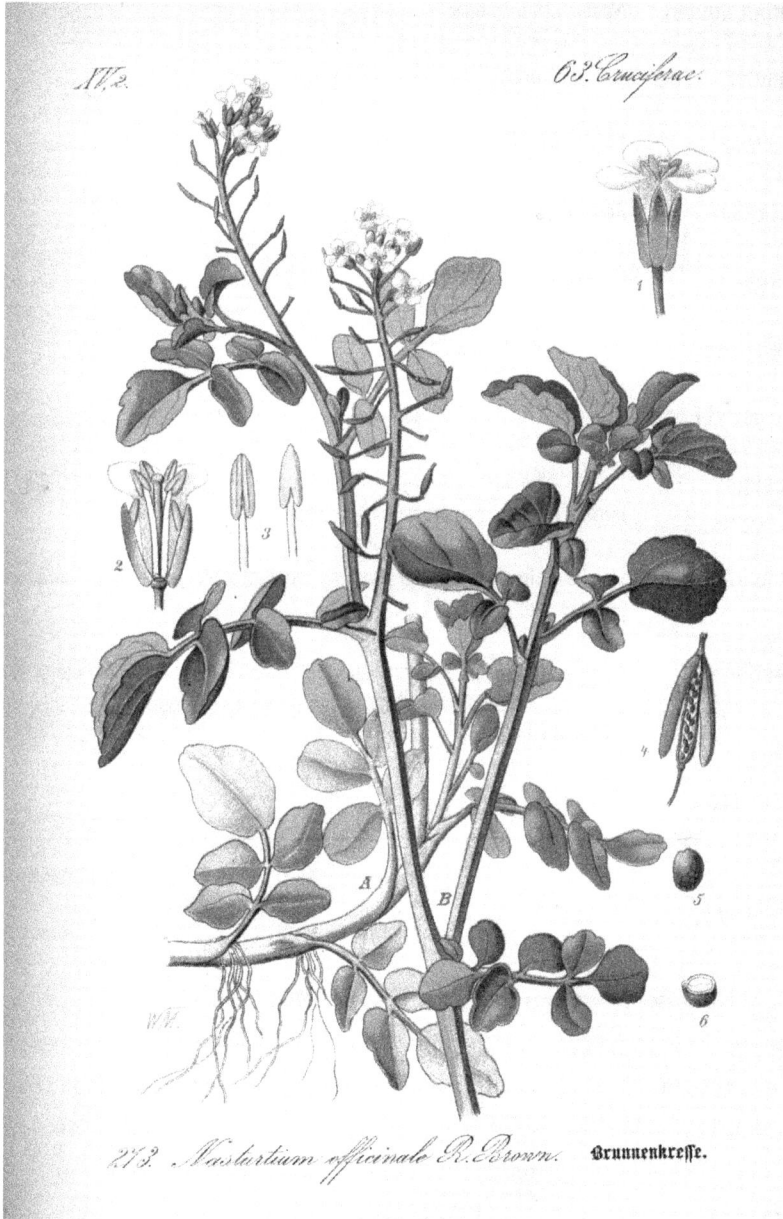

273. *Nasturtium officinale R. Brown.* **Brunnenkreſſe.**

Quick Facts

Latin/Linnaen:	*Nasturtium officinale*
Family:	*Brassicaceae*
Old English :	Faencyrse
Synonyms:	Fen-Cress
Action:	Unknown
Parts Used:	Above ground plant parts
Indicated For:	Catarrh of respiratory tract
Dosage:	Unless otherwise prescribed: Daily dosage: 4-6g dried herb; 20-30g fresh herb; 60-150g fresh pressed juice; equivalent preparations
Preparation:	Cut herb, freshly pressed juice, as well as other galenical preparations for internal use.
Cautions:	Contraindications: Gastric and intestinal ulcers, inflammatory kidney diseases. No application for children under age of four. Side Effects: In rare cases, gastrointestinal complaints
Other Uses:	Culinary

Description

Watercresses (*Nasturtium officinale, N. microphyllum*; formerly *Rorippa nasturtium-aquaticum, R. microphylla*) are fast-growing, aquatic or semi-aquatic, perennial plants native from Europe to central Asia, and one of the oldest known leaf vegetables consumed by human beings. These plants are members of the *Family Brassicaceae* or cabbage family, botanically related to garden cress, mustard and radish -- all noteworthy for a peppery, tangy flavour.

The hollow stems of watercress are floating, and the leaves are pinnately compound. Watercresses produce small, white and green flowers in clusters.

Cultivation

Hardiness Zone:	9-10
Soil pH:	6.5-7.5
Soil type:	Compost rich, sandy soil submerged in water.
Cultivation:	By seed or cuttings
Sunlight:	Full sun
Habitat:	Native to Europe and parts of Asia

Watercress is related to the cabbage family. It is a semi aquatic plant. It can be grown for sprouts also.

Cultivation of watercress is practical on both a large scale and a garden scale. Being semi-aquatic, watercress is well-suited to hydroponic cultivation, thriving best in water that is slightly alkaline. It is frequently produced around the headwaters of chalk streams. In many local markets, the demand for hydroponically grown watercress exceeds supply, partly because cress leaves are unsuitable for distribution in dried form, and can only be stored fresh for a short period.

Watercress can be sold in supermarkets inside sealed plastic bags, containing a little moisture and lightly pressurised to prevent crushing of contents. This has allowed national availability with a once-purchased storage life of one to two days in chilled/refrigerated storage.

Also sold as sprouts, the edible shoots are harvested days after germination. If unharvested, watercress can grow to a height of 50–120 cm. Like many plants in this family, the foliage of watercress becomes bitter when the plants begin producing flowers.

In the United States in the 1940s, New Market, Alabama was known as the "Watercress Capital of the World".

Watercress is grown in a number of counties of the United Kingdom, most notably Hertfordshire, Hampshire, Wiltshire and Dorset, although the first commercial cultivation was along the River Ebbsfleet in Kent grown by William Bradbery (horticulturist) in 1808. Alresford, near Winchester, is often considered the watercress capital of Britain (to the extent that a steam railway line is named after the famous local crop). In recent years, watercress has become more widely available in the UK, at least in the South-East, being stocked pre-packed in some supermarkets, as well as fresh by the bunch at farmers' markets and greengrocers. Value-added products, such as the traditional watercress soup and pesto, are increasingly easy to source.

Historical Notes

A hardy perennial found in abundance near springs and open running watercourses, of a creeping habit with smooth, shining, brownish-green, pinnatifid leaves and ovate, heart-shaped leaflets, the terminal one being larger than the rest. Flowers small and white, produced towards the extremity of the branches in a sort of terminal panicle.

The true nasturtium or Indian Cress cultivated in gardens as a creeper has brilliant orange-red flowers and produces the seeds which serve as a substitute for capers in pickles.

The poisonous Marshwort or 'Fool's Cress' is often mistaken for Watercress, with which it is sometimes found growing. It may readily be distinguished by its hemlock-like white flowers, and when out of flower, by its finely toothed and somewhat pointed leaves, much longer than those of the watercress and of a paler green. The Latin name 'Nasturtium' is derived from the words nasus tortus (a convulsed nose) on account of its pungency.

Constituents: A sulpho-nitrogenous oil, iodine iron, phosphates, potash, with other mineral salts, bitter extract and water. Its volatile oil rich in nitrogen combined with some sulphur in the sulpho-cyanide of allyl.

Historical Medicinal Uses - For Entertainment ONLY

Watercress is particularly valuable for its antiscorbutic (preventing or relieving scurvy) qualities and has been used as such from the earliest times. As a salad it promotes appetite. Culpepper says that the leaves bruised or the juice will free the face from blotches, spots and blemishes, when applied as a lotion.

Dosage: Expressed juice, 1 to 2 fluid ounces.

Wormwood

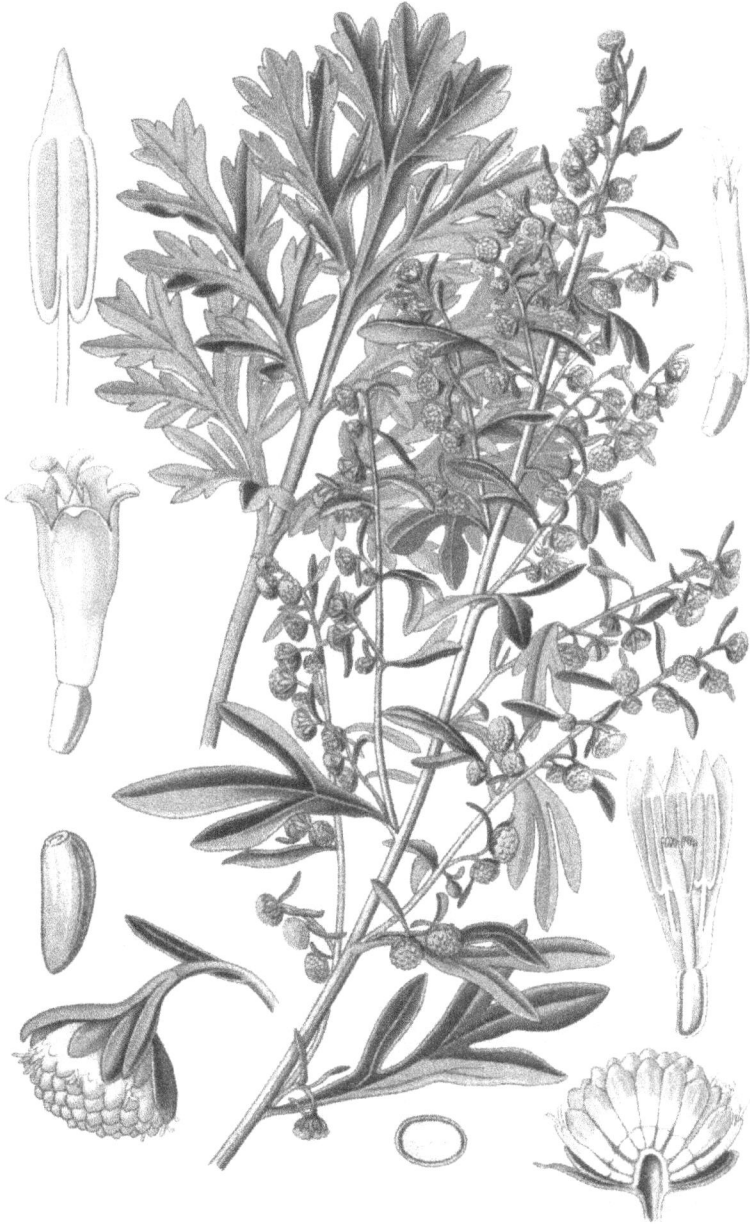

Quick Facts

Latin/Linnaen:	*Artemisia absinthium*
Family:	*Asteraceae*
Old English :	Wermod, Wormwode or Wermode.
Synonyms:	Green Ginger.
Action:	The effectiveness as an aromatic bitter is based on the bitter principles and volatile oil. Useful experimental pharmacological data of recent years are not available.
Parts Used:	Upper shoots and leaves
Indicated For:	Loss of appetite, dyspepsia, biliary dyskinesia
Dosage:	Unless otherwise prescribed: Daily dosage: 2-3g of herb as water infusion.
Preparation:	Cut herb for infusions and decoctions, herb powder, also extracts and tinctures as liquid or solid forms of medications for oral administration.
Cautions:	Warning: Combinations with other bitters or aromatics may be advantageous. In toxic doses, thujone, the active component of the oil, acts as a convulsant poison. Therefore, the essential oil must not be used except in combinations.
Other Uses:	**Beverage:** Most notably it's an ingredient in the spirit absinthe, and also used for flavouring in some other spirits and wines, including bitters, vermouth and pelinkovac. It's also added in mint tea in Moroccan tea culture.
	In the Middle Ages, it was used to spice mead. In 18th century England, wormwood was sometimes used instead of hops in beer.
	Culinary: Wormwood is the traditional colour and flavour agent for green songpyeon, a type of dduk / tteok (Korean rice cake), eaten during the Korean thanksgiving festival of chuseok in the autumn. Wormwood is picked in the spring when it is still young. The juice from macerated fresh (or reconstituted dry) leaves provides the colouring and flavouring ingredient in the dough prepared to make green songpyeon.

Description

Artemisia absinthium (absinthium, absinthe wormwood, wormwood, common wormwood, green ginger or grand wormwood) is a species of wormwood, native to temperate regions of Eurasia and northern Africa.

It is an herbaceous, perennial plant with fibrous roots. The stems are straight, growing to 0.8-1.2 m (rarely 1.5m, but, sometimes even larger) tall, grooved, branched, and silvery-green. The leaves are spirally arranged, greenish-grey above and white below, covered with silky silvery-white trichomes, and bearing minute oil-producing glands; the basal leaves are up to 25 cm long, bipinnate to tripinnate with long petioles, with the cauline leaves (those on the stem) smaller, 5–10 cm long, less divided, and with short petioles; the uppermost leaves can be both simple and sessile (without a petiole). Its flowers are pale yellow, tubular, and clustered in spherical bent-down heads (capitula), which are in turn clustered in leafy and branched panicles. Flowering is from early summer to early autumn; pollination is anemophilous. The fruit is a small achene; seed dispersal is by gravity.

It grows naturally on uncultivated, arid ground, on rocky slopes, and at the edge of footpaths and fields.

The leaves and flowering tops are gathered when the plant is in full bloom, and dried naturally or with artificial heat. Its active substances include silica, two bitter substances (absinthin and anabsinthine), thujone, tannic and resinous substances, malic acid, and succinic acid. It is used medicinally as a tonic, stomachic, antiseptic, antispasmodic, carminative, cholagogue, febrifuge and anthelmintic. It has also been used to remedy indigestion and gastric pain. Wormwood tea is used as a remedy for labor pain. A dried, encapsulated form of the plant is used as an anthelmintic. Extracts of the plant have shown to exhibit strong antimicrobial activity, especially against Gram-positive pathogenic bacteria.

A wine can also be made by macerating the herb. It is also available in powder form and as a tincture. The oil of the plant can be used as a cardiac stimulant to improve blood circulation. Pure wormwood oil is very poisonous, but with proper dosage poses little or no danger. The oil is a potential source of novel agents for the treatment of leishmaniasis.

Cultivation

Hardiness Zone:	4-8
Soil pH:	6.1-7.5
Soil type:	Dry mid weight soil high in nitrogen.
Cultivation:	Root divisions, cuttings or by seed
Sunlight:	Shade-partial sun
Habitat:	Native to temperate regions of Africa and Eurasia.

Harvest Wormwood on a dry day after the dew is gone from the leaves.

The plant can easily be cultivated in dry soil. It should be planted under bright exposure in fertile, mid-weight soil. It prefers soil rich in nitrogen. It can be propagated by growth (ripened cuttings taken in March or October in temperate climates) or by seeds in nursery beds. It is naturalised in some areas away from its native range, including much of North America.

Wormwood likes a shady situation, and is easily propagated by division of roots in the autumn, by cuttings, or by seeds sown in the autumn soon after they are ripe. No further care is needed than to keep free from weeds. Plant about 2 feet apart each way.

The plant's characteristic odor can make it useful for making a plant spray against pests. It is used in companion planting to suppress weeds, because its roots secrete substances that inhibit the growth of surrounding plants. It can repel insect larvae when planted on the edge of the cultivated area. It has also been used to repel fleas and moths indoors.

Historical Notes

Artemisia comes from the Ancient Greek name Artemis. In Hellenistic culture, Artemis was a goddess of the hunt, and protector of the forest and children.

Absinthium comes from Ancient Greek apsinthion. Alternatively, it might possibly mean "unenjoyable", and probably refer to the bitter nature of the derived beverage. Consider the following quote by Lucretius in De Rerum Natura, I, 936-8:

"And as physicians when they seek to give

A draught of bitter wormwood to a child,

First smearing along the edge that rims the cup

The liquid sweets of honey, golden-hued,"

The word "wormwood" comes from Middle English wormwode or wermode. The form "wormwood" is influenced by the traditional use as a cure for intestinal worms. Webster's Third New International Dictionary attributes the etymology to Old English wermōd (compare with German Wermut and the derived drink vermouth), which the OED (s.v.) marks as "of obscure origin". An alternative explanation dubiously combines the Old English wer, meaning "man" (as in "werewolf"), with Old English mōd, meaning "mood".

Wormwood is mentioned seven times in the Jewish Bible and once in the New Testament, always with the implication of bitterness.

The Common Wormwood held a high reputation in medicine among the Ancients. Tusser (1577), in July's Husbandry, says:

'While Wormwood hath seed get a handful or twaine

To save against March, to make flea to refraine:

Where chamber is sweeped and Wormwood is strowne,

What saver is better (if physick be true)

For places infected than Wormwood and Rue?

It is a comfort for hart and the braine

And therefore to have it it is not in vaine.'

Besides being strewn in chambers as Tusser recommended, it used to be laid among stuffs and furs to keep away moths and insects.

According to the Ancients, Wormwood counteracted the effects of poisoning by hemlock, toadstools and the biting of the sea dragon. The plant was of some importance among the Mexicans, who celebrated their great festival of the Goddess of Salt by a ceremonial dance of women, who wore on their heads garlands of Wormwood.

With the exception of Rue, Wormwood is the bitterest herb known, but it is very wholesome and used to be in much request by brewers for use instead of hops. The leaves resist putrefaction, and have been on that account a principal ingredient in antiseptic fomentations.

An Old Love Charm

'On St. Luke's Day, take marigold flowers, a sprig of marjoram, thyme, and a little Wormwood; dry them before a fire, rub them to powder; then sift it through a fine piece of lawn, and simmer it over a slow fire, adding a small quantity of virgin honey, and vinegar. Anoint yourself with this when you go to bed, saying the following lines three times, and you will dream of your partner "that is to be":

"St. Luke, St. Luke, be kind to me,

In dreams let me my true-love see." '

Culpepper, writing of the three Wormwoods most in use, the Common Wormwood, Sea Wormwood and Roman Wormwood, tells us: 'Each kind has its particular virtues' . . . the Common Wormwood is 'the strongest,' the Sea Wormwood, 'the second in bitterness,' whereas the Roman Wormwood, 'to be found in botanic gardens' - the first two being wild - 'joins a great deal of aromatic flavour with but little bitterness.'

The Common Wormwood grows on roadsides and waste places, and is found over the greater part of Europe and Siberia, having been formerly much cultivated for its qualities. In Britain, it appears to be truly indigenous near the sea and locally in many other parts of England and Scotland, from Forfar southwards. In Ireland it is a doubtful native. It has become naturalized in the United States.

The root is perennial, and from it arise branched, firm, leafy stems, sometimes almost woody at the base. The flowering stem is 2 to 2 1/2 feet high and whitish, being closely covered with fine silky hairs. The leaves, which are also whitish on both sides from the same reason, are about 3 inches long by 1 1/2 broad, cut into deeply and repeatedly (about three times pinnatifid), the segments being narrow (linear) and blunt. The leaf-stalks are slightly winged at the margin. The small, nearly globular flowerheads are arranged in an erect, leafy panicle, the leaves on the flower-stalks being reduced to three, or even one linear segment, and the little flowers themselves being pendulous and of a greenish-yellow tint. They bloom from July to October. The ripe fruits are not crowned by a tuft of hairs, or pappus, as in the majority of the *Compositae* family.

The leaves and flowers are very bitter, with a characteristic odour, resembling that of thujone. The root has a warm and aromatic taste.

Parts Used: The whole herb - leaves and tops - gathered in July and August, when the plant is in flower and dried.

Collect only on a dry day, after the sun has dried off the dew. Cut off the upper green portion and reject the lower parts of the stems, together with any discoloured or insect-eaten leaves. Tie loosely in bunches of uniform size and length, about six stalks to a bunch, and spread out in shape of a fan, so that the air can get to all parts. Hang over strings, in the open, on a fine, sunny, warm day, but in half-shade, otherwise the leaves will become tindery; the drying must not be done in full sunlight, or the aromatic properties will be partly lost. Aromatic herbs should be dried at a temperature of about 70 degrees. If no sun is available, the bunches may be hung over strings in a covered shed, or disused greenhouse, or in a sunny warm attic, provided there is ample ventilation, so that the moist heated air may escape. The room may also be heated with a coke or anthracite stove, care being taken that the window is kept open during the day. If after some days the leaves are crisp and the stalks still damp, hang the bunches over a stove, when the stalks will quickly finish drying. Uniformity in size in the bunches is important, as it facilitates packing. When the drying process is completed, pack away at once in airtight boxes, as otherwise the herbs will absorb about 12 per cent moisture from the air. If sold to the wholesale druggists in powdered form, rub through a sieve as soon as thoroughly dry, before the bunches have had time to absorb any moisture, and pack in tins or bottles at once.

Constituents: The chief constituent is a volatile oil, of which the herb yields in distillation from 0.5 to 1.0 per cent. It is usually dark green, or sometimes blue in colour, and has a strong odour and bitter, acrid taste. The oil contains thujone (absinthol or tenacetone), thujyl alcohol (both free and combined with acetic, isovalerianic, succine and malic acids), cadinene, phellandrene and pinene. The herb also contains the bitter glucoside absinthin, absinthic acid, together with tannin, resin, starch, nitrate of potash and other salts.

Historical Medicinal Uses - For Entertainment ONLY

Medicinal Action and Uses: Tonic, stomachic, febrifuge, anthelmintic.

A nervine tonic, particularly helpful against the falling sickness and for flatulence. It is a good remedy for enfeebled digestion and debility.

Preparations: Fluid extract, 1/2 to 1 drachm. Wormwood Tea, made from 1 oz. of the herb, infused for 10 to 12 minutes in 1 pint of boiling water, and taken in wineglassful doses, will relieve melancholia and help to dispel the yellow hue of jaundice from the skin, as well as being a good stomachic, and with the addition of fixed alkaline salt, produced from the burnt plant, is a powerful diuretic in some dropsical cases. The ashes yield a purer alkaline salt than most other vegetables, except Beanstalks and Broom.

The juice of the larger leaves which grow from the root before the stalk appears has been used as a remedy for jaundice and dropsy, but it is intensely nauseous. A light infusion of the tops of the plant, used fresh, is excellent for all disorders of the stomach, creating an appetite, promoting digestion and preventing sickness after meals, but it is said to produce the contrary effect if made too strong.

The flowers, dried and powdered, are most effectual as a vermifuge, and used to be considered excellent in agues. The essential oil of the herb is used as a worm-expeller, the spirituous extract being preferable to that distilled in water. The leaves give out nearly the whole of their smell and taste both to spirit and water, but the cold water infusions are the least offensive.

The intensely bitter, tonic and stimulant qualities have caused Wormwood not only to be an ingredient in medicinal preparations, but also to be used in various liqueurs, of which absinthe is the chief, the basis of absinthe being absinthol, extracted from Wormwood. Wormwood, as employed in making this liqueur, bears also the name 'Wermuth' - preserver of the mind - from its medicinal virtues as a nervine and mental restorative. If not taken habitually, it soothes spinal irritability and gives tone to persons of a highly nervous temperament. Suitable allowances of the diluted liqueur will promote salutary perspiration and may be given as a vermifuge. Inferior absinthe is generally adulterated with copper, which produces the characteristic green colour.

The drug, absinthium, is rarely employed, but it might be of value in nervous diseases such as neurasthenia, as it stimulates the cerebral hemispheres, and is a direct stimulant of the cortex cerebri. When taken to excess it produces giddiness and attacks of epileptiform convulsions. Absinthium occurs in the British Pharmacopoeia in the form of extract, infusion and tincture, and is directed to be extracted also from *A. maritima*, the Sea Wormwood, which possesses the same virtues in a less degree, and is often more used as a stomachic than the Common Wormwood. Commercially this often goes under the name of Roman Wormwood, though that name really belongs to *A. Pontica*. All three species were used, as in Culpepper's time.

Dr. John Hill (1772) recommends Common Wormwood in many forms. He says:

'The Leaves have been commonly used, but the flowery tops are the right part. These, made into a light infusion, strengthen digestion, correct acidities, and supply the place of gall, where, as in many constitutions, that is deficient. One ounce of the Flowers and Buds should be put into an earthen vessel, and a pint and a half of boiling water poured on them, and thus to stand all night. In the morning the clear liquor with two spoonfuls of wine should be taken at three draughts, an hour and a half distance from one another. Whoever will do this regularly for a week, will have no sickness after meals, will feel none of that fulness so frequent from indigestion, and wind will be no more troublesome; if afterwards, he will take but a fourth part of this each day, the benefit will be lasting.'

He further tells us that if an ounce of these flowers be put into a pint of brandy and let to stand six weeks, the resultant tincture will in a great measure prevent the increase of gravel - and give great relief in gout.

'The celebrated Baron Haller has found vast benefit by this; and myself have very happily followed his example.'

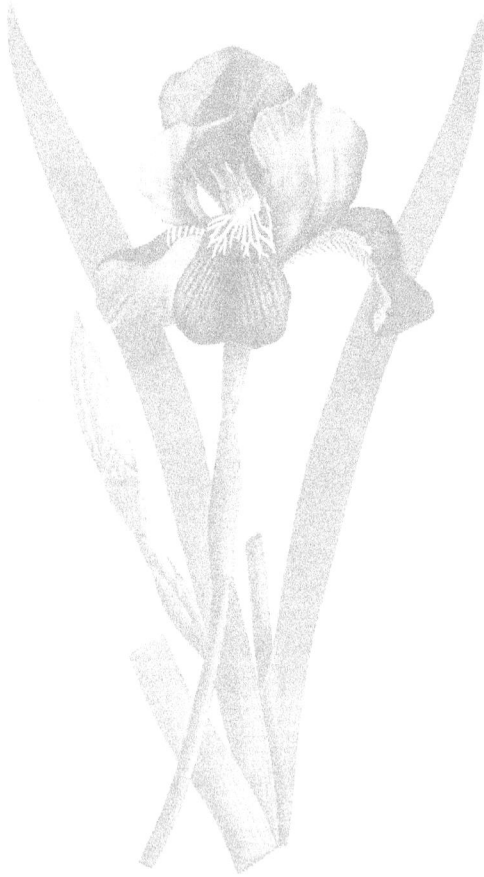

Yarrow

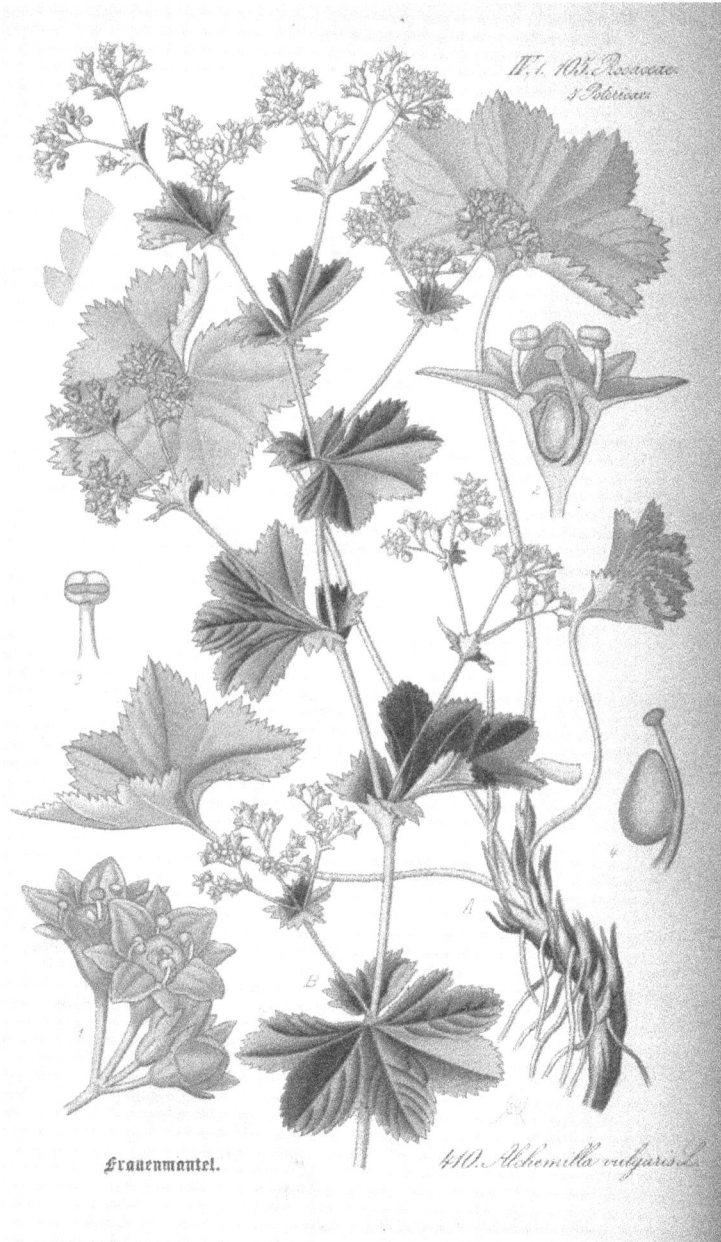

Frauenmantel.   410. Alchemilla vulgaris L.

Quick Facts

Latin/Linnaen: *Achillea Millefolium*

Family: *Asteraceae*

Old English : Gearwe

Synonyms: Milfoil, Old Man's Pepper, Soldier's Woundwort, Knight's Milfoil, Herbe Militaris, Thousand Weed, Nose Bleed, Carpenter's Weed, Bloodwort, Staunchweed, Sanguinary, Devil's Nettle, Devil's Plaything, Bad Man's Plaything, Yarroway, (Saxon) Gearwe, (Dutch) Yerw, (Swedish) Field Hop.

Action: Choleritic, Antibacterial, Astringent, Antispasmodic

Parts Used: Above ground plant parts.

Indicated For: Internal: Loss of appetite, dyspeptic ailments, such as mild, spastic discomforts of the gastrointestinal tract. As sitz bath: Painful, cramp like conditions in the lower part of the female pelvis.

Dosage: Unless otherwise prescribed: Daily dosage: 4.5g yarrow herb; 3tsp pressed juice from fresh plants; 3 g yarrow flowers; equivalent preparations. For sitz baths: 100g yarrow per 20L of water.

Preparation: Comminuted drug for teas and other galenical preparations for internal use and for sitz baths, pressed juice of fresh plants for internal use.

Cautions: Contraindications: Allergy to yarrow and other composites.

Other Uses:

Culinary: In the seventeenth century it was an ingredient of salads.

Beverages: In Sweden it is called 'Field Hop' and has been used in the manufacture of beer. Linnaeus considered beer thus brewed more intoxicating than when hops were used. It is said to have a similar use in Africa.

Misc: It has been employed as snuff, and is also called Old Man's Pepper, on account of the pungency of its foliage. Both flowers and leaves have a bitterish, astringent, pungent taste.

Descripton

Achillea millefolium or yarrow is a flowering plant in the family *Asteraceae*, native to the Northern Hemisphere. In New Mexico and southern Colorado, it is called plumajillo, or "little feather", for the shape of the leaves. In antiquity, yarrow was known as herbal militaris, for its use in staunching the flow of blood from wounds. Other common names for this species include common yarrow, gordaldo, nosebleed plant, old man's pepper, devil's nettle, sanguinary, milfoil, soldier's woundwort, thousand-leaf (as its binomial name affirms), and thousand-seal.

Common yarrow is an erect herbaceous perennial plant that produces one to several stems (0.2 to 1m tall) and has a rhizomatous growth form. Leaves are evenly distributed along the stem, with the leaves near the middle and bottom of the stem being the largest. The leaves have varying degrees of hairiness (pubescence). The leaves are 5–20 cm long, bipinnate or tripinnate, almost feathery, and arranged spirally on the stems. The leaves are cauline and more or less clasping. The inflorescence has 4 to 9 phyllaries and contains ray and disk flowers which are white to pink. There are generally 3 to 8 ray flowers that are ovate to round. Disk flowers range from 15 to 40. The inflorescence is produced in a flat-topped cluster. The fruits are small achenes.

Yarrow grows at low or high altitudes, up to 3500m above sea level. The plant commonly flowers from May through June, and is a frequent component in butterfly gardens. Common yarrow is frequently found in the mildly disturbed soil of grasslands and open forests. Active growth occurs in the spring.

In North America, there are both native and introduced genotypes, and both diploid and polyploid plants. The plant has a strong, sweet scent, similar to chrysanthemums.

Cultivation

Hardiness Zone:	3-9
Soil pH:	6.0-6.5
Soil type:	Well drained soil, tolerant of poor soil on roadsides.

Cultivation:	Root division, cuttings or by seed
Sunlight:	Full sun-part shade
Habitat:	Native to Europe and Asia

Avoid planting Yarrow near downspouts where they will get too much water. Yarrow can do well in pots, given its preference for dry soil.

Historical Notes

Yarrow grows everywhere, in the grass, in meadows, pastures, and by the roadside. As it creeps greatly by its roots and multiplies by seeds it becomes a troublesome weed in gardens, into which it is seldom admitted in this country, though it is cultivated in the gardens of Madeira.

The name Yarrow is a corruption of the Anglo-Saxon name for the plant - gearwe; the Dutch, yerw.

The stem is angular and rough, the leaves alternate, 3 to 4 inches long and 1 inch broad, clasping the stem at the base, bipinnatifid, the segments very finely cut, giving the leaves a feathery appearance.

It flowers from June to September, the flowers, white or pale lilac, being like minute daisies, in flattened, terminal, loose heads, or cymes. The whole plant is more or less hairy, with white, silky appressed hairs.

Yarrow was formerly much esteemed as a vulnerary, and its old names of Soldier's Wound Wort and Knight's Milfoil testify to this. The Highlanders still make an ointment from it, which they apply to wounds, and Milfoil tea is held in much repute in the Orkneys for dispelling melancholy. Gerard tells us it is the same plant with which Achilles stanched the bleeding wounds of his soldiers, hence the name of the genus, Achillea. Others say that it was discovered by a certain Achilles, Chiron's disciple.

Its specific name, *millefolium*, is derived from the many segments of its foliage, hence also its popular name, Milfoil and Thousand Weed. Another popular name for it is Nosebleed, from its property of stanching bleeding of the nose, though another reason given for this name is that the leaf, being rolled up and applied to the nostrils, causes a bleeding from the nose, more or less copious, which will thus afford relief to headache. Parkinson tells us that 'if it be put into the nose, assuredly it will stay the bleeding of it' - so it seems to act either way.

It was one of the herbs dedicated to the Evil One, in earlier days, being sometimes known as Devil's Nettle, Devil's Plaything, Bad Man's Plaything, and was used for divination in spells.

Yarrow, in the eastern counties, is termed Yarroway, and there is a curious mode of divination with its serrated leaf, with which the inside of the nose is tickled while the following lines are spoken. If the operation causes the nose to bleed, it is a certain omen of success:

'Yarroway, Yarroway, bear a white blow,

If my love love me, my nose will bleed now.'

An ounce of Yarrow sewed up in flannel and placed under the pillow before going to bed, having repeated the following words, brought a vision of the future husband or wife:

'Thou pretty herb of Venus' tree,

Thy true name it is Yarrow;

Now who my bosom friend must be,

Pray tell thou me to-morrow.'

---(Halliwell's Popular Rhymes, etc.)

Parts Used: The whole plant, stems, leaves and flowers, collected in the wild state, in August, when in flower.

Constituents: A dark green, volatile oil, a peculiar principle, achillein, and achilleic acid, which is said to be identical with aconitic acid, also resin, tannin, gum and earthy ash, consisting of nitrates, phosphates and chlorides of potash and lime.

Historical Medicinal Uses - For Entertainment ONLY

Medicinal Action and Uses: Diaphoretic, astringent, tonic, stimulant and mild aromatic.

Yarrow Tea is a good remedy for severe colds, being most useful in the commencement of fevers, and in cases of obstructed perspiration. The infusion is made with 1 oz. of dried herb to 1 pint of boiling water, drunk warm, in wineglassful doses. It may be sweetened with sugar, honey or treacle, adding a little Cayenne Pepper, and to each dose a teaspoonful of Composition Essence. It opens the pores freely and purifies the blood, and is recommended in the early stages of children's colds, and in measles and other eruptive diseases.

A decoction of the whole plant is employed for bleeding piles, and is good for kidney disorders. It has the reputation also of being a preventative of baldness, if the head be washed with it.

Preparations: Fluid extract, 1/2 to 1 drachm. An ointment made by the Highlanders of Scotland of the fresh herb is good for piles, and is also considered good against the scab in sheep.

An essential oil has been extracted from the flowers, but is not now used.

Linnaeus recommended the bruised herb, fresh, as an excellent vulnerary and styptic. It is employed in Norway for the cure of rheumatism, and the fresh leaves chewed are said to cure toothache.

Culpepper spoke of Yarrow as a profitable herb in cramps, and Parkinson recommends a decoction to be drunk warm for ague.

The medicinal values of the Yarrow and the Sneezewort (*A. millefolium* and *A. ptarmica*), once famous in physic, were discarded officially in 1781.

Woolly Yellow Yarrow (*A. tomentosa*) is very rare, and a doubtful native; its leaves are divided and woolly, the flowers bright yellow.

Index

A

B

C

D

E

H

I

J

K

L

L

M

N

O

P

Q

R

S

V

W

Y

Short Bibliography

Grieves, M. (1971). A modern herbal (volume 1, a-h): The medicinal, culinary, cosmetic and economic properties, cultivation and folk-lore of herbs, grasses, fungi, shrubs . (Vol. 1). Dover Publications.

Grieves, M. (1971). A modern herbal (volume 2, i-z): The medicinal, culinary, cosmetic and economic properties, cultivation and folk-lore of herbs, grasses, fungi, shrubs . (Vol. 2). Dover Publications.

Pollington, S. (2000). *Leechcraft - Early English Charms, Plant Lore, and Healing.* Norfolk: Anglo-Saxon Books.

Rister, R. (1998). The complete german commission e monographs: Therapeutic guide to herbal medicines. (p. 684). The American Botanical Council.

Other Great Books by the Author

Buy directly from the Author or available worldwide via Amazon

Northern Lore

A Field Guide to the Northern Mind, Body, & Spirit

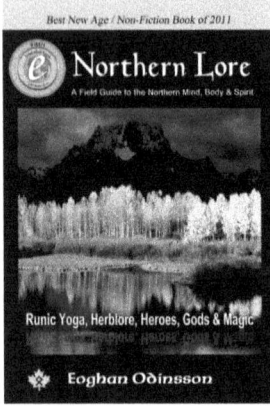

Winner of the Global eBook Award for Best *New Age / Non-Fiction* Book in 2011

Northern Lore is a Field Guide to the Northern Mind-Body-Spirit, and will help you re-discover the Folk-Lore & Traditions of North Western Europe, and acquaint you with modern practices inspired by that lore.

In today's exciting cosmopolitan society, we tend to discard the old in favor of the new; and while discovering new traditions is a wonderful experience, it's important to also reflect on the traditions that have shaped our culture, and see where they've taken us.

Together we'll take an incredible journey back in time, and forward, embracing a synthesis of ancestral riches, and modern sensibilities. My hope is that after reading this, you'll go and dig deeper into your history - read the Eddas, harvest some herbs, practice runic yoga and cook a viking feast!

In Northern Lore you will:

- Practice "Runic Yoga" for Health and Well Being
- Learn Ancient Herblore for Holistic Healing
- Meet your Animal Spirit Guide, or Fylgia
- Discover Lost Meaning in the Days of the Week
- Explore Modern Holidays & connections to Ancestral Festivals
- Unlock the Mysteries of the Runes
- Sample Viking and Anglo-Saxon cuisine

Buy directly from the Author at:

https://www.createspace.com/3451960/

Save 15% - Use Coupon Code: **E8GSAJTG** When checking out

Northern Wisdom

The Havamal, Tao of the Vikings

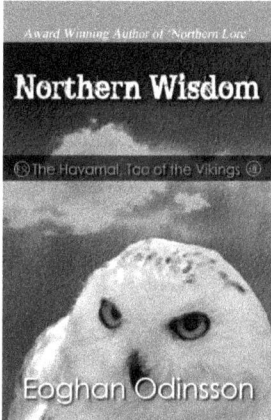

The Orient has long shared its ancient wisdom, and so now do the Northmen.

Northern Wisdom presents ancient Viking parables and knowledge in a delightfully accessible modern format.

Combining Teachings on par with Buddha, Sun-Tzu, Myamoto Musashi, Nicollo Machiavelli & Lao Tzu, The Havamal sheds light on forgotten lore of the dark ages.

In the days of the shield-wall, there yet lived poets, scribes and philosophers.

In Northern Wisdom you will:

- Journey through the Mundane and the Mystical passages of the Havamal
- Discover the famed Hospitality of the Northmen
- Learn Maxims for respectable conduct
- Develop the Leadership traits of Heroes
- Explore tips for safe travel in Dark Ages Europe
- Uncover lessons for the bravest Warriors
- Share in the secrets of Odin's Love Quests
- Tap into the power of Viking Magic

Buy directly from the Author at:

https://www.createspace.com/3711599

Save 15% - Use Coupon Code: **E8GSAJTG** When checking out

The Runes in 9 minutes

Start using the runes in 9 minutes!

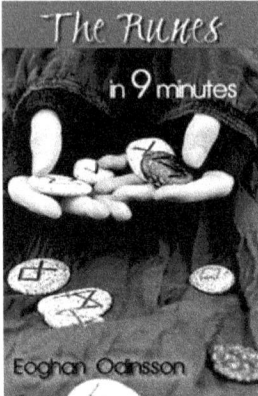

In 9 minutes you will be using the runes for personal development and exploration. Of course you aren't going to master the runes in 9 minutes, but you can start!

We'll even teach you how to create your own set of runes. All you need, in addition to this book, is a sheet of paper and something to write with.

This is a book of runes for beginners, and as such, I designed it to be a concise and inexpensive introduction. If you like what you see and the runes are for you, then you can extend your studies. If the runes aren't your thing, then you haven't invested much time or money. Call it a runic sampler if you will.

In The Runes in 9 minutes you will:

* Make your own set of 24 Elder Futhark Runes
* Learn how to use the runes in 3 essential layouts
* Discover a Never Before Published way to use the runes!
* Interpret their meanings in the context of your life
* Study the symbolism of each ancient symbol
* Explore different types of runes such as the Elder Futhark, Anglo-Saxon Futhorc, and Younger Futhork
* Uncover the history and culture behind the runes

Buy directly from the Author at

https://www.createspace.com/3777299

Save 15% - Use Coupon Code: **E8GSAJTG** When checking out

A Door in the Woods (ages 9-12)

What would you do if you found a magical door in the woods?

When twelve year old Connor Jones discovers a magical door in the woods leading to other worlds, he starts a series of amazing adventures, meets incredible friends, and soon discovers that he's destined to save Earth!

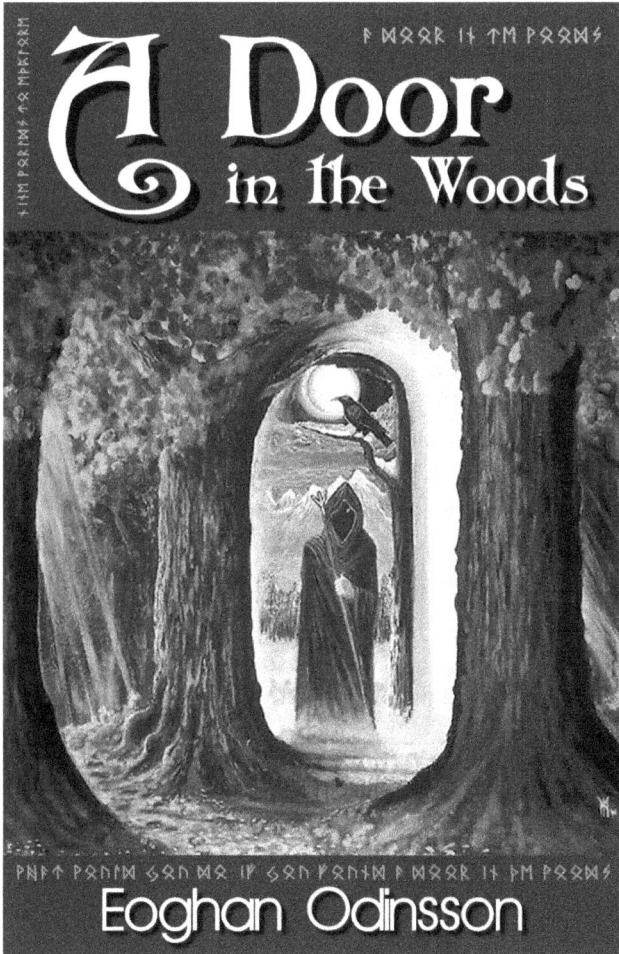

Coming Spring 2012 - Keep up to date at:

http://www.eoghanodinsson.com/my-books/a-door-in-the-woods.html

Leechcraft - Early English Charms, Plantlore and Healing - By Stephen Pollington

One of the Key Resources Referenced in this Book, **Stephen Pollington's** "Leechcraft - Early English Charms, Plantlore and Healing" deserves a place of honor on your bookshelf.

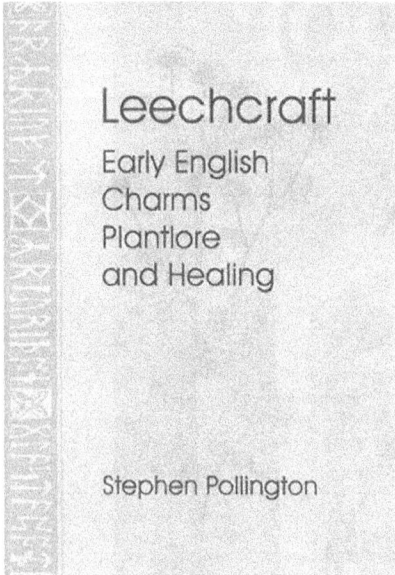

Leechcraft

Early English
Charms
Plantlore
and Healing

Stephen Pollington

An unequaled examination of every aspect of early English healing, including the use of plants, amulets, charms, and prayer. Other topics include: Anglo-Saxon witchcraft, shaminism, tree-lore, omens, dreams, runes, gods, elves, dwarfs, and theories of magic. The author has brought together a wide range of evidence for the English healing tradition, and presented it in a clear and readable manner. The three key Old English texts are reproduced in full, accompanied by new translations: - *Bald's Third Leechbook - Old English Herbarium Apulei - Lacnunga*

28 illustrations 544 pages 9.5" x 6.5" (248mm x 170mm) soft covers ISBN 1-898281-47-4

Buy from Amazon at: http://amzn.to/IA24n0

www.ingramcontent.com/pod-product-compliance
Lightning Source LLC
Chambersburg PA
CBHW050447270326
41927CB00009B/1647